MACHINERY PROGNOSTICS AND PROGNOSIS ORIENTED MAINTENANCE MANAGEMENT

MACHINERY PROGNOSTICS AND PROGNOSIS ORIENTED MAINTENANCE MANAGEMENT

Jihong Yan

Harbin Institute of Technology, P.R.China

WILEY

This edition first published 2015

Registered office
John Wiley & Sons Singapore Pte. Ltd., 1 Fusionopolis Walk, #07-01 Solaris South Tower, Singapore 138628.

For details of our global editorial offices, for customer services and for information about how to apply for permission to reuse the copyright material in this book please see our website at www.wiley.com.

Library of Congress Cataloging-in-Publication Data
Yan, Jihong.
Machinery prognostics and prognosis oriented maintenance management / Jihong Yan.
pages cm
Includes bibliographical references and index.
ISBN 978-1-118-63872-9 (hardback)
1. Machinery–Maintenance and repair. 2. Machinery–Service life. 3. Machinery–Reliability. I. Title.
TJ174.Y36 2014
621.8′16–dc23

2014022259

Set in 11/13pt, TimesLTStd by Laserwords Private Limited, Chennai, India

Printed and bound in Singapore by Markono Print Media Pte Ltd

1 2015

Contents

About the Author

Jihong Yan is a full-time Professor (since 2005) in Advanced Manufacturing at Harbin Institute of Technology (HIT), China and is head of the Department of Industrial Engineering, who received her Ph.D. degree in Control Engineering from HIT in 1999. Professor Yan has been working in the area of intelligent maintenance for over 10 years, starting from 2001 when she worked for the Centre for Intelligent Maintenance Systems (IMS) funded by NSF in the US as a researcher for 3 years, mainly focused on prognosis algorithm development and application. Then she joined Pennsylvania State University in 2004 to work on personnel working performance related topics. As a Principal Investigator, she has worked on and completed more than 10 projects in the maintenance-related area, funded by the NSF of China, National High-tech "973" project, the Advanced Research Foundation of the General Armament Department, the Astronautics Supporting Technology Foundation, High-tech funding from industries, and so on. Specifically, her research is focused on the area of advanced maintenance of machinery, such as online condition monitoring, signal data pre-processing, feature extraction, reliability and performance evaluation, fault diagnosis, fault prognosis and remaining useful life prediction, maintenance scheduling, and sustainability-based maintenance management. She has authored and co-authored over 80 research papers and edited 2 books.

Preface

Prognostics-based maintenance, which is a typical pattern of predictive maintenance (PdM) has been developed rapidly in recent years. Prognosis, which is defined as a systematic approach that can continuously track health indicators to predict risks of unacceptable behavior over time, can serve the purpose of assessing the degradation of a facility's quality based on acquired online condition monitoring data. The existing prognostics models can be divided into two main categories, mechanism-based models and data-driven models. Although the real-life system mechanism is often too stochastic and complex to model, a physics-based model might not be the most practical solution. Artificial intelligence based algorithms are currently the most commonly found data-driven technique in prognostics research.

Prognostics provides the basic information for a maintenance management system where the maintenance decision is made by predicting the time when reliability or remaining life of a facility reaches the maintenance threshold. However, inappropriate maintenance time will result in waste of energy and a heavier environmental load. Nowadays, more efficient maintenance strategies, such as sustainability-oriented maintenance management are put forward. Sustainability-based maintenance management not only benefits manufacturers and customers economically but also improves environmental performance. Therefore, from both environmental and economic perspectives, improving the energy efficiency of maintenance management is instrumental for sustainable manufacturing. Sustainability-based maintenance management will be one of the important strategies for sustainable development.

This book aims to present a state-of-the-art survey of theories and methods of machinery prognostics and prognosis-oriented maintenance management, and to reflect current hot topics: feature fusion, on-line monitoring, residual life prediction, prognosis-based maintenance and decision-making, as well as related case studies.

The book is intended for engineers and qualified technicians working in the fields of maintenance, systems management, and shop floor production line maintenance. Topics selected to be included in this book cover a wide range of issues in the area of prognostics and maintenance management to cater for all those interested in maintenance, whether practitioners or researchers. It is also suitable for use as a textbook for postgraduate programs in maintenance, industrial engineering, and applied mathematics.

This book contains eight chapters covering a wide range of topics related to prognostics and maintenance management, and is organized as introduced briefly below.

Chapter 1 presents a systems view of prognostic- and sustainability-based maintenance management.

Chapter 2 introduces widely used probability distribution functions, such as uniform distribution, geometric distribution, normal distribution, and binomial distribution, for processing discrete data, and is illustrated with several examples.

Chapter 3 presents a systematic and in-depth study of signal processing and the application to mechanical condition monitoring and fault identification.

Chapter 4 introduces the reader to the health monitoring concept. In addition, the degradation process, the main parts of a typical real-time monitoring system, and fault prognosis and the methods for remaining useful life prediction are discussed.

Chapter 5 addresses different prediction methods in machine prognosis.

Chapter 6 focuses on maintenance planning and scheduling techniques, including maintenance scheduling modeling, grouping technology (GT) based maintenance, and so on.

Chapter 7 provides an overview of prognosis-oriented maintenance decision-making issues and shows how the prognosis plays an important role in the development of maintenance management.

Chapter 8 presents five significant case studies on prognostics and maintenance management to demonstrate the application of the contents of the previous chapters. These are extracted from some published papers of the author's research group.

This book is a valuable addition to the literature and will be useful to both practitioners and researchers. It is hoped that this book will open new views and ideas to researchers and industry on how to proceed in the direction of sustainability-based maintenance management. I hope the readers find this book informative and useful.

Jihong Yan
Harbin, China
March 2014

Acknowledgements

I wish to thank specific people and institutions for providing help during 2013–2014, making the publication of this book possible. I would like to acknowledge the contributors for their valuable contributions. This book would not have been possible without their enthusiasm and cooperation throughout the stages of this project. I also would like to express my gratitude to all the reviewers who improved the quality of this book through their constructive comments and suggestions. Also, I want to thank my students Lin Li, Chaozhong Guo, Lei Lu, Fenyang Zhang, Weicheng Yang, Bohan Lv, Jing Wen, Yue Meng, Chunhua Feng, and Dongwei Liu for editing and typing the manuscript.

The work presented in this book is funded by the National Science Foundation of China (#70971030, #71271068).

Finally, I would like to express my gratitude to my family, especially my little son Richard, for their patience, understanding, and assistance during the preparation of this book. Work on this book has sometimes been at the expense of their time.

1

Introduction

1.1 Historical Perspective

With the rapid development of industrial technology, machine tools have become more and more complex in response to the need for higher production quality. While a significant increase in failure rate due to the complexity of machine tools is becoming a major factor which restricts the improvement of production quality and efficiency.

Before 1950, maintenance was basically unplanned, taking place only when breakdowns occurred. Between1950 and 1960, a time-based preventive maintenance (PM) (also called planned maintenance) technique was developed, which sets a periodic interval to perform PM regardless of the health status of a physical asset. In the later 1960s, reliability centered maintenance (RCM) was proposed and developed in the area of aviation. Traditional approaches of reliability estimation are based on the distribution of historical time-to-failure data of a population of identical facilities obtained from in-house tests. Many parametric failure models, such as Poisson, exponential, Weibull, and log-normal distributions have been used to model machine reliability. However, these approaches only provide overall estimates for the entire population of identical facilities, which is of less value to an end user of a facility [1]. In other words, reliability reflects only the statistical quality of a facility, which means it is likely that an individual facility does not necessarily obey the distribution that is determined by a population of tested facilities of the same type. Therefore, it is recommended that on-line monitoring data should also be used to reflect the quality and degradation severity of an individual facility more specifically.

In the past two decades, the maintenance pattern has been developing in the direction of condition-based maintenance (CBM), which recommends maintenance actions based on the information collected through on-line monitoring. CBM attempts to avoid unnecessary maintenance tasks by taking maintenance actions only when there is evidence of abnormal behavior of a physical asset. A CBM program, if properly established and effectively implemented, can significantly reduce maintenance cost by eliminating the number of unnecessary scheduled PM operations.

Machinery Prognostics and Prognosis Oriented Maintenance Management, First Edition. Jihong Yan.

Prognostics-based maintenance, which is a typical pattern of predictive maintenance (PdM) has been developed rapidly in recent years. Despite the fact that fault diagnosis and prediction are related to the assessment of the status of equipment, and generally considered together, the goals of the decision-making are obviously different. The diagnosis results are commonly used for passive maintenance decision-making, but the prediction results are used for initiative maintenance decision-making. Its goal is minimum use risk and maximum life. By means of fault prediction, the opportune moment from initial defect to functional fault could be estimated. The failure rate of the whole system or some of the components can be modified, so prognostic technology has become a hot research issue. Now fault prediction techniques are classified into three categories according to the recent literature: failure prediction based on an analytical model, failure prediction based on data, and qualitative knowledge-based fault prediction. Artificial-intelligence-based algorithms are currently the most commonly found data-driven technique in prognostics research [1, 2].

Recently, a new generation of maintenance, e-maintenance, is emerging with globalization and fast growth of communication technologies, computer, and information technologies. e-Maintenance is a major pillar in modern industries that supports the success of the integration of e-manufacturing and e-business, by which manufactures and users can benefit from the increased equipment and process reliability with optimal asset performance and seamless integration with suppliers and customers.

1.2 Diagnostic and Prognostic System Requirements

Diagnostics deals with fault detection, isolation, and identification when it occurs. Fault detection is a task to indicate whether something is going wrong in the monitored system; fault isolation is a task to locate the component that is faulty; and fault identification is a task to determine the nature of the fault when it is detected. In recent years, technological development in areas like data mining (DM), data transmission, and databases has provided the technical support for prognostics. Prognostics deals with fault prediction before it occurs. Fault prediction is a task to determine whether a fault is impending and to estimate how soon and how likely it is that a fault will occur. Diagnostics is post-event analysis, and prognostics is prior event analysis. Prognostics is much more efficient than diagnostics in achieving zero-downtime performance. Diagnostics, however, is required when the fault prediction of prognostics fails and a fault occurs.

As a minimum, the basic technical requirements of diagnostics mainly include

1. Sensor location, which has a significant impact on the measurement accuracy.
2. Feature extraction to obtain the parameter which characterizes equipment performance by utilizing signal processing methods including a fast Fourier Transform (FFT) algorithm, a wavelet transform (WT), and so on.
3. Method of fault classification to increase the accuracy of equipment failure classification.

In addition to those technical requirements mentioned above, to specify prognostics accuracy requirements we also need

1. Data on performance degradation, which indicates the decline of equipment performance in the working process.
2. Methods for life prediction to guarantee the safe operation of equipment and improve economic benefits.
3. A confidence interval to estimate the bounds of parameters in the model-based prediction.

Commonly, some aspects of hardware technology, such as the accuracy of sensors, the selection of the location of sensors, and data acquisition provide the technological foundations of prognostics. Also, computer-assisted software techniques, including data transmission, database, and signal processing methods are essential components of a prognostics system.

1.3 Need for Prognostics and Sustainability-Based Maintenance Management

Any organization that owns any large capital assets will eventually face a crucial decision whether to repair or replace those assets, and when. This decision can have far reaching consequences, replacing too early can mean a waste of resources, and replacing too late can mean catastrophic failure. The first is becoming more unacceptable in today's sustainability-oriented society, and the second is unacceptable in the competitive marketplace.

Equipment degradation and unexpected failures impact the three key elements of competitiveness – quality, cost, and productivity [3]. Maintenance has been introduced to reduce downtime and rework and to increase consistency and overall business efficiency. However, traditional maintenance costs constitute a large portion of the operating and overhead expenses in many industries [4]. More efficient maintenance strategies, such as prognostics-based maintenance are being implemented to handle the situation. It is said that prognostics-based maintenance can reduce the maintenance costs by approximately 25% [5]. Generally, machines go through degradation before failure occurs, monitoring the trend of machine degradation and assessing performance allow the degraded behavior or faults to be corrected before they cause failure and machine breakdowns. Therefore, advanced prognostics focuses on performance degradation monitoring and prediction, so that the failures can be predicted and prevented [6].

If large capital assets are analyzed as repairable systems, additional significant information can be incorporated into maintenance optimization models. When these assets break down, but have not yet reached their end-of life, they can be repaired and returned to operating condition. However, sometimes malfunctioning equipment cannot be properly fixed or repaired to its original healthy condition. In this case, the application of prognostics will help solve this problem and avoid irreparable and irreversible damage. Prognostics provides the basic information for a maintenance management system where a maintenance decision is made by predicting the time when the reliability or the remaining life of a facility reaches the maintenance threshold. However, inappropriate maintenance time will result in waste of resources and a heavier environmental load. Nowadays, more efficient maintenance strategies, such as sustainability oriented maintenance management, are put forward. Sustainability-based maintenance management (SBMM) not only benefits manufacturers and customers economically but also improves environmental performance. Therefore, from both environmental and economic perspectives, improving the energy efficiency of maintenance management is instrumental for sustainable manufacturing. SBMM will be one of the important strategies for sustainable development.

1.4 Technical Challenges in Prognosis and Sustainability-Based Maintenance Decision-Making

In order to implement prognostics, three main steps are needed. (i) Feature extraction and selection: feature extraction is the process of transforming the raw input data acquired from mounted or built-in sensors into a concise representation that contains the relevant information on the health condition. Feature selection is the selection of typical features which reflect an overall degradation trend from the extracted features. (ii) Performance assessment: how to effectively evaluate the performance based on the selected features is crucial to prognostics. A good performance assessment method ought to be capable of fusing different information on multiple features for system degradation assessment. (iii) Remaining life prediction: this is a process using prediction models to forecast future performance and obtain the residual useful life of machinery. Remaining life prediction is the most important step in prognostics; it appears to be a hot issue attracting the most attention.

The key point in carrying out intelligent prognostics is the conversion of all kinds of raw data into useful information which indicates the equipment/components performance degradation process. The proposed framework is shown in Figure 1.1, it consists of two modules, a model training module and a real-time prognostics module. The performance assessment model M_E and the life prediction model M_P are the outputs of the model training module, which are employed in the real-time prognostics module. The model training module consists of four major parts: data pre-processing, feature extraction, performance assessment, and remaining life prediction. The real-time prognostics module consists of five components: real-time data acquisition, data pre-processing, feature extraction, performance assessment, and dynamic life prediction. If degradation appears, then early stage diagnosis/prognosis would be conducted.

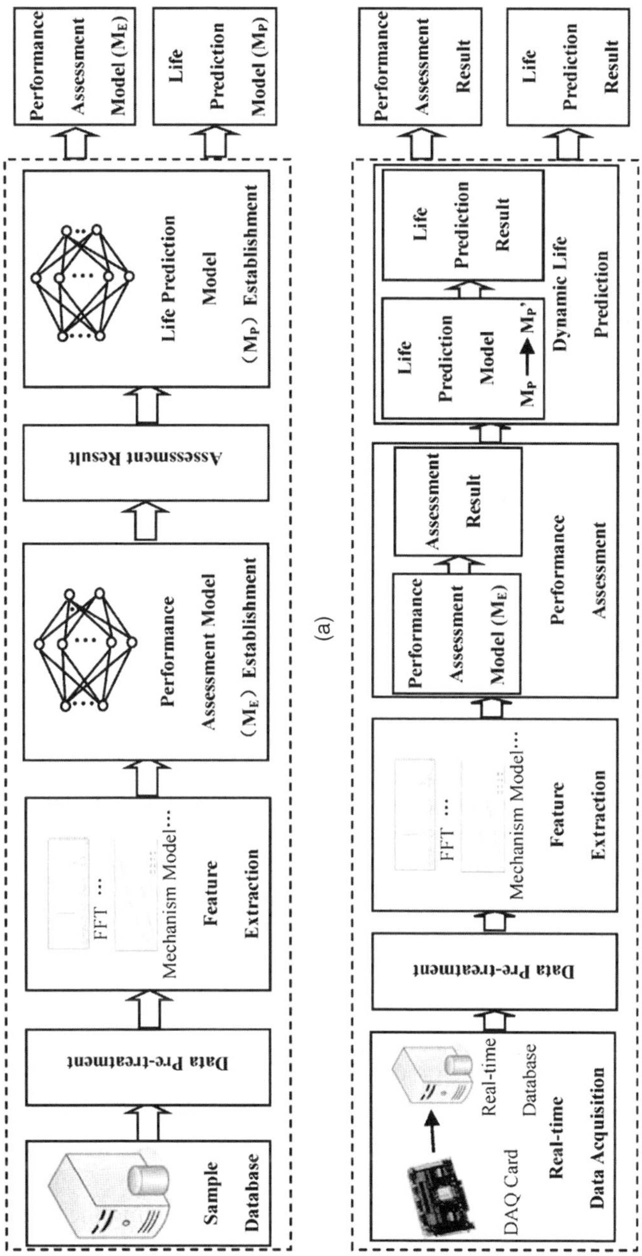

Figure 1.1 Framework of intelligent prognostics methods. (a) Model training, (b) real-time prognostics

Several aspects need to be further investigated before prognostics systems can be reliably applied in real-life situations, such as the incorporation of CM data into reliability analyses; the utilization of incomplete trending data; the consideration of effects from maintenance actions and variable operating conditions; the deduction of the non-linear relationship between the measured condition and the actual degradation; the considerations of failure interactions; the accuracy of assumptions and practicability of requirements, as well as the development of performance measurement frameworks. Repair and maintenance decisions for repairable systems are often based on the remaining useful life (RUL), also known as the residual life. Accurate RUL predictions are of interest particularly when the repairable system in question is a large capital asset. In addition, in a business setting, the economic and strategic life for complex and expensive equipment must be taken into account. This can make maintenance decision-making for such systems difficult.

Since environmental issues are involved in maintenance management, the relationship between energy consumption and performance of maintenance facilities should be taken into consideration during the decision-making process. In order to achieve energy reduction in facilities, it is necessary to study the relationship between energy consumption and the performance of maintenance facilities. For example, energy consumption will vary with wear or reliability of maintenance facilities in the use stage.

Existing research on maintenance planning and scheduling to reduce environmental impacts is quite limited. Normally, only one scheduling objective, such as maintenance cost, is solved in the maintenance planning and scheduling problem. Since sustainability is considered in maintenance management, it is necessary to incorporate the energy models of maintenance facilities into the objective function and constraints. Inevitably, energy consumption models of maintenance facilities become more complex and difficult to solve. Optimization methods could be of significant importance to effectively and efficiently solve these "sustainability" challenges. In addition, models and solution approaches are essential to decide on strategic and tactical plans and to ensure that economic, environmental, and societal aspects are balanced. This demands new solution methods and technology to provide the kind of tools that maintenance decision-making needs. For example, improved algorithms should be employed to optimize multiple scheduling objectives, such as maintenance cost and total energy consumption.

The technical challenges of sustainability-based maintenance decision-making mainly consists of three aspects: (i) energy consumption modeling of maintenance facilities, (ii) establishing the relationship between energy consumption and performance of maintenance facilities, and (iii) solving the sustainability-based maintenance planning and scheduling problem.

In order to propose efficient and realistic strategies for reducing the consumption of energy and resources, it is imperative to develop methods for estimating the energy consumption of maintenance facilities. Maintenance can manage product quality and quality of services during the use phase. It also decreases environmental impacts since equipment in good condition can use energy efficiently and its physical life can be extended. However, when a maintenance system is not properly constructed, the efficiency of maintenance can be lower and might harm life-cycle management. Moreover, energy consumption models are the inputs of sustainability-based maintenance planning and scheduling problems. It is, therefore, important to establish reliable energy consumption models of maintenance facilities with a high accuracy.

1.5 Data Processing, Prognostics, and Decision-Making

Data acquisition, data processing, prognostics, and maintenance decision-making are the four key elements of a prognostics-based maintenance management flowchart (see Figure 1.2).

Data acquisition is the process of collecting, converting, and recording useful data from targeted physical assets. The hardware of data acquisition systems typically includes sensors, an amplifier circuit, an analog-to-digital (A/D) converter, a data transmission device, and a data recording circuit. A sensor is a converter that measures a physical quantity and converts it into a signal which can be read by an observer or by a (nowadays mostly electronic) instrument. An electronic amplifier, amplifier, or (informally) amp is an electronic device that increases the power of a signal by taking energy from a power supply and controlling the output to match the input signal shape but with a larger amplitude. An A/D converter is a device that converts a continuous physical quantity (usually voltage) to a digital number that represents the quantity's amplitude. In real-time monitoring systems, the control computers are far from the targeted assets. The digital signals indicating the health state of the assets need to transmit from the on-site plant to the control computer.

Data processing plays a crucial role in machinery prognostics and maintenance management. The first step of data processing is data cleaning. This is an important step since data, especially event data, which is usually entered manually, always contains errors. Data cleaning ensures, or at least increases the chance, that clean (error-free) data are used for further analysis and modeling. Without the data cleaning step, one may get into the so-called "garbage in garbage out" situation. Data errors are caused by many factors including the human factor mentioned above. For condition monitoring data, data errors may be caused by sensor faults. In this case, sensor fault isolation is the right way to go. In general, however, there is no simple way to clean data. Sometimes it requires manual examination. Graphical tools would be very helpful in finding and removing data errors. The next step of data processing is data analysis. A variety of models, algorithms, and tools are available in the literature to analyze data for

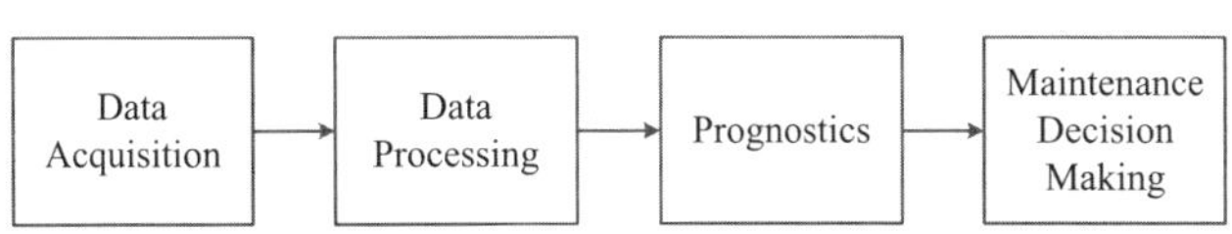

Figure 1.2 Four elements in a prognostics oriented maintenance management flowchart

better understanding and interpretation. The models, algorithms, and tools used for data analysis depend mainly on the types of data collected.

Data processing for waveform and multidimensional data is also called signal processing. Various signal processing techniques have been developed to analyze and interpret waveform and multidimensional data to extract useful information for further diagnostic and prognostic purposes. The procedure of extracting useful information from raw signals is the so-called feature extraction.

There are numerous signal processing techniques and algorithms in the literature for diagnostics and prognostics of mechanical systems. Case-dependent knowledge and investigation are required to select appropriate signal processing tools from among a number of possibilities.

The most common waveform data in condition monitoring are vibration signals and acoustic emissions. Other waveform data are ultrasonic signals, motor current, partial discharge, and so on. In the literature, there are three main categories of waveform data analysis: time-domain analysis, frequency-domain analysis, and time–frequency analysis.

The real-time monitoring systems provide fundamental information representing the health states of the monitored systems. The information helps to identify if the asset health has deviated from the normal. Then fault diagnostics and prognostics can be implemented. Fault diagnostics is used to detect, isolate, and identify the abnormal phenomenon. However, the more important question is how to utilize the health information to predict how long the machine can operate safely and perform its function, in order to optimize the maintenance schedules and ultimately maximize organizational efficiency. That is the relatively new research topic – prognostics which provides critical information such as early stage fault recognition and remaining life prediction for diagnostics.

Prognostics, the real issues involved with predicting life remaining, have been defined in the literature. ISO 13381–1(3) [7] defines prognosis as a "Technical process resulting in determination of remaining useful life". Jardine *et al.* [8] define two main prediction types in machine prognosis. The most widely used prognosis is "To predict how much time is left before a failure (or, one or more faults) occurs given the current machine condition and past operation profile". The time left before observing a failure is usually called remaining useful life or sometimes just the term useful life is used. The second prediction type is for situations when a failure is catastrophic (e.g., in nuclear power plants). The probability that a machine operates without a failure up to the next inspection interval, when the current machine condition and the past operation profile are known, is predicted. Damage prognosis is a frequently used term in structural safety and reliability. It is defined, as the estimate of an engineered system's remaining useful life [9].

Rule-based prognostic systems detect and identify incipient faults in accordance with the rules representing the relation of each possible fault to the actual monitored equipment condition. Case-based prognostic systems use historical records of maintenance cases to provide an interpretation for the actual monitored conditions of the equipment. The case library of maintenance is required to record all previous incidents, faults, and malfunctions of equipment which are used to identify the historical case that is most similar to the current condition. If a previous equipment fault occurs again, a case-based prognostic system will automatically pick up the maintenance advice, including trouble–cause–remedy, from the case library. A model-based prognostic system uses different mathematical, neural network, and logical methods to improve prognostic reasoning based on the structure and properties of the equipment system. A model-based prognostic system compares the real monitored condition with the model of the object in order to predict the fault behavior.

Maintenance managers deal with manufacturing systems that are subject to deteriorations and failures. One of their major concerns is the complex decision-making problem when they consider the availability aspect as well as the economic issue of their maintenance activities. They are continuously looking for a way to improve the availability of their production machines in order to ensure given production throughputs at the lowest cost.

This decision-making problem concerns the allocation of the right budget to the appropriate equipment or component. The objective is to minimize the total expenditure and to maximize the effective availability of production resources.

Proper instrumentation of critical systems and equipment plays a vital role in the acquisition of necessary technical data, while the support of analytical software with embedded mathematical models is crucial for the decision-making process.

The intelligent predictive decision support system (IPDSS) for maintenance integrates the concepts of:

1. Equipment condition monitoring.
2. Intelligent condition-based fault diagnosis.
3. Prediction of the trend of equipment deterioration.

Through integrating these three elements, the quality of maintenance decisions could be improved.

1.6 Sustainability-Based Maintenance Management

SBMM is a maintenance program that implements maintenance actions (diagnostics, PM, CBM, and prognostics) to obtain sustainability oriented maintenance strategies that minimize negative environmental impacts, conserve energy and natural resources, are safe for employees, communities, and consumers and increase the availability, reliability, and life span of facilities to keep high productivity and reduce maintenance cost, which will make maintenance actions balance with respect to economic, environmental, and societal aspects.

A traditional maintenance management system includes decision processes, such as selection of end of life options, including reuse and recycle. Decisions are made based

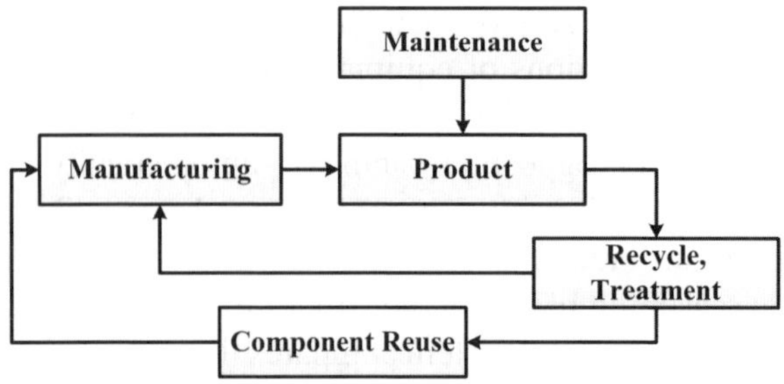

Figure 1.3 Maintenance and manufacturing

on the conditions of the products which are subject to maintenance. If such SBMM works, component reuse can be promoted.

Figure 1.3 shows the relation between maintenance and manufacturing. Maintenance can improve the quality of the collected components and reduce the work required for quality assurance.

A SBMM system can be interpreted as a life-cycle management process. It includes environment-based maintenance service providers and a monitoring system connected to the equipment. A SBMM system, if properly established and effectively implemented, can significantly reduce maintenance cost, environmental burden, and societal impacts to improve the competitiveness of an enterprise.

The concept of SBMM has become increasingly important as a measure to reduce environmental impact and resource consumption in manufacturing. Figure 1.4 shows the circular manufacturing with maintenance in the product use stage. As depicted, the life-cycle options, such as maintenance, upgrade, reuse, and recycling, which correspond to various paths in circular manufacturing, are means to reduce environmental load and resource consumption.

We use technologies such as condition diagnosis, residual life estimation, disassembly, restoration (including cleaning, adjustment, repair, and replacement), inspection, and re-assembly to achieve maintenance management. When products continue to be used by the same user, the activities to maintain or enhance the original functionality of the product are called maintenance and upgrade. The maintenance technologies are

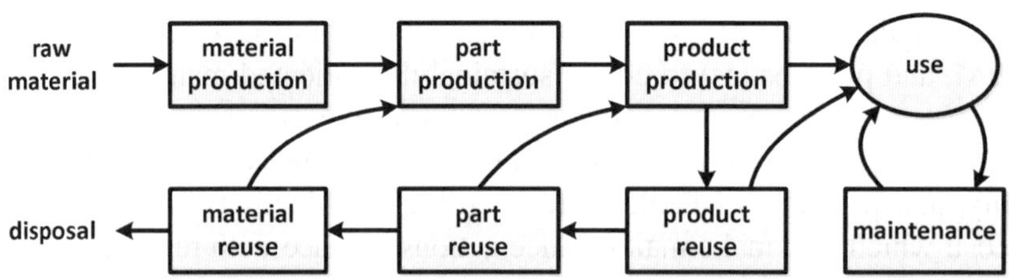

Figure 1.4 Conventional architecture of maintenance management

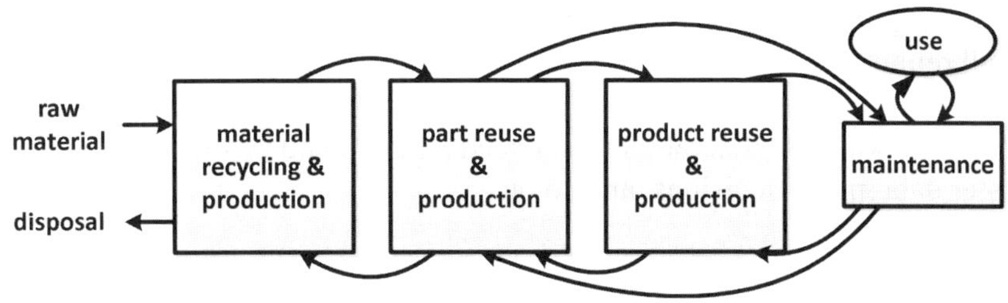

Figure 1.5 Life-cycle maintenance management

necessary to exhaust the item's life to the fullest extent possible through restoration and upgrade.

The maintenance strategies in Figure 1.4 have been selected without regard for reuse, and reuse has been discussed without regard for recycling. To make effective use of maintenance, we need to plan the product life-cycle maintenance management [10]. For example, reused products should be recycled at the end. According to the concept of the product life-cycle planning, the implementation of life-cycle options should be discussed in an integrated way. However, in the conventional architecture of maintenance management illustrated in Figure 1.4, maintenance, reuse, and recycling are represented as supplemental processes.

On the basis of the recognition that the purpose of life-cycle maintenance is to provide the required function to users, there is no reason to discriminate between newly produced products and reused products as far as they satisfy user needs. In this sense, we should integrate maintenance into life-cycle manufacturing as indicated in Figure 1.5. We call such a system life-cycle maintenance management because the innermost loop that is, maintenance, is prioritized as the most efficient circulation.

1.7 Future of Prognostics-Based Maintenance

The definition of prognostics has already been put forward and prognostic techniques are developing rapidly in some areas. However, prognostics-based maintenance still needs further research, in particular:

1. The development of smart sensors and other low-cost on-line monitoring systems that will permit the cost-effective continuous monitoring of key equipment items. An example is the micro-electro-mechanical sensor (MEMS), an accelerometer that is produced in silicon using the same processes as integrated circuit manufacture. It allows the sensor and amplifier electronics to be integrated into a single chip to replace traditional piezoelectric accelerometers.
2. The increasing provision of built-in sensors as standard features in large motors, pumps, turbines, and other large equipment and critical components.

3. The development of fusion techniques in the complete maintenance to improve overall reliability.
4. Increasing integration and acceptance of common standards for integrating maintenance software. A general platform needs these standards to share information, transfer data, make decisions, and so on.

Diagnostic and preventive maintenance are not, however, the terminal goals of our research and obviously will not meet the fast development of high-tech in the near future. For the sake of higher flexibility and lower maintenance cost, biotechnology is the main area to consider for future scientific research. Bio-mechanisms of self-recovery and self-healing are worth further research and will have broad application prospects in maintaining the performance of equipment. By utilizing biotechnology, prognostics-based maintenance will eventually implement true continuous production.

References

1. Heng, A., Zhang, S., Tan, A.C.C. *et al.* (2009) Rotating machinery prognostics: state of the art, challenges and opportunities. *Mechanical Systems and Signal Processing*, **23**, 724–739.
2. Lee, J., Ni, J., Djurdjanovic, D. *et al.* (2006) Intelligent prognostics tools and e-maintenance. *Computers in Industry*, **57**, 476–489.
3. Yan, J., Koc, M. and Lee, J. (2004) A prognostic algorithm for machine performance assessment and its application. *Production Planning and Control*, **15**, 796–801.
4. Gebraeel, N. and Lawley, M. (2004) Residual life predictions from vibration-based degradation signals: a neural network approach. *IEEE Transactions on Industrial Electronics*, **51**, 694–699.
5. Camci, F. (2005) Process monitoring, diagnostics and prognostics using support vector machines and Hidden Markov Model. PhD thesis. Department of Industry Engineering, Wayne State University, Detroit, Michigan.
6. Huang, R., Xi, L., Li, X. *et al.* (2007) Residual life predictions for ball bearings based on self-organizing map and back propagation neural network methods. *Mechanical Systems and Signal Processing*, **21**, 193–207.
7. ISO ISO 13381-1. (2004) *Condition Monitoring and Diagnostics of Machines Prognostics Part1: General Guidelines*, International Organization for Standardization, Geneva.
8. Jardine, A.K.S., Lin, D. and Banjevic, D. (2006) A review on machinery diagnostics and prognostics implementing condition-based maintenance. *Mechanical Systems and Signal Processing*, **20**, 1483–1510.
9. Farrar, C.R. and Lieven, N. (2006) Damage prognosis: the future of structural health monitoring. *Philosophical Transactions of the Royal Society, Series A*, **365**, 623–632.
10. Umeda, Y., Takata, S., Kimura, F. *et al.* (2012) Toward integrated product and process life cycle planning – An environmental perspective. *CIRP Annals – Manufacturing Technology*, **61** (2), 681–702.

2

Data Processing

2.1 Probability Distributions

The classical probability definition originates from the days when probability calculus was founded by Pascal and Fermat. The inspiration for this theory can be found in the games of cards and dice. The classical definition of the probability of the event A can be formulated as [1],

$$P(A) = \frac{n_A}{N} \tag{2.1}$$

where n_A is the number of equally likely ways by which an experiment may lead to A, N is the total number of equally likely ways in the experiment. The properties of probability are as follows:

1. For two possible events A and B, if A happens B cannot happen and vice versa (that is, they are mutually exclusive), then the probability of either A or B happening is the sum of the probabilities of the two events: $P(A \text{ or } B) = P(A) + P(B)$.
2. For mutually exclusive events of a trial, the sum of probabilities of all possible events is unity, because the result of every trial must be one of all the events: $P(A) + P(B) + P(C) = 1$.
3. For two independent events, the probability that both of them will happen is the product of the probability of each event: $P(A \text{ and } B) = P(A) \times P(B)$.

The following conclusions are drawn from the above three rules:

1. For n mutually exclusive events with different outcomes, the a priori probability of each event happening is equivalent, and then the probability of the outcome of each trial is equal to $1/n$.
2. When all the outcomes of the events are classified into different classes, and if m outcomes of events belong to the same class, then the probability of the event in that class happening is equal to m/n.

Machinery Prognostics and Prognosis Oriented Maintenance Management, First Edition. Jihong Yan.

Probability distribution describes the probability value of the possible outputs of a random experiment of statistical inference, which is one of the basic concepts of probability theory.

Suppose space Ω is either a finite or countable set, a probability distribution P on space Ω is a real-valued function defined on subsets (events) of Ω, when the following conditions are satisfied,

1. $0 \leq P(A) \leq 1$, for all $A \subseteq \Omega$.
2. $P(\Omega) = 1$.
3. For a finite or infinite collection of disjoint events $\{A_i\}_i$, for $i \neq j, A_i \cap A_j \neq \emptyset$, then

$$P(\underset{i}{\cup} A_i) = \sum_i P(A_i) \tag{2.2}$$

Different types of random variables result in different forms of probability distribution. The probability distribution would be a categorical statistical result when the sample space is non-numerical. It would be discrete when the sample space only consists of a finite or countable infinite number of distinct values, and it can be specified by a continuous probability function where the experiments with sample spaces are encoded by continuous random variables.

A random variable is a variable with real-valued outcomes on a random event, and is usually written as capital letters, such as X, Y, or Z. The corresponding outcome of random variables is denoted as x, y, and z. In this text, statistical functions of random variable X, such as probability, density, and distribution, are expressed as $P(X = x)$, $f(X = x)$, and $F(X = x)$, and abbreviated to $P(x), f(x)$, and $F(x)$.

2.1.1 Uniform Distribution

Consider a continuous random variable X with uniform probability density function over the interval $[a, b]$, that is the probability is represented in proportion to the length of the interval. As illustrated in Figure 2.1, the probability density function can be obtained as,

$$f(x) = \begin{cases} \dfrac{1}{b-a}, & a \leq x \leq b \\ 0, & x < a \quad or \quad x > b \end{cases} \tag{2.3}$$

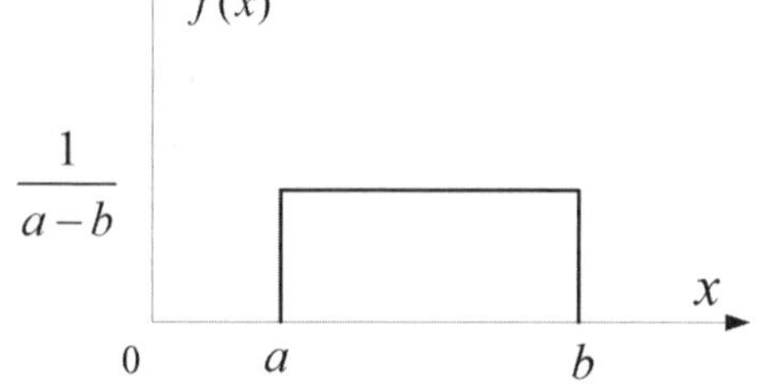

Figure 2.1 Uniform density function over interval $[a, b]$

The expectation and variance of a random variable with uniform distribution can be calculated as

$$
\begin{aligned}
E(X) &= \int_{-\infty}^{\infty} xf(x)\mathrm{d}x = \int_a^b x\frac{1}{b-a}\mathrm{d}x = \frac{1}{2(b-a)}x^2|_a^b \\
&= \frac{b^2-a^2}{2(b-a)} \\
&= \frac{b+a}{2}
\end{aligned} \tag{2.4}
$$

$$
\begin{aligned}
V(X) &= E(X^2) - [E(X)]^2 \\
&= \int_a^b x^2\frac{1}{b-a}\mathrm{d}x - \left(\frac{b+a}{2}\right)^2 = \frac{1}{3(b-a)}x^3|_a^b - \left(\frac{b+a}{2}\right)^2 \\
&= \frac{b^3-a^3}{3(b-a)} - \left(\frac{b+a}{2}\right)^2 \\
&= \frac{b^2+ab+a^2}{3} - \frac{b^2+2ab+a^2}{4} \\
&= \frac{(b-a)^2}{12}
\end{aligned} \tag{2.5}
$$

The distribution function of the random variable is

$$
F(x) = \begin{cases} 0, & x \leq a \\ \displaystyle\int_a^x \frac{1}{b-a}dx = \frac{x-a}{b-a}, & a \leq x \leq b \\ 1, & x \geq b \end{cases} \tag{2.6}
$$

Example 2.1

For a random variable X over the interval [0, 25], which follows a uniform distribution, calculate the probability density function $f(x)$, the mean value and the variance of the distribution, and then find the cumulative distribution function $F(x)$.

The probability density function $f(x)$ can be calculated by the formula,

$$
f(x) = \begin{cases} \dfrac{1}{25-0} = 0.04, & 0 \leq x \leq 25 \\ 0, & \text{otherwise} \end{cases}
$$

The mean and variance of a random variable X gives,

$$
E(X) = \frac{25+0}{2} = 12.5
$$

$$
V(X) = \frac{(25-0)^2}{12} = 52.08
$$

For a random variable X over the interval [0, 25], it can be divided into three distinct regions $x < 0$, $0 \leq x \leq 25$, and $x > 25$, then the probability density function gives:

$$F(x) = \begin{cases} 0, & x < 0 \\ \dfrac{x}{25}, & 0 \leq x \leq 25 \\ 1, & x > 25 \end{cases}$$

2.1.2 Normal Distribution

The normal probability distribution is one of the most frequently used distributions for describing a continuous random variable. It has wide applications for probabilistic modeling of uncertain phenomena in signal processing, scientific measurements, statistical inference, and so on. The formula for the normal probability density function of random variable X is abbreviated as $X \sim N(\mu, \sigma^2)$ and given as

$$f(x) = \frac{1}{\sqrt{2\pi}\sigma} \exp\left(\frac{-(x-\mu)^2}{2\sigma^2}\right) \tag{2.7}$$

where, exp is the notation of the mathematical constant e, π is the mathematical constant, μ is the mean value, and σ is the standard deviation.

Standard normal distribution is a special version of the normal distribution that should be mentioned. For a continuous random variable Z, which is said to be a standard normal random variable when the expectation value $E(z) = 0$ and the standard deviation $V(z) = 1$, and the notation is $Z \sim N(0, 1)$. Then the density function can be written as,

$$f(z) = \frac{1}{\sqrt{2\pi}} \exp\left(\frac{-z^2}{2}\right) \tag{2.8}$$

Normal distribution (with any mean and standard deviation) can be transformed into the standard normal distribution through the following transform function. Figure 2.2 illustrates different normal distributions obtained from standard normal distribution by varying the two parameters μ and σ.

$$Z = \frac{x-\mu}{\sigma} \tag{2.9}$$

An important characteristic of normal distribution is that the probability of all variables is equal to 1, no matter what the values of the mean value μ and the standard deviation σ,

$$\int_{-\infty}^{+\infty} \frac{1}{\sqrt{2\pi}\sigma} \exp\left(\frac{-(x-\mu)^2}{2\sigma^2}\right) dx = 1 \tag{2.10}$$

It should be noted that, no matter what the values of the mean value μ and the standard deviation σ, the area between $\mu - \sigma$ and $\mu + \sigma$ is about 68%; the area

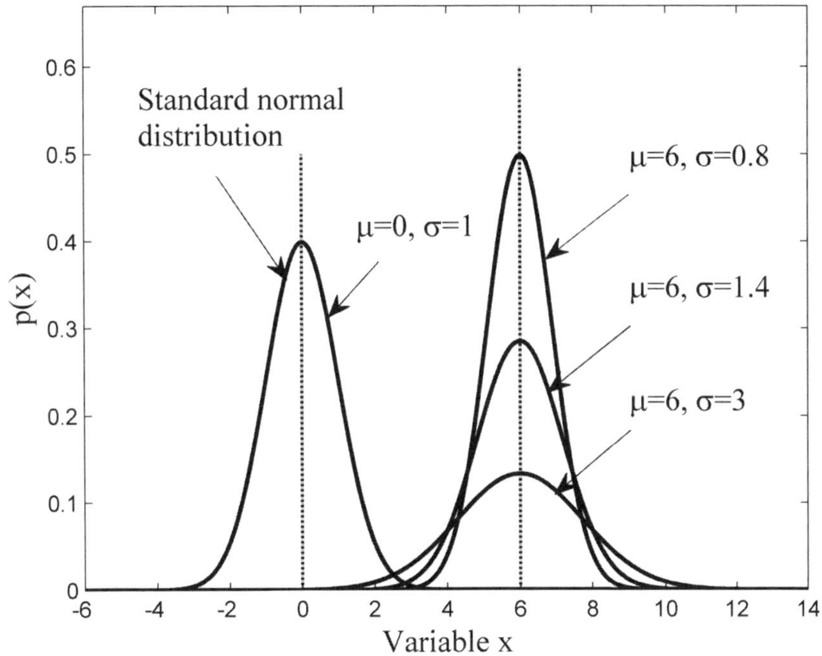

Figure 2.2 Normal distributions for different μ and σ

between $\mu - 2\sigma$ and $\mu + 2\sigma$ is about 95%; and the area between $\mu - 3\sigma$ and $\mu + 3\sigma$ is about 99.7%.

Example 2.2

Suppose the examination results of college students are restricted to 200–800, and they roughly follow a normal distribution, it is known that the average score is 500 and the standard deviation is 50, then it can be calculated that,

1. 68% of students will have scores in the range

$$\begin{aligned} R_1 &= [\mu - \sigma,\ \mu + \sigma] \\ &= [500 - 50,\ 500 + 50] \\ &= [450, 550] \end{aligned}$$

2. 95% will have scores in the range

$$\begin{aligned} R_2 &= [\mu - 2\sigma,\ \mu + 2\sigma] \\ &= [500 - 100,\ 500 + 100] \\ &= [400, 600] \end{aligned}$$

3. 99.7% will have scores in the range,

$$\begin{aligned} R_3 &= [\mu - 3\sigma,\ \mu + 3\sigma] \\ &= [500 - 150,\ 500 + 150] \\ &= [350, 650] \end{aligned}$$

2.1.3 Binomial Distribution

A binomial random variable X is defined as the number of "successes" in n independent trials where the P ("success") $= p$ is constant. In the definition, the following conditions need to be satisfied for a binomial experiment:

1. The number of trials carried out is a fixed number.
2. The outcome of a given trial is either a "success" or "failure".
3. The probability of success remains constant from trial to trial.
4. The trials are independent and the outcome of a trial is not affected by the outcome of any other trials.

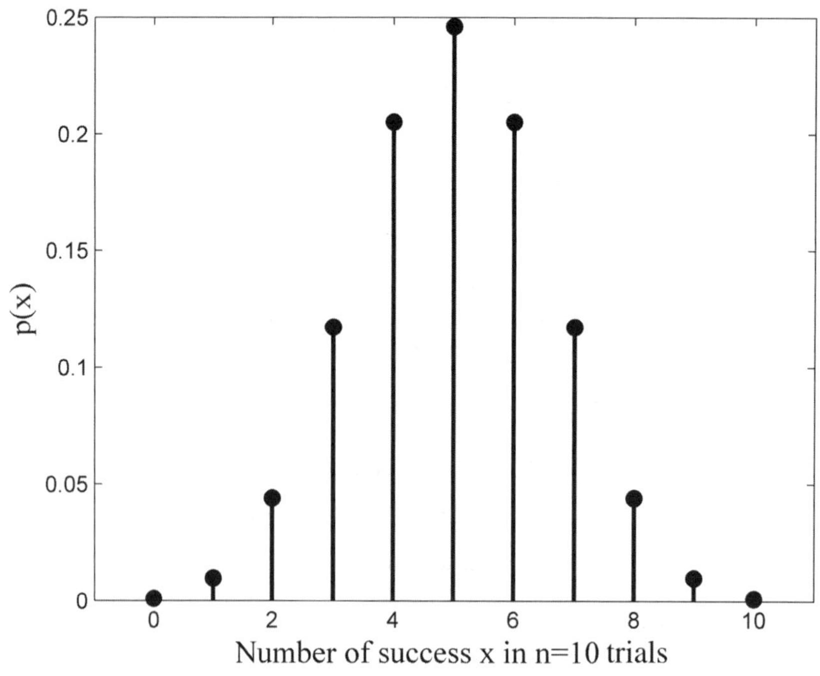

Figure 2.3 Binomial distribution with $n = 10$ and $p = 0.5$

For a binomial random variable X following binomial distribution, abbreviated as $B(n, p)$, the formula function is as in Equation 2.11. Some examples of the binomial distribution are shown in Figure 2.3 for the number of trials $n = 10$ and $P = 0.5$.

$$P(x) = \binom{n}{x} p^x (1-p)^{n-x} = \frac{n!}{x!(n-x)!} p^x (1-p)^{n-x} \tag{2.11}$$

where, $n! = n \times (n-1) \times (n-2) \times \ldots \times 1$, $\binom{n}{x}$ means "n choose x," the number of ways to obtain x "successes" in n trials, P ("success") $= p$, and $x = 0, 1, \ldots, n$.

If X follows a binomial distribution with parameters n and p, $X \sim B(n, p)$, then the expectation value, variance, and standard deviation can be calculated as,

$$E(x) = \mu_x = np \tag{2.12}$$

$$\mathrm{Var}(x) = {\sigma_x}^2 = np(1-p) \tag{2.13}$$

$$\mathrm{SD}(x) = \sigma_x = \sqrt{np(1-p)} \tag{2.14}$$

Example 2.3

Apples are packed in bags of 12. The probability of each apple in the bag being decayed is 0.35. Find the probability of less than 3 rotten apples in a random bag,

$$\begin{aligned} P(X < 3) &= P(X = 0) + P(X = 1) + P(X = 2) \\ &= \binom{12}{0} 0.35^0 \times 0.65^{(12)} + \binom{12}{1} 0.35^1 \times 0.65^{(11)} + \binom{12}{2} 0.35^2 \times 0.65^{(10)} \\ &= 1 \times 1 \times 0.005688 + 12 \times 0.35^1 \times 0.65^{11} + 66 \times 0.1225 \times 0.01346 \\ &= 0.0151 \end{aligned}$$

2.1.4 *Geometric Distribution*

A situation is said to be a "geometric distribution" if the following four conditions are met:

1. Each observation falls into one of two categories.
2. The probability of success is the same for each observation.
3. The observations are all independent.
4. The variable of interest is the number of trials required to obtain the first success.

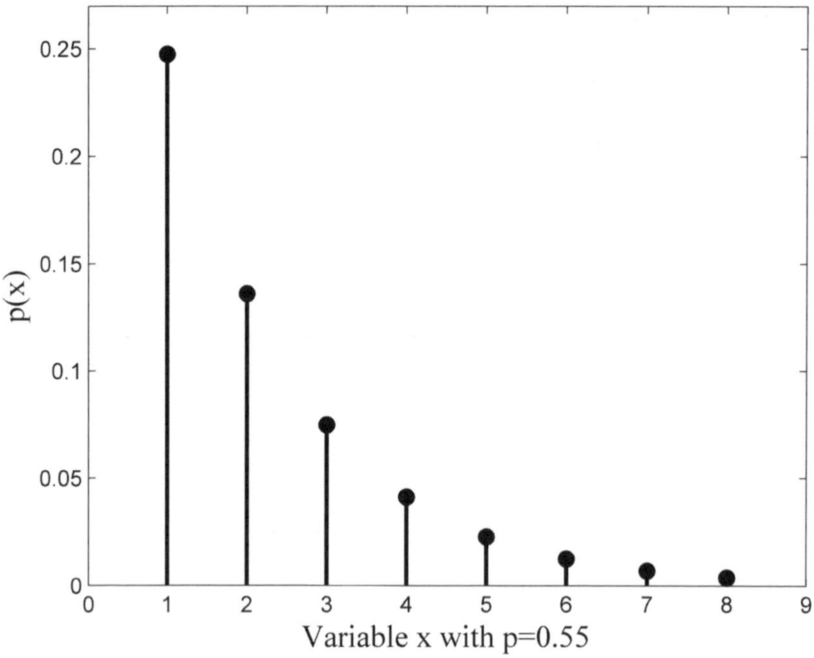

Figure 2.4 Geometric distribution of a random variable

If a discrete random variable X has a geometric distribution with probability p of success and $(1 - p)$ of failure on each observation, the possible values of X are $1, 2, 3, \ldots$. If n is any one of these values, the probability that the first success occurs on the nth trial is calculated as Equation 2.15 [2]. As illustrated in Figure 2.4, the probability is strictly decreasing with the increasing nth trial $n = 1, 2, 3, \ldots$

$$P(X = n) = (1 - p)^{n-1}p \tag{2.15}$$

For a discrete random variable X with a geometric distribution with probability p, the expected value, variance, and standard deviation can be calculated as,

$$E(x) = \mu_x = \frac{1}{p} \tag{2.16}$$

$$\mathrm{Var}(x) = {\sigma_x}^2 = \frac{1 - p}{p^2} \tag{2.17}$$

$$\mathrm{SD}(x) = \sigma_x = \frac{\sqrt{1 - p}}{p} \tag{2.18}$$

The probability of waiting more than n observations for a first success can be calculated as,

$$P(X > n) = (1 - p)^n \tag{2.19}$$

Example 2.4

A tester normally hits the balloon 70% of the time, the probability of the tester's first successful hit of the balloon follows a geometric distribution, then the probability that the man's first hit is on the second balloon is,

$$P(x = 2) = p(1 - p)^{n-1} = 0.7 \cdot (1 - 0.3)^{2-1} = 0.21$$

The expected value of the tester's successful hits of the balloon is,

$$\mu = \frac{1}{p} = \frac{1}{0.7} = 1.43$$

The standard deviation of the tester's successful hits of the balloon is,

$$\sigma_x = \frac{\sqrt{1-p}}{p} = \frac{\sqrt{1-0.7}}{0.7} = 0.78$$

2.1.5 Hyper-Geometric Distribution

The hypergeometric distribution, $h(N, k, n, x)$, arises in the following way.

Suppose there are N balls k of which are red and $N - k$ are blue, n balls without replacement are taken to form a sample. Let X equal the number of red balls in our sample of size n. Then

$$P(X = x) = h(N, k, n, x) = \frac{({}_kC_x)({}_{(N-k)}C_{(n-x)})}{{}_NC_n} = \frac{\binom{k}{n}\binom{N-k}{n-k}}{\binom{N}{n}}, \quad x = 0, 1, 2, \ldots, n \tag{2.20}$$

The probability distribution of a hypergeometric random variable is called a hypergeometric distribution. The following notation is helpful when we talk about hypergeometric distributions and hypergeometric probability.

N: The number of items in the population.
k: The number of items in the population that are classified as successes.

n: The number of items in the sample.
x: The number of items in the sample that are classified as successes.
${}_kC_x$ is the number of combinations of k things taken x at a time.

Example 2.5

A worker packs 15 bulbs with 5 defective ones and 10 non-defective ones. If 7 bulbs are randomly selected without replacement, what is the probability that at least 3 defective bulbs will be taken?

$$P(X \geq 3) = 1 - P(X \leq 2) = 1 - [P(0) + P(1) + P(2)] = 0.4267$$

$$P(0) = \frac{\binom{5}{0}\binom{10}{7}}{\binom{15}{7}} = 0.0186$$

$$P(1) = \frac{\binom{5}{1}\binom{10}{6}}{\binom{15}{7}} = 0.1631$$

$$P(2) = \frac{\binom{5}{2}\binom{10}{5}}{\binom{15}{7}} = 0.3916$$

2.1.6 *Poisson Distribution*

The Poisson distribution is a discrete function to model the number of events in a given time interval. It can be regarded as a special case of the binomial distribution. The Poisson distribution does not have a fixed number of trials, instead employing a specified interval of time, area, or space in which the number of successes is recorded.

Suppose X is the number of events in a fixed time interval and λ is the average number of events per interval, then the probability of observing x events in a specified interval can be calculated as,

$$P(X = x) = \mathrm{e}^{-\lambda}\frac{\lambda^x}{x!}, \qquad x = 0, 1, 2, 3, 4, \ldots \tag{2.21}$$

where, e is the mathematical constant and the n factorial is expressed as $n! = n \times (n-1) \times \cdots 2 \times 1$.

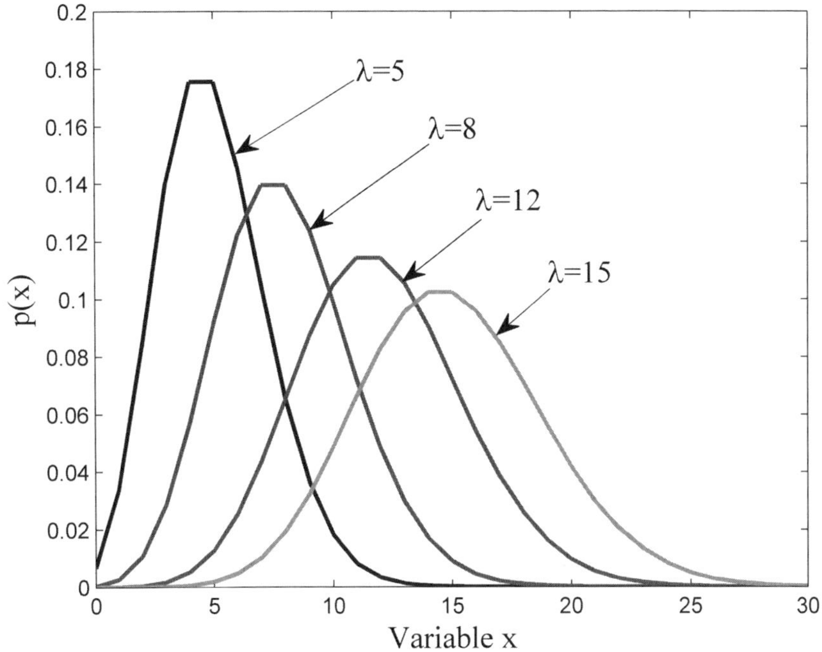

Figure 2.5 Poisson distribution of a random variable

If the probabilities of X are distributed in this way, we say X follows a Poisson distribution with parameter λ, and it can be written, $X \sim \text{Pois}(\lambda)$. It should be pointed out that a Poisson random variable can take on any positive integer value. In contrast, in binomial distribution it has a finite upper limit. As illustrated in Figure 2.5, the mean value λ greatly affects the shape of the Poisson distribution, the larger the mean values, the flatter the Poisson distribution.

Example 2.6

Births in a child care service center occur randomly with statistical records of an average 1.8 births per hour. For a given hour, calculate the probability of 4 births in the center. Calculate the probability of more than or equal to 2 births in a fixed hour in the center.

Let X be the number of births in a fixed hour. It is known that (i) events occur randomly and (ii) the mean rate $\lambda = 1.8$, thus the probabilities of X can be regarded as following a Poisson distribution, $X \sim \text{Pois}(1.8)$.

Then, the probability of 4 births in a fixed hour can be calculated as

$$P(X = 4) = \mathrm{e}^{-1.8}\frac{1.8^4}{4!} = 0.0723.$$

The probability of more than or equal to 2 births can be calculated as

$$\begin{aligned} P(X \geq 2) &= P(X = 2) + P(X = 3) + \ldots \\ &= 1 - P(X < 2) \\ &= 1 - P(X = 0) + P(X = 1) \\ &= 1 - \left(\mathrm{e}^{-1.8}\frac{1.8^0}{0!} + \mathrm{e}^{-1.8}\frac{1.8^1}{1!}\right) \\ &= 1 - (0.16529 + 0.29753) \\ &= 0.537 \end{aligned}$$

2.1.7 Chi-Squared Distributions

Suppose random variables $Z_1^2, Z_2^2, \ldots, Z_k^2$ are all standard normal random variables (i.e., each $Z_i \sim N(0, 1)$), and they are independent, then the sum of the random variables follows a chi-squared distribution with k degrees of freedom,

$$Z_1^2 + Z_2^2 + \ldots + Z_k^2 \sim \chi^2(k) \tag{2.22}$$

For random samples $y_1, y_2, \ldots, y_k$ with normal distribution $N(\mu, \sigma)$, let Y_i be the random variable with y_i, then it can be calculated that each $\frac{Y_i-\mu}{\sigma}$ follows standard normal, and $\frac{Y_1-\mu}{\sigma}, \frac{Y_2-\mu}{\sigma}, \ldots, \frac{Y_k-\mu}{\sigma}$ are independent, thus

$$\frac{Y_1 - \mu}{\sigma} + \frac{Y_2 - \mu}{\sigma} + \ldots + \frac{Y_k - \mu}{\sigma} \sim \chi^2(k) \tag{2.23}$$

The probability density function of chi-squared distribution can be written as

$$f(x) = \frac{x^{k/2-1}\mathrm{e}^{-x/2}}{\Gamma(k/2)2^{k/2}} \tag{2.24}$$

where, $x \in [0, \infty)$ is the random variable, k is the parameter, and $\Gamma(x)$ is the gamma function, (i) $\Gamma(x) = (x - 1)!$ when x is an integer and (ii) $\Gamma(x) = \int_0^\infty t^{x-1}\mathrm{e}^{-t}\mathrm{d}t$ for non-integers. A few examples with varying parameter values can be found in Figure 2.6, it can be seen that when k is small, the shape of the curve is very sharp, while when k is large, the curve tends to be flat.

The cumulative distribution function for the chi-squared distribution is

$$F(x, k) = \frac{\gamma(k/2, x/2)}{\Gamma(k/2)} \tag{2.25}$$

where $\gamma(a, x)$ is the lower incomplete gamma function defined by $\gamma(a, x) = \int_0^x t^{a-1}\mathrm{e}^{-t}\mathrm{d}t$.

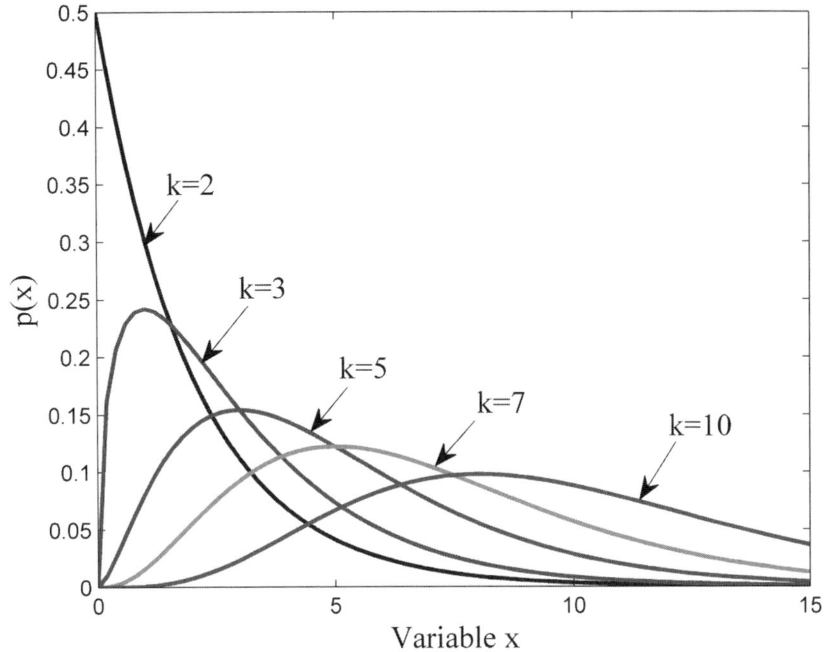

Figure 2.6 Chi-squared distribution of a random variable

The mean, median, and mode values for the chi-squared distribution can be calculated as, Mean $= k$, Median $= k(1 - \frac{2}{9k})^2$, Mode $= \max(k - 2, 0)$.

Example 2.7

For a random variable X that follows chi-squared distribution with three degrees of freedom, calculate the probability $P(0.35 \leq X \leq 7.81)$. From the chi-square distribution table, one can find the values $F_X(7.81) = 0.95$, $F_X(0.35) = 0.05$.

$$\begin{aligned} P(0.35 \leq X \leq 7.81) &= P(X \leq 7.81) - P(X \leq 0.35) \\ &= F_X(7.81) - F_X(0.35) \\ &= 0.95 - 0.05 = 0.9 \end{aligned}$$

2.2 Statistics on Unordered Data

For many modern data sets (financial and consumer data, text documents, and internet web pages), the collected data are high-dimensional, noisy, and unordered, with no particular meaning to the given order of the variable. Thus, it should be possible to achieve good discrimination by using only a small fraction of the original feature vector (which contains all the expression data) [3, 4].

2.2.1 Treelets Analysis

Treelets is a relatively novel method based on hierarchical clustering and local principal component analysis (PCA), and developed for multi-scale representation and eigen analysis of data where the variables can occur in any given order [5]. This method has two advantages, first, it finds a "natural" system of coordinates that reflects the underlying internal structure of the data and that is robust to noise. Secondly, it improves the performance of conventional regression and classification techniques by finding a reduced representation of the data prior to learning. The details of the algorithm are as follows [3, 5, 6]:

1. Define the clustering levels $l = 0, 1, 2, \ldots, L$ (where L is the highest level). At level $l = 0$, each observation is represented by the original variables, initialize the basis matrix B as an identity matrix whose size is $L \times L$, compute the correlation coefficient matrix M, which contains the correlation coefficients of all pairs of sum variables s_i and s_j. The matrix M can be calculated from

$$M_{ij} = \frac{C_{ij}}{\sqrt{C_{ii}C_{jj}}} \tag{2.26}$$

   where, $i,j = 1,2, \ldots, L$, and $i < j$, $C_{ij} = E[(s_i - E(s_i)) \cdot (s_j - E(s_j))]$, and $E(\cdot)$ stands for mathematical expectation.
2. At each level of the tree, we find the most similar variables according to the similarity matrix M, we denote the two variables which have the maximum correlation coefficients as α and β,

$$(\alpha,\ \beta) = \arg\max_{i,\ j \in S} M_{ij} \tag{2.27}$$

   where, S is the sum variable subscript set, initialized as $S = \{1, 2, \ldots, L\}$, the operator argmax returns values of α and β that make the similarity M_{ij} a maximum.
3. Perform a local PCA on (α, β), and find a Jacobian rotation matrix J, then update matrix B and M by the following equation

$$B_l = J(\alpha,\ \beta,\ \theta) \cdot B_{l-1} \tag{2.28}$$

   where, $J(\alpha,\ \beta,\ \theta) = \begin{bmatrix} 1 & \cdots & 0 & \cdots & 0 & \cdots & 0 \\ 0 & \cdots & c & \cdots & -s & \cdots & 0 \\ 0 & \cdots & s & \cdots & c & \cdots & 0 \\ 0 & \cdots & 0 & \cdots & 0 & \cdots & 1 \end{bmatrix}$, $c = \cos(\theta)$, $s = \sin(\theta)$, and $-\pi/4 \leq \theta \leq \pi/4$.

4. Repeat the above steps until the highest level $l = L - 1$ is reached. Then we get a final orthogonal matrix B that reflects the internal structure of the data.

For a random vector with distribution F, mean 0, and covariance matrix $\Sigma = \sigma_1^2 1_{p\times p}$, where $1_{p\times p}$ denotes a $p \times p$ matrix with all entries equal to 1. Then, at any level $1 \leq l \leq p-1$ of the tree, the treelet operator T_l returns an orthogonal decomposition,

$$T_l(\Sigma) = \sum_{i=1}^{p-l} s_{l,i}\phi_{l,i} + \sum_{i=1}^{l} d_i \psi_i \tag{2.29}$$

With sum variables $s_{l,i} = \frac{1}{\sqrt{A_{l,i}}}\sum_{j\in A_{l,i}} x_j$ and scaling functions $\phi_{l,i} = \frac{1}{\sqrt{A_{l,i}}} \times I_{s_{l,i}}$, which are defined on disjoint index subsets $A_{l,i} \subseteq \{1, \ldots, p\}(i = 1, \ldots, p-l)$ with lengths $|A_{l,i}|$ and $\sum_{i=1}^{p-l}|A_{l,i}| = p$. The expansion coefficients have variances $V\{s_{l,i}\} = |A_{l,i}|\sigma_1^2$ and $V\{d_i\} = 0$. In particular, for $l = p-1$,

$$T_{p-1}(\Sigma) = s\phi + \sum_{i=1}^{p-1} d_i \psi_i \tag{2.30}$$

where, $s = \frac{1}{\sqrt{p}}(x_1 + \ldots + x_p)$ and $\phi = \frac{1}{\sqrt{p}}[1, \ldots, 1]^{\mathrm{T}}$.

The output of the algorithm can be summarized in terms of a hierarchical tree with a height $L \leq p-1$ and an ordered set of rotations and pairs of indices. Figure 2.7 shows an example of a treelet construction for a signal of length $P = 5$, with the data representations $x^{(l)}$ at different levels of the tree.

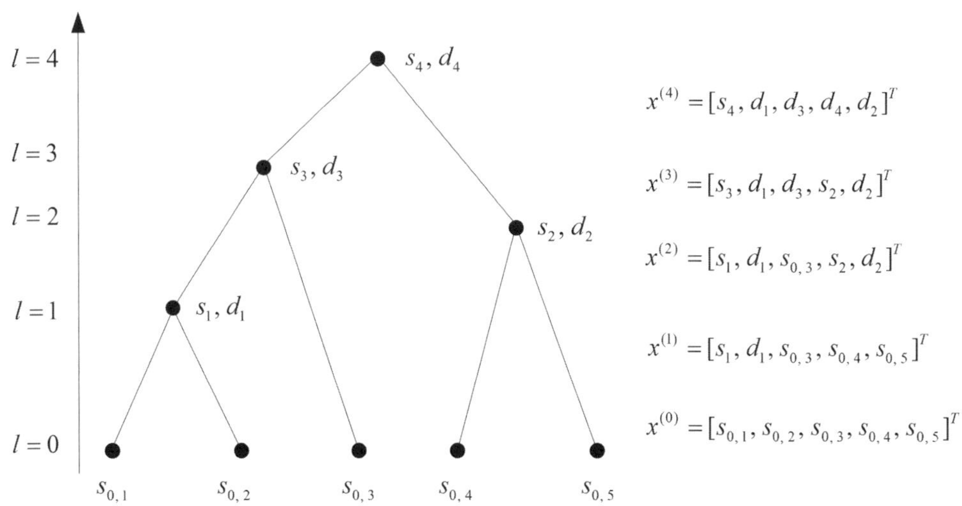

Figure 2.7 An example of a hierarchical tree data of dimension $p = 5$

2.2.2 *Clustering Analysis*

The goal of clustering is to identify structure in an unlabeled sample or unordered data by objectively organizing data into homogeneous groups where the within-group-object similarity is minimized and the between-group-object dissimilarity is maximized. Clustering is necessary when no labeled data are available, regardless of whether the data are binary, categorical, numerical, interval, ordinal, relational, textual, spatial, temporal, spatiotemporal, image, multimedia, or mixtures of the above data types. Data are called static if all their feature values do not change with time, or only change negligibly [7]. Most examples of clustering analyses have been performed on static data, and most are developed as an independent program or as part of data mining software to deal with static data.

Given a set of data objects (entities, input patterns, instances, observances, units), the objective of clustering is to partition them into a certain number of clusters (categories, groups, or subsets) in order to explore the underlying structure and provide useful insights for further analysis. However, there exists no universally agreed-upon and precise definition of the term cluster, partially due to the inherent subjectivity of clustering, which precludes an absolute judgment as to the relative efficacy of all clustering techniques. The best definition differs from problem to problem and depends on the desired goal and the data properties. In spite of this difficulty, several operational or working definitions are still available, for example, we have the following [8]:

1. A cluster is a set of data objects that are similar to each other, while data objects in different clusters are different from one another.
2. A cluster is a set of data objects such that the distance between an object in a cluster and the centroid of the cluster is less than the distance between this object and the centroids of any other clusters.
3. A cluster is a set of data objects such that the distance between any two objects in the cluster is less than the distance between any object in the cluster and any object not in it.
4. A cluster is a continuous region of data objects with a relatively high density, which is separated from other such dense regions by low-density regions.

Clearly, the definitions are closely related to internal homogeneity and external separation are not clearly elucidated. Here, we give some simple mathematical descriptions of two types of clustering, known as hierarchical and partitional clustering [9, 10]. Hierarchical clustering considers grouping data objects with a sequence of nested partitions, while partitional clustering directly divides data objects into some number of clusters without the hierarchical structure. In the following we briefly describe some widely used clustering algorithms/procedures.

2.2.2.1 Relocation Clustering

The relocation clustering procedure has the following three steps [7, 11],

Step 1: Start with an initial clustering, denoted by C, having the prescribed k number of clusters.
Step 2: For each time point, compute the dissimilarity matrix and store all resultant matrices computed for all time points for the calculation of trajectory similarity.
Step 3: Find a clustering C', such that C' is better than C in terms of the *generalized Ward criterion function*. The clustering C' is obtained from C by relocating one member of C_p to C_q or by swapping two members between C_p and C_q, where C_p, $C_q \in C$, $p, q = 1, 2, \ldots, k$, and $p \neq q$. If no such clustering exists, then stop; else replace C by C' and repeat *Step 3*.

2.2.2.2 K-Means Algorithm

The most popular and the simplest clustering algorithm is K-means. Since partitional algorithms are preferred in pattern recognition due to the nature of the available data, our coverage here is focused on these algorithms. K-means has a rich and diverse history as it was independently discovered in different scientific fields. Even though K-means was first proposed over 50 years ago, it is still one of the most widely used algorithms for clustering. Ease of implementation, simplicity, efficiency, and empirical success are the main reasons for its popularity [12, 13].

Let $X = \{x_i\}$, $i = 1, 2, \ldots, n$ be the set of n d-dimensional points to be clustered into a set of K clusters $C = \{c_k, k = 1, 2, \ldots, K\}$. The K-means algorithm finds a partition such that the squared error between the empirical mean of a cluster and the points in the cluster is minimized. Let μ_k be the mean of cluster c_k. The squared error between μ_k and the points in cluster c_k is defined as,

$$J(c_k) = \sum_{x_i \in c_k} \|x_i - \mu_k\|^2 \tag{2.31}$$

The goal of the K-means algorithm is to minimize the sum of the squared error over all K clusters,

$$J(c) = \sum_{k=1}^{K} \sum_{x_i \in c_k} \|x_i - \mu_k\|^2 \tag{2.32}$$

Minimizing this objective function is known to be an NP-hard problem (even for $K = 2$). Thus K-means, which is a greedy algorithm, can only converge to a local minimum, even though recent study has shown with a large probability that K-means could converge to the global optimum when clusters are well separated. K-means starts with an initial partition with K clusters and assigns patterns to clusters so as to reduce the squared error. Since the squared error always decreases with an increase in the number of clusters K, it can be minimized only for a fixed number of clusters. The main steps of the K-means algorithm are:

Step 1: Select an initial partition with K clusters; repeat *steps 2* and *3* until the cluster membership stabilizes.
Step 2: Generate a new partition by assigning each pattern to its closest cluster center.
Step 3: Compute new cluster centers.

An illustration of the K-means algorithm on a two-dimensional dataset with two clusters is shown in Figure 2.8.

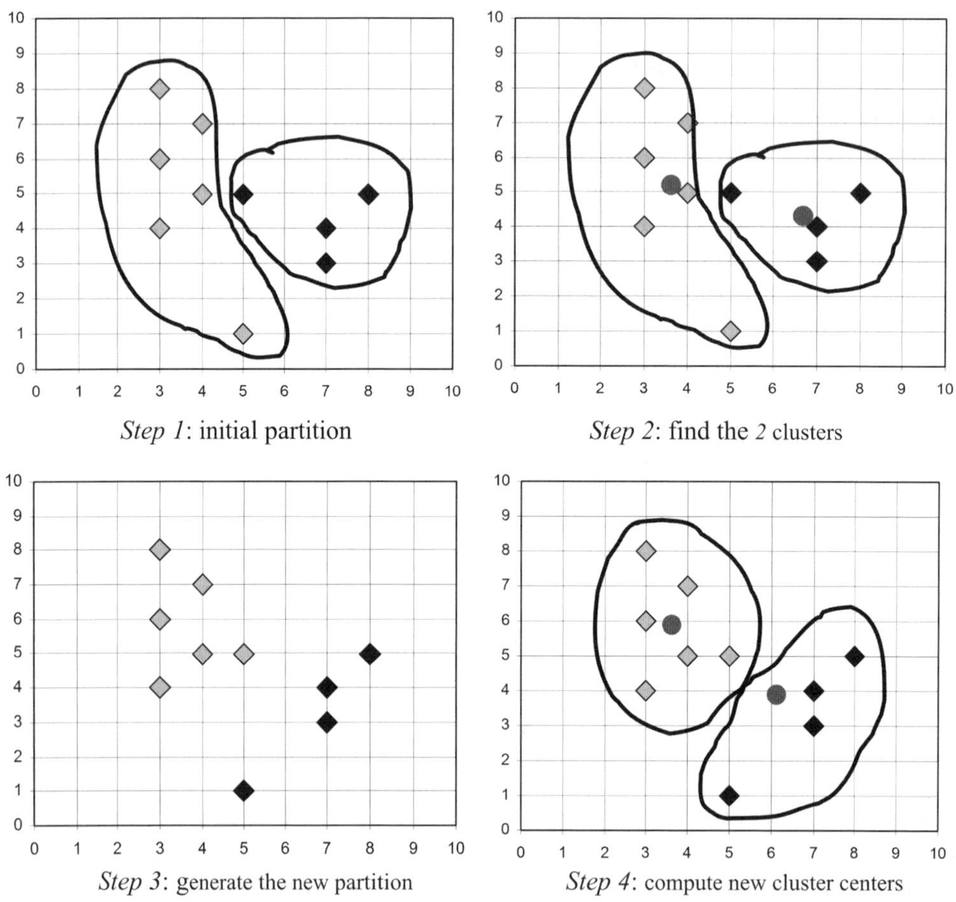

Figure 2.8 Illustration of the K-means algorithm

2.2.2.3 Self-Organizing Maps

Self-organizing maps (SOMs) are a class of neural networks with neurons arranged in a low-dimensional (often two-dimensional) structure and trained by an iterative unsupervised or self-organizing procedure. The training algorithm proposed by Kohonen [14] for forming a feature map is:

Step 1: Initialization. Choose random values for the initial weights w_i.

Step 2: Winner Finding. Find the winning neuron c at time t, using the minimum Euclidean distance criterion.

$$c = \arg\min_i \|x - w_i\|, \qquad i = 1, 2, \ldots, M \tag{2.33}$$

where, the operator argmin returns values of the winning neuron c that minimize the Euclidean distance criterion. $x = [x_1, x_2, \ldots, x_m]$ represents an input vector at time t, M is the total number of neurons, and $\|\cdot\|$ indicates the Euclidean norm.

Step 3: Weights Updating. Adjust the weights of the winner and its neighbors, using the following rule,

$$w_i(t+1) = w_i(t) + \eta(t) h_{ci}(t)[x_j(t) - w_i(t)] \tag{2.34}$$

$$h_{ci}(t) = \exp\left(-\frac{\|r_c - r_i\|^2}{2\sigma^2(t)}\right) \tag{2.35}$$

where $x_j(t)$ represents an input data at time t, $h_{ci}(t)$ is the topological neighborhood function of the winner neuron c at time t, $\eta(t)$ is a positive constant called the learning-rate factor, $r_c \in R^2$ and $r_i \in R^2$ are the location vectors of nodes c and i, respectively. $\sigma(t)$ defines the width of the kernel. Both $\eta(t)$ and $\sigma(t)$ will decrease with time. It should be emphasized that the success of the map formation is critically dependent on the values of the main parameters, the initial values of the weight vectors, and the pre-specified number of iterations.

In the case of a discrete data set and fixed neighborhood kernel, the sum of the squared-error of SOM can be defined as follows:

$$SSE = \sum_{j=1}^{n} \sum_{i=1}^{M} h_{ci} \|x_j - w_i\|^2 \tag{2.36}$$

where n is the number of training samples and M is the number of map units. The neighborhood kernel h_{ci} is centered at unit c, which is the best matching unit of input vector x_j, and evaluated for the ith unit.

2.3 Statistics on Ordered Data

Ordered data are a collection of observations made chronologically. The characteristics of ordered data, especially time series, include: large data size, high dimensionality, and the necessity to update continuously. Moreover, ordered data, which are characterized by their numerical and continuous nature, are always considered as a whole instead of as individual numerical fields. To seek useful knowledge in these processes, this section presents an experience based on the use of association rules from multiple time series captured from industrial processes [15, 16].

Association rule mining (ARM) is an unsupervised learning method that discovers significant relationships among items in a given data set. It is widely used in various research areas, such as pattern recognition [17], explaining mechanical failure [15], and bio-medical data analysis [18]. ARM can be applied to the case without target variables, and the results can be easily understood since they are expressed in if–then formats. Association rules are sentences of the type $X \Rightarrow Y$ (X implies Y, X is called the antecedent and Y is the consequent), where X and Y are sets of frequent items in a given database, whereby $X \cap Y = \emptyset$.

The three general measurements for association rules are expressed as below [19]. First, the support ($X \rightarrow Y$) is defined as the ratio of the number of transactions that include both items X and Y to the total number of transactions. It represents the usefulness of discovered rules by the probability of co-occurrence of item X and Y. Secondly, the confidence ($X \rightarrow Y$) measures the ratio of the number of transactions containing item Y to the number of transactions containing item X. It denotes the conditional probability of Y given X, representing the certainty of the rule. Finally, the lift ($X \rightarrow Y$) is calculated by dividing the confidence by the probability of Y. The lift ($X \rightarrow Y$) shows the statistical dependence between items X and Y, indicating the positive correlation if the value is less than one.

$$\text{Support}\,(X \rightarrow Y) \,:= P(X \cap Y) = \frac{N(X \cap Y)}{N} \tag{2.37}$$

$$\text{Confidence}\,(X \rightarrow Y) \,:= \frac{P(X \cap Y)}{P(X)} = P(Y|X) = \frac{N(X \cap Y)}{N(X)} \tag{2.38}$$

$$\text{Lift}\,(X \rightarrow Y) \,:= \frac{P(Y|X)}{P(Y)} = \frac{N(X \cap Y) \cdot N}{N(X) \cdot N(Y)} \tag{2.39}$$

The basic procedure of ARM consists of two steps [19, 20]: (i) identification of the frequently co-occurring item set and (ii) generation of association rules. Specifically, the item sets having support ($X \rightarrow Y$) greater than the user-specified threshold are first identified, and the association rules are then generated among frequently co-occurring item sets by selecting ones whose confidence ($X \rightarrow Y$) is higher than the user-specified threshold. Finally, the association rules with the lift $(X \rightarrow Y) > 1$ are selected as useful rules.

2.4 Technologies for Incomplete Data

Most of the real world databases are characterized by an unavoidable problem of incompleteness, in terms of missing or erroneous values. Varieties of different reasons result in the introduction of incompleteness in the data. Examples include manual data entry procedures, incorrect measurements, equipment errors, and many others. The existence of errors, and in particular missing values, makes it often difficult to generate useful knowledge from investigated data [21].

Many technologies have been used to solve the incompleteness or missing data problem: case deletion, prediction rules, linear regression, and so on. There are also many references to data analysis approaches of rough sets in an incomplete information system [21–23]. In general, the tolerance relation is used to create a tolerance matrix and a discernibility matrix for dealing with incomplete data in rough sets.

An information system (IS) is a quadruple IS $=< U, A, V, f >$, where U is a non-empty finite set of objects. A is a non-empty finite set of attributes, V is the union of attribute domains, $V = \cup_{a\in A} V_a$, where V_a is the value set of attribute a, called the domain of $a, f : U \times A \rightarrow V$ is an information function which assigns particular values from domains of attribute to objects such as $\forall a \in A$, $x \in U$, $f(a,x) \in V_a$, where $f(a,x)$ denotes the value of attribute a for object x [22].

A decision system (DS) is a quadruple DS $=< U, C \cup D, V, f >$, where C is a conditional attribute set, D is a decision attribute set, and $C \cap D = \emptyset$, V is the union of attribute domains, $V = V_C \cup V_D = \cup\{V_a|a \in C\} \cup \{V_d|d \in D\}$. Unlike an IS that contains no decision attribute, a DS contains the decision attribute set D. Hence, a labeled data set is a DS. It should also be noticed that the attributes are supposed to be symbolic. The concept of indiscernibility is central to rough set theory. Let IS $=< U, A, V, f >$ be an information system, for any $R \subseteq A$, the associated indiscernibility relation IND(R) is

$$\text{IND}(R) = \{(x, y)|\forall a \in R, f(a, x) = f(a, y)\} \tag{2.40}$$

Obviously, IND(R) is an equivalence relation, which is reflexive, symmetric, and transitive. The family of all equivalence classes of IND(R) will be denoted by $U/\text{IND}(R)$, or simply U/R. An equivalence class of IND(R) containing x will be denoted by $[x]_R$. For $X \subseteq U$, the lower and upper approximations of X with respect to R can be defined as,

$$R_l(X) = \{x|[x]_R \subseteq X\} \tag{2.41}$$

$$R_U(X) = \{x|[x]_R \cap X \neq \emptyset\} \tag{2.42}$$

An information system is a pair $S = (U, A)$, where U is a non-empty finite set of objects, A is a non-empty finite set of attributes [24], and for every $a \in A$, there is a mapping a, $a : U \rightarrow V_a$, where V_a is called the value set of a. However, it may happen that some of the attribute values for an object are missing. For this situation, a

Table 2.1 Incomplete information system

U	a_1	a_2	a_3	a_4	D
x_1	3	2	1	0	y
x_2	2	3	2	0	y
x_3	*	1	3	2	n
x_4	2	*	*	3	y
x_5	1	*	*	*	y
x_6	*	2	*	*	n
x_7	3	2	1	*	y

null value is usually assigned to those attributes denoted by $*$. If V_a contains a null value for at least one attribute $a \in A$, then S is called an incomplete information system, otherwise it is a complete one [25]. If all the attributes in an incomplete IS are nominal or symbolic, then it is an incomplete symbolic IS. Similarly, for a DS $= < U,\ C \cup D,\ V, f >$, if $* \notin V_D$, but $* \in V_C$, then the DS is called an incomplete decision system. If all the attributes in an incomplete DS are nominal or symbolic, then it is an incomplete symbolic DS. An incomplete symbolic DS is shown in Table 2.1, where $U = \{x_1, x_2, x_3, x_4, x_5, x_6, x_7\}$, $C = \{a_1, a_2, a_3, a_4\}$, and decision $D = \{y, n\}$.

In an incomplete IS, the equivalence relation is not suitable because of some missing values. Kryszkiewicz [25] proposed a rough set approach to learning rules directly from incomplete data sets without guessing unknown attribute values. For any subset of attributes $B \subseteq A$, let $T(B)$ denote the binary tolerance relation between objects that are possibly indiscernible in terms of values of attribute B. Then the tolerance relation between objects for the attribute subset is defined as follows,

$$T(\{a\}) = \{(x, y)|f(a, x) = f(b, x) \vee f(a, x) = * \vee f(b, x) = *\} \tag{2.43}$$

$T(\{a\})$ is reflexive and symmetric, but may not be transitive.

$$T(B) = \underset{a \in B}{\cap} T(\{a\}) \tag{2.44}$$

The tolerance class of an object x with respect to an attribute set B is denoted as $T_B(x) = \{y|(x, y) \in T(B)\}$. It shows that the tolerance relation can deal with symbolic data sets with missing values. The lower approximation and the upper approximation are then derived from the generalized decisions. Rules possibly with disjunctive conclusions are then derived from the lower and the upper approximations.

References

1. Faber, M.H. (2012) *Statistics and Probability Theory*, Springer, Dordrecht.
2. Ling, K.D. (1990) On geometric distributions of order (k1, … ,km). *Statistics and Probability Letters*, **9** (2), 163–171.

3. Lee, A.B., Nadler, B. and Wasserman, L. (2008) Treelet – An adaptive multi-scale basis for sparse unordered data. *The Annals of Applied Statistics*, **2** (2), 435–471.
4. Sheng, L., Ortega, A., Pique-Regi, R. *et al.* (2009) Treelets as a feature transformation tool for block diagonal linear discrimination. IEEE International Workshop on Genomic Signal Processing and Statistics, 2009. GENSIPS 2009, Minneapolis, MN, pp. 1–4.
5. Wang, G., Min, Z., Tian, X. *et al.* (2011) Unsupervised change detection for remote sensing images using multiscale decomposition and treelet fusion: a level set approach. 2011 IEEE CIE International Conference on Radar, pp. 1558–1561.
6. Tuglus, C. and van der Laan, M.J. (2008) Discussion of: treelets – An adaptive multi-scale basis for sparse unordered data. *The Annals of Applied Statistics*, **2** (2), 489–493.
7. Warren Liao, T. (2005) Clustering of time series data – a survey. *Pattern Recognition*, **38** (11), 1857–1874.
8. Rui, X. and Wunsch, D.C. (2010) Clustering algorithms in biomedical research: a review. *IEEE Reviews in Biomedical Engineering*, **3**, 120–154.
9. Hansen, P. and Jaumard, B. (1997) Cluster analysis and mathematical programming. *Mathematical Programming*, **79** (1–3), 191–215.
10. Jain, A.K., Murty, M.N. and Flynn, P.J. (1999) Data clustering: a review. *ACM Computing Surveys*, **31** (3), 264–323.
11. Grotkjær, T., Winther, O., Regenberg, B. *et al.* (2006) Robust multi-scale clustering of large DNA microarray datasets with the consensus algorithm. *Bioinformatics*, **22** (1), 58–67.
12. Jain, A.K. (2010) Data clustering: 50 years beyond K-means. *Pattern Recognition Letters*, **31** (8), 651–666.
13. Liao, K., Liu, G., Xiao, L. *et al.* (2013) A sample-based hierarchical adaptive K-means clustering method for large-scale video retrieval. *Knowledge-Based Systems*, **49**, 123–133.
14. Kohonen, T. (1990) The self-organizing map. *Proceedings of the IEEE*, **78** (9), 1464–1480.
15. Martínez-de-Pisón, F.J., Sanz, A., Martínez-de-Pisón, E. *et al.* (2012) Mining association rules from time series to explain failures in a hot-dip galvanizing steel line. *Computers & Industrial Engineering*, **63** (1), 22–36.
16. Fu, T.-c. (2011) A review on time series data mining. *Engineering Applications of Artificial Intelligence*, **24** (1), 164–181.
17. Chen, G., Liu, H., Yu, L. *et al.* (2006) A new approach to classification based on association rule mining. *Decision Support Systems*, **42** (2), 674–689.
18. Nahar, J., Imam, T., Tickle, K.S. *et al.* (2013) Association rule mining to detect factors which contribute to heart disease in males and females. *Expert Systems with Applications*, **40** (4), 1086–1093.
19. Lee, C., Song, B. and Park, Y. (2012) Design of convergent product concepts based on functionality: an association rule mining and decision tree approach. *Expert Systems with Applications*, **39** (10), 9534–9542.
20. Agrawal, R., Imielinski, T., and Swami, A. (1993) Mining association rules between sets of items in large databases. SIGMOD '93 Proceedings of the 1993 ACM SIGMOD International Conference on Management of Data, New York, pp. 207–216.
21. Sadiq, A.T., Duaimi, M.G., and Shaker, S.A. (2012) Data missing solution using rough set theory and swarm intelligence. 2012 International Conference on Advanced Computer Science Applications and Technologies (ACSAT), pp. 173–180
22. Dai, J. (2013) Rough set approach to incomplete numerical data. *Information Sciences*, **241**, 43–57.
23. Zou, Y. and Xiao, Z. (2008) Data analysis approaches of soft sets under incomplete information. *Knowledge-Based Systems*, **21** (8), 941–945.
24. Qian, Y., Liang, J., Pedrycz, W. *et al.* (2011) An efficient accelerator for attribute reduction from incomplete data in rough set framework. *Pattern Recognition*, **44** (8), 1658–1670.
25. Kryszkiewicz, M. (1998) Rough set approach to incomplete information systems. *Information Sciences*, **112** (1–4), 39–49.

3

Signal Processing

3.1 Introduction

The level of industrial automization is constantly increasing and any unforeseen downtime resulting from equipment damage or failure may lead to significant economic losses and potentially disastrous consequences for the machine itself [1]. Cost-effective detection of mechanical faults will go a long way towards improving the availability of industrial equipment. Consequently, there is an increasing need for condition monitoring and fault diagnostics methods aiming to detect in advance symptoms warning of failure, giving the lead time to make alternative arrangements and, more importantly, avoid product deterioration, performance degradation, major damage to the machinery itself and damage to human health or even loss of life.

With the advances in digital signal processing methods, there has been an increasingly strong interest in the application of signal analysis techniques for the detection of fault features of machinery elements [2]. Owing to the advantage of direct association with the rotating characteristics, spectral analysis has been the most used signal processing tool in vibration analysis of rotating machinery [3]. The primary advantage of time domain methods is that they use directly the measured vibration signal in signal processing. However, signal analysis methods in the frequency domain average out the vibration signals over the time period and smear the local characteristics. Moreover, their effectiveness is quite limited when applied to the identification of highly damped systems and systems with severe modal interference. Noise and random vibrations may be suppressed from the vibration signal using time domain signal processing techniques, such as filtering, averaging, correlation, convolution, and so on. However, sometimes random vibrations are also important because they are related to some types of machine faults.

Time–frequency analysis approaches introduced in the past few decades have perfectly solved those shortcomings. Owing to the advantage of multi-scale resolution in time–frequency analysis for characterizing the transitory features of non-stationary signals, wavelet transform can decompose an inspected signal into several elementary

Machinery Prognostics and Prognosis Oriented Maintenance Management, First Edition. Jihong Yan.

functions with different levels. This ability renders the analysis of the inspected signal easier for machine operators. Extensive research has been conducted on applying wavelet transform in machine fault diagnosis [4–7], and the recent advances of wavelet transform analysis have derived a new set of techniques of time–frequency analysis that have been shown to be powerful in the field of transient signal processing, such as wavelet coefficients analysis [8], wavelet ridge method [9], undecimated discrete wavelet transform (DWT) [10], and so on.

A newly proposed signal processing method, the Hilbert–Huang transform (HHT) developed by Huang *et al.* [11], was demonstrated to be superior to wavelet analysis in many applications [12–14], As we know, time scale and the corresponding energy distribution are the two most important parameters of a signal in signal processing [15], by employing empirical mode decomposition (EMD) the key part of HHT, the complicated dataset can be decomposed into a series of mono-component modes, defined as intrinsic mode functions (IMFs), with local characteristic time scales of the investigated signal, then the instantaneous frequency could be obtained through the Hilbert transform, which could represent the physical meaning of the local phase change [12]. Moreover, the frequency components contained in each IMF not only relate to the sampling frequency, but also change with the signal itself. Furthermore, unlike Fourier transform analysis and wavelet transform, the whole transform process does not lead to energy diffusion and leakage [11]. Therefore, EMD is suitable for the analysis of non-linear and non-stationary processes. It is most remarkable that this technique has been applied in many fields, such as signal processing, wind engineering, biomedical engineering, ocean waves, and earthquake engineering.

After extracting fault features from investigated data, pattern recognition techniques were employed to evaluate the performance of mechanical equipment. The Bayesian network (BN) and support vector machines (SVMs) are two widely used statistical pattern recognition algorithms. The prominent ability of the BN is to support probabilistic reasoning from uncertainty data, and probabilistic inference can be conducted to predict the values of some variables based on observed values of other variables via a well trained network. While SVMs, based on statistical learning theory, are introduced into machine fault diagnosis due to their high accuracy and good generalization for a smaller number of samples [16].

3.2 Signal Pre-Processing

3.2.1 Digital Filtering

Digital filters are used in numerous applications from control systems, systems for audio and video processing, and communication systems to systems for medical applications, to name just a few [17]. They are typically considered in two categories: infinite impulse response (IIR) and finite impulse response (FIR) [18]. FIR filters are commonly known as non-recursive filters and IIR filters as recursive filters. Implementation of FIR filters is easy, but they are slower than IIR filters. Though IIR filters are fast, practical implementation is complicated compared to FIR filters [19]. An FIR filter is an attractive choice because of the ease in design and stability, and they are known to have many desirable features, such as guaranteed stability, the possibility of an exact linear phase characteristic at all frequencies and digital implementation as non-recursive structures [17].

The general difference equation of an FIR digital filter is,

$$y(n) = \sum_{k=0}^{N} b_k x(n-k), \qquad n = 0, 1, \ldots, N \tag{3.1}$$

where, $y(n)$ is the filter output, $x(n-k)$ is the input data delayed by k samples, b_k is the filter coefficient, and N is the order of the filter. The frequency response of an FIR digital filter with N taps specified by a real-valued impulse response $h(n)$ is given by Kidambi [20]

$$H(\mathrm{e}^{\mathrm{j}\omega}) = \sum_{n=0}^{N-1} h(n)\mathrm{e}^{-\mathrm{j}n\omega} \tag{3.2}$$

For the desired filter output $D(n)$ with frequency response $D(\mathrm{e}^{\mathrm{j}\omega})$. Then the mean-square error E_{MSE} is defined as

$$E_{\mathrm{MSE}} = \sum_{l=1}^{M} W(\omega_l)|D(\mathrm{e}^{\mathrm{j}\omega_l}) - H(\mathrm{e}^{\mathrm{j}\omega_l})|^2 \tag{3.3}$$

where, $W(\omega)$ is a non-negative frequency-dependent weighting function and M is the number of sample points. In minimizing E_{MSE}, a system of linear equations can be obtained when the derivative $\partial E_{\mathrm{MSE}}/\partial h$ is set as zero, this can be solved by a computationally efficient and robust Levinson method [21].

A vibration signal contaminated by white Gaussian noise was used to investigate the performance of the FIR filter. As shown in Figure 3.1a, a vibration signal was collected from a Bently test-bed with rotation speed 3000 rev/min, the fundamental frequency and frequency-doubled were represented as 50 and 100 Hz, respectively. A fifth-order lower-pass Butterworth filter was designed with normalized cut-off frequency of 0.24, and the stop-band corner normalized frequency was 0.3. The frequency spectrum of filter magnitude and phase is shown in Figure 3.2. The filtered vibration signal is shown in Figure 3.1b, with the high frequency noise effectively removed.

3.2.2 Outlier Detecting

Outlier analysis has been considered quite significant in identifying atypical observations from a given set of data. Usually, outliers deviate markedly from other data samples and can highly influence the predictive accuracy of several commonly used data mining algorithms [22]. In simple terms, outliers represent the observations that fail to follow the general pattern of the majority of data samples. Thus, it is critical to

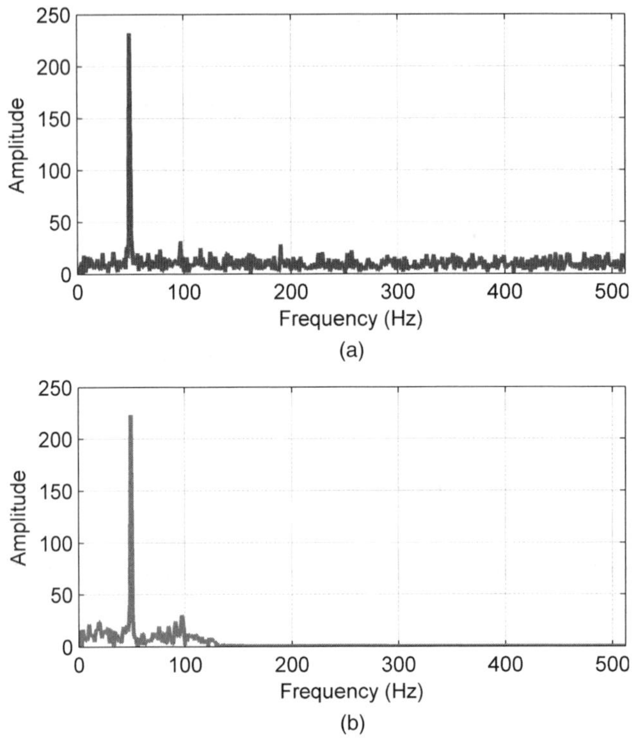

Figure 3.1 (a) Noisy vibration signal and (b) filtered vibration signal

detect and appropriately treat such anomalous observations, contributing to undesired performance degradation, or suggesting unexpected but interesting patterns [23].

A widely used outlier identification method is established on the distance-based model, this method aims to detect outliers by computing a measure of how far a particular point is from the center of the data. Let the data matrix $X = (x_1, x_2, \ldots, x_n)^T$, where $x_i (i = 1, 2, \ldots, n)$ is a column vector with p dimensionality that represents the ith observation.

The data are assumed to be independently sampled from a multivariate normal distribution $N_p\left(\mu, \sum\right)$. A general measure of squared distance from an observation x_i to the centroid of the p-dimensional space μ, for $i = 1, 2, \ldots, n$, can thus be written as [23, 24]

$$d_i = (x_i - \mu)^T \cdot M \cdot (x_i - \mu) \tag{3.4}$$

where, M is a $p \times p$ symmetrical matrix. It can be easily noted that Equation 3.4 is a squared Euclidean distance if $M = I$, where, I is the identity matrix, and a weighted Euclidean distance if $M = W$, where, W is a symmetric weight matrix. Moreover, if $M = \sum^{-1}$ where $\sum$ is the population covariance matrix, the squared Mahalanobis

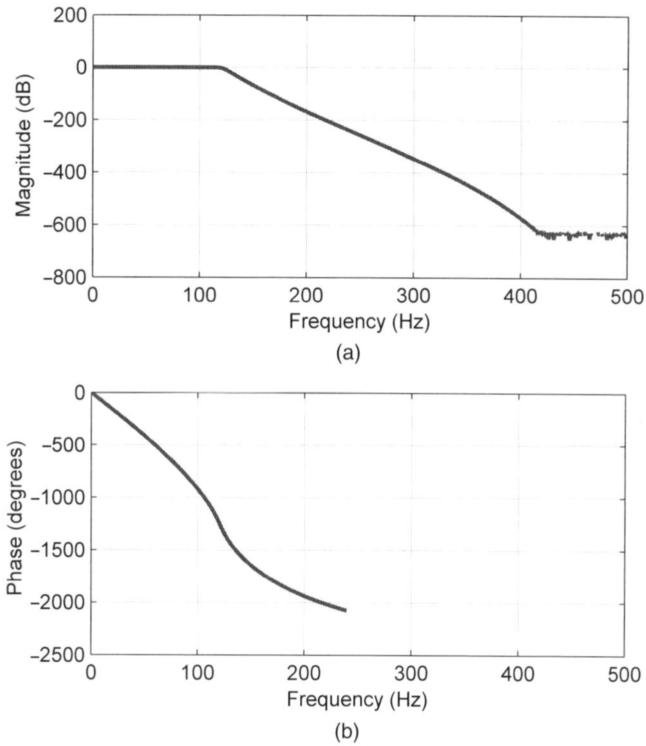

Figure 3.2 (a) Magnitude of low-pass filter and (b) phase of low-pass filter

distance is obtained as,

$$d_i = (x_i - \mu)^{\mathrm{T}} \cdot \sum^{-1} \cdot (x_i - \mu) \tag{3.5}$$

These distances are distributed according to χ_p^2 and if the parameters μ and $\sum$ are estimated by the arithmetic mean $\overline{x}$ and the sample covariance matrix $S = 1/(n-1) \cdot \sum_{i=1}^{n}(x_i - \overline{x})(x_i - \overline{x})^{\mathrm{T}}$ respectively, the squared Mahalanobis distances are,

$$D_i = (x_i - \overline{x})^{\mathrm{T}} \cdot S^{-1} \cdot (x_i - \overline{x}) \tag{3.6}$$

This deviation statistic, D_i is then compared to threshold value D_{th}. Herein, if $D_i > D_{\mathrm{th}}$ then x_i is an outlier. The threshold value, D_{th} can be established with a certain confidence level, outliers can be detected from the signal with the results of the comparison [24].

3.2.3 Signal Detrending

A vibration signal is often affected by disturbance, and presents with varying mean and standard deviation (SD). These effects have to be well distinguished from the intrinsic fluctuations and correlations of the system in order to find the correct scaling behavior. Sometimes, we do not know the reasons for underlying non-stationarity in collected data and, even worse, we do not know the type of the underlying non-stationarity [25].

In a simple approach, the trend of a time series is identified by fitting a deterministic component, usually linear. The trend is then subtracted in order to guarantee stationarity of the resulting time series. More generally, detrending is the process by which a trend is removed from a time series. The residue after this operation can be called variability or fluctuation. One common constraint on this process is that the detrended series must be a zero-mean process for the time span considered in the detrending [25, 26]. In this approach, assuming a simple additive superposition of trend and variability, a time series can be decomposed as:

$$y(t) = T(t) + r(t) \tag{3.7}$$

where, $r(t)$ is a residual, variability, or fluctuation around the trend $T(t)$, $y(t)$ is the output of the time series. The fluctuation component can have both stochastic and deterministic components. Then, a uniform model of $y(t)$ becomes $\widehat{y}(t) = T(t) + m_{\mathrm{CI}}(t)$, where, the first component is the overall trend and the second component is the model of the fluctuations around the overall trend [26, 27].

3.3 Techniques for Signal Processing

3.3.1 Time-Domain Analysis

The simplest method of signal analysis is plotting a sequence of data points in a time domain. It is advisable to always inspect the signal in this way before further processing in order to identify possible abnormalities, for example, due to deviating behavior or problems with the data acquisition [28]. Statistical features [29, 30] in the time domain are widely used to mine useful information. Defined as follows, time domain features are calculated to represent a characteristic of collected data.

1. Root mean square (RMS)

$$\mathrm{RMS} = \sqrt{\frac{1}{n}\sum_{i=1}^{n}(x_i)^2} \tag{3.8}$$

2. Peak-to-peak (PP)

$$\mathrm{PP} = \max(x_i) - \min(x_i) \tag{3.9}$$

3. Pulse index (PI)

$$\mathrm{PI} = \frac{x_{\max}}{\overline{x}} \tag{3.10}$$

4. Kurtosis (KR)

$$\mathrm{KR} = \frac{n\sum_{i=1}^{n}(x_i - \overline{x})^4}{\left(\sum_{i=1}^{n}(x_i - \overline{x})^2\right)^2} \tag{3.11}$$

Then the following additional time-domain features are extracted, which were specifically developed for gear damage detection and reported in several NASA technical reports [29, 31, 32].

5. FM0

$$\mathrm{FM0} = \frac{\mathrm{PP}}{\sum_{h=0}^{H} P_h} \tag{3.12}$$

where, P_h is the amplitude of the hth harmonic of the meshing frequency and H is the total number of harmonics considered.

6. FM4

$$\mathrm{FM4} = \frac{n\sum_{i=1}^{n}(d_i - \overline{d})^4}{\left(\sum_{i=1}^{n}(d_i - \overline{d})^2\right)^2} \tag{3.13}$$

where, d_i is the ith measurement of the difference signal of the time series and $\overline{d}$ is the average of the difference signal.

7. NA4

$$\mathrm{NA4} = \frac{\frac{1}{n}\sum_{i=1}^{n}(r_i - \overline{r})^4}{\left(\frac{1}{N}\sum_{j=1}^{N}\left(\frac{1}{n}\sum_{k=1}^{n}(r_{jk} - \overline{r_j})^2\right)\right)^2} \tag{3.14}$$

where, x_i $(i = 1, 2, \ldots, n)$ is the ith sampling point of the time series, n is the number of points in the signal, and $\overline{x}$ is the average of the signal. r_i is the ith measurement of the residual signal of the time record, $\overline{r}$ is the average of r_i, r_{jk} is the kth measurement in the jth time record residual signal r_j, $\overline{r_j}$ is the average of r_j, and N is the number of time records in a run ensemble.

An example of analyzing a degradation process using time-domain features is shown in Figures 3.3 and 3.4, which is implemented on a Bently test-bed. Figure 3.3 shows

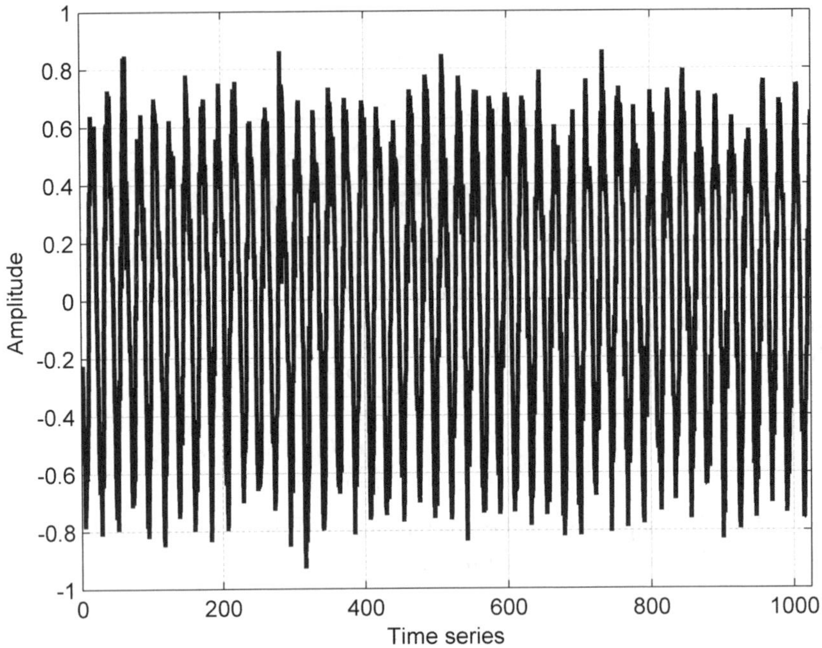

Figure 3.3 Vibration signal of Bently test-bed during a degradation process

the signal probed by eddy current sensors fixed on the mass wheel. The rotor speed is 2700 rpm, and the sampling frequency is 1000 Hz. The degradation process is simulated by gradually adding weights to the screw holes of the mass wheel. As can be seen from Figure 3.4, the degradation process is effectively represented by a maximum value and SD extracted from the time-domain signal.

3.3.2 Spectrum Analysis

Spectral analysis is a common tool for investigating a mechanical vibration signal, and aims at obtaining dominant frequencies present in the time-series and assigning them to various physical phenomena. This type of analysis is typically carried out through a Fourier transform, which is an important method in the analysis of digital signals and systems, and is defined as follows [33].

$$X(k) = \sum_{n=0}^{N-1} x(n) W_N^{kn} \tag{3.15}$$

where, $W_N^{kn} = e^{-i\frac{2\pi kn}{N}}$. $x(n)$ stands for the input data array, while $X(k)$ represents the output array.

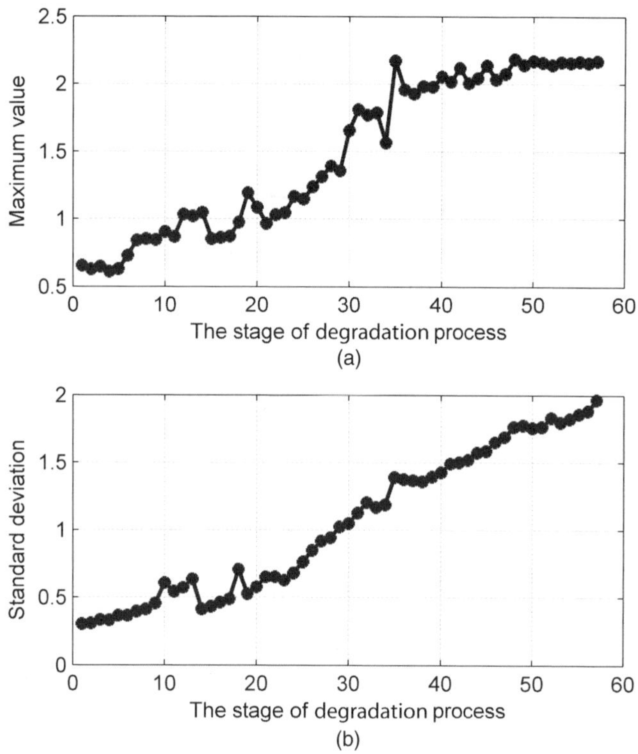

Figure 3.4 (a) Maximum value and (b) standard deviation for the degradation process

Similarly, an inverse discrete Fourier transform (DFT) is defined as,

$$x(k) = \sum_{n=0}^{N-1} X(n) W_N^{-kn} \tag{3.16}$$

In the frequency-domain, feature parameters are extracted from the spectrum of the investigated signal, which contain information that is not present in the time-domain features parameters. They are defined as follows [29, 34],

1. Mean frequency *(*MF*)*

$$MF = \frac{1}{K} \sum_{k=1}^{K} X_k \tag{3.17}$$

where, X_k is the kth measurement of the frequency spectrum of the signal and K is the total number of the signal in the frequency domain.

2. Frequency center (FC)

$$\mathrm{FC} = \frac{\sum_{k=1}^{K} f_k X_k}{\sum_{k=1}^{K} X_k} \tag{3.18}$$

where, f_k is the frequency value of the kth spectrum line.

3. Root mean square frequency (RMSF)

$$\mathrm{RMSF} = \sqrt{\frac{\sum_{k=1}^{K} f_k^2 X_k}{\sum_{k=1}^{K} X_k}} \tag{3.19}$$

4. Standard deviation frequency (STDF)

$$\mathrm{STDF} = \sqrt{\frac{\sum_{k=1}^{K} (f_k - \mathrm{FC})^2 X_k}{\sum_{k=1}^{K} X_k}} \tag{3.20}$$

MF indicates the vibration energy in the frequency domain. FC and RMSF show the position changes of the main frequencies. STDF describes the convergence degree of the spectrum power.

In order to improve its computational speed, DFT is widely implemented using the fast Fourier transform (FFT) algorithm, which effectively improves the computational speed. Figure 3.5 shows the frequency spectrum of the vibration signal that was investigated above, which clearly indicates the main frequency during the rotation process. While, as shown in Figure 3.6, the 3D frequency spectrum of the signal represents the degradation process.

3.3.3 Continuous Wavelet Transform

The wavelet transform has attracted great interest in applied mathematics for signal processing. This new technique has been demonstrated to be fast in computation with localization and quickly reveals properties in contrast to existing popular methods,

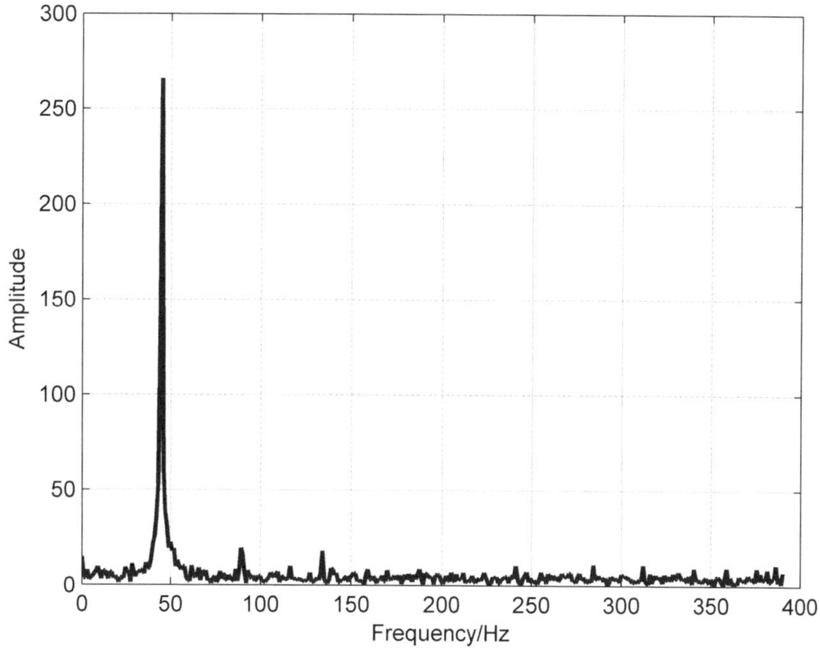

Figure 3.5 Frequency spectrum analysis

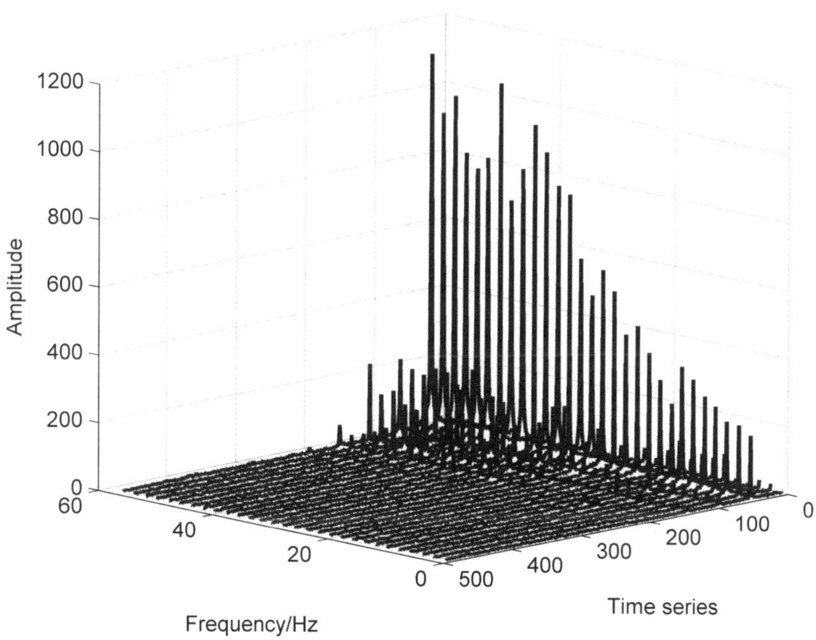

Figure 3.6 3D frequency spectrum

especially the FFT. It may be viewed as a synthesis of ideas originating from engineering (sub-band coding), physics (coherent states and renormalization group), and pure mathematics. The wavelet transform became a tool widely used for signal analysis. From 1989 onwards, the wavelet transform has been applied for signal processing in engineering owing to its efficiency, large number of basis functions available, and high speed in data treatment [35].

The wavelet transform can be considered as a mathematical tool that converts a signal in the time domain into a different form, that is, a series of wavelet coefficients, in a time-scale domain. A wavelet function, which is a small wave, possessing oscillating wavelike characteristics and concentrating its energy in a short time, is needed to implement the wavelet transform. Traditionally, the wavelet transform can be categorized as a continuous wavelet transform (CWT), aDWT, and a wavelet packet transform (WPT) [36].

The CWT of a signal $x(t)$ can be performed through a convolution operation between the signal $x(t)$ and the complex conjugate of a family of wavelets, which is expressed as

$$\mathrm{cwt}(s,\tau) = \frac{1}{\sqrt{s}}\int x(t)\psi^*\left(\frac{t-\tau}{s}\right)\mathrm{d}\tau \tag{3.21}$$

where, the symbols s and τ denote scale and translation parameters, respectively. $\psi^*(\bullet)$ is the complex conjugate of the scaled and shifted wavelet function $\psi(\bullet)$. Equation 3.21 indicates that the CWT is similar to the Fourier transform except that the family of wavelets is used as the basis function to replace the sine and cosine functions. Since the family of wavelets contains two parameters, transforming a signal with the family of wavelets means such a signal will be projected into a two-dimensional, time-scale plane, instead of the one-dimensional plane in the Fourier transform. Furthermore, computation of Equation 3.21 can be achieved by a pair of a Fourier transform and an inverse Fourier transform as below.

$$\begin{aligned}\mathrm{CWT}(s,f) &= F\{\mathrm{cwt}(s,\tau)\}\\ &= \frac{1}{\sqrt{s2\pi}}\int_{-\infty}^{\infty}\left(\int_{-\infty}^{\infty}x(t)\,\psi^*\left(\frac{t-\tau}{s}\right)\mathrm{d}t\right)\mathrm{e}^{-j2\pi f\tau}\mathrm{d}\tau\\ &= \sqrt{s}X(f)\psi^*(sf)\end{aligned} \tag{3.22}$$

where, the symbol $F(\bullet)$ denotes the operator of the Fourier transform. $X(f)$ denotes the Fourier transform of $\psi^*(\bullet)$. By taking the inverse Fourier transform, Equation 3.22 is converted back onto the time domain as

$$\mathrm{cwt}(s,\tau) = F^{-1}\{\mathrm{CWT}(s,f)\} = \sqrt{s}F^{-1}\{X(f)\psi^*(sf)\} \tag{3.23}$$

where, the symbol $F^{-1}(\bullet)$ denotes the operator of the inverse Fourier transform. Equation 3.23 indicates that the CWT of a signal $x(t)$ can work as a band-pass filter with the wavelet function itself and its scale parameter s controls the filtering performance.

3.3.4 Discrete Wavelet Transform

Performing CWT on a signal will lead to redundant information generation, as the scale parameter τ changes continuously. Although redundancy is useful in some applications, such as signal denoising and feature extraction where the desired performance is achieved at the cost of increased computational time, other applications may need to emphasize computational efficiency. It turns out that dyadic scales (i.e., $s = 2,\ \tau = k2^j$) can achieve such a requirement, while at the same time avoiding sacrificing information contained in the signal. Mathematically, after such scale discretization, the DWT can be realized as

$$\mathrm{dwt}(j,k) = \frac{1}{\sqrt{2^j}} \int x(t)\psi^* \left(\frac{t-k2^j}{2^j}\right) \mathrm{d}t \tag{3.24}$$

Practically, DWT can be implemented by means of a pair of low-pass and high-pass wavelet filters, denoted as $h(k)$ and $g(k) = (-1)^k h(1-k)$, respectively. These filters are constructed from the selected wavelet function $\psi(t)$ and its corresponding scaling function $\phi(t)$, expressed as

$$\begin{cases} \phi(t) = \sqrt{2}\sum\limits_k h(k)\phi(2t-k) \\ \psi(t) = \sqrt{2}\sum\limits_k g(k)\phi(2t-k) \end{cases} \tag{3.25}$$

With $\sum\limits_k h(k) = \sqrt{2}$ and $\sum\limits_k g(k) = 0$. Using the wavelet filters, the signal is decomposed into a set of low and high-frequency components as

$$\begin{cases} a_{j,k} = \sum\limits_m h(2k-m)\, a_{j-1,m} \\ d_{j,k} = \sum\limits_m g(2k-m) a_{j-1,m} \end{cases} \tag{3.26}$$

In Equation 3.26, $a_{j,k}$ the approximation coefficient, which represents the signal's low-frequency components, and $d_{j,k}$ the detail coefficient at wavelet scale 2^j (with j denoting the level) are obtained by convolving the approximation coefficients at the previous level $(j-1)$ with the low-pass and high-pass filter coefficients, respectively.

An illustration of DWT analysis can be found in Figure 3.7a, and an example of DWT analysis is shown in Figure 3.7b. The investigated signal $s(x)$ was decomposed into five layers by Daubechies wavelet of the fourth order (db4 wavelet). The relationship between the original signal and the decomposed sub-bands is:

$$\begin{aligned} s(x) &= a_1 + d_1 \\ &= a_2 + d_2 + d_1 \\ &= a_3 + d_3 + d_2 + d_1 \\ &= a_4 + d_4 + d_3 + d_2 + d_1 \\ &= a_5 + d_5 + d_4 + d_3 + d_2 + d_1 \end{aligned} \tag{3.27}$$

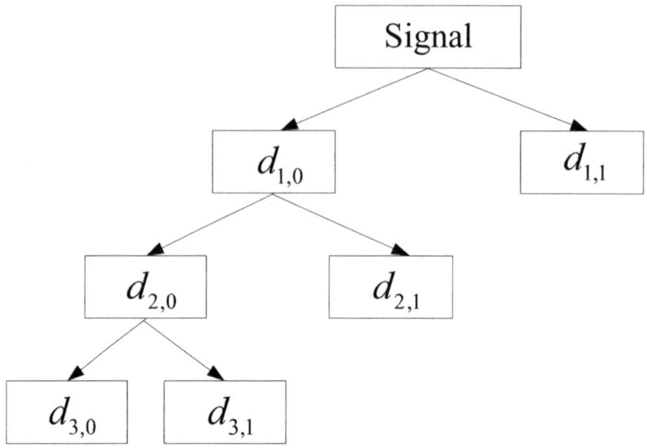

(a)

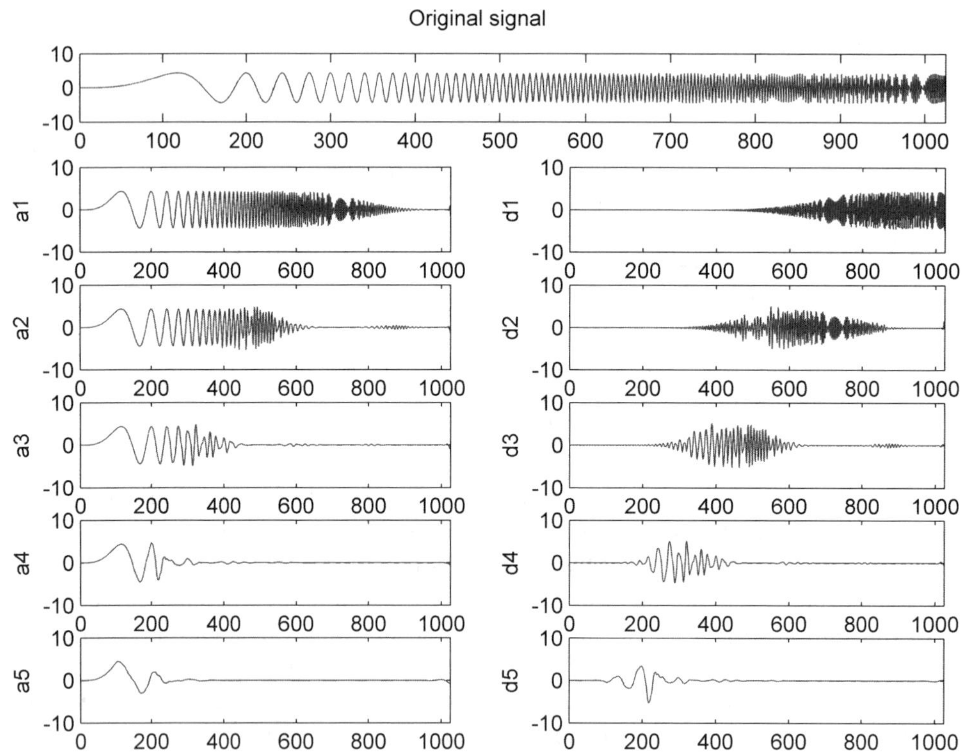

(b)

Figure 3.7 (a) Illustration of discrete wavelet transforms and (b) example of discrete wavelet transforms where, symbol a represents the approximation part of the signal and d the detail part of the signal.

3.3.5 Wavelet Packet Transforms

The WPT can further decompose the detail information of the signal in the high frequency region. To perform WPT of a signal at a certain level (e.g., level 3), the functions in Equation 3.25 are unified as

$$\begin{cases} u_{2n}(t) = \sqrt{2}\sum_k h(k)u_n(2t-k) \\ u_{2n+1}(t) = \sqrt{2}\sum_k g(k)u_n(2t-k) \end{cases} \tag{3.28}$$

where $u_0(t) = \phi(t)$, and $u_1(t) = \psi(t)$. Correspondingly, the signal is decomposed as

$$\begin{cases} d_{j+1,2n}(t) = \sum_k h(m-2k)d_{j,n} \\ d_{j+1,2n+1}(t) = \sum_k g(m-2k)d_{j,n} \end{cases} \tag{3.29}$$

where, $d_{j,n}$ denotes the wavelet coefficients at the j level, n sub-band, $d_{j+1,2n}$ and $d_{j+1,2n+1}$ denote the wavelet coefficients at the $j+1$ level, $2n$ and $2n+1$ sub-bands, respectively, and m is the number of the wavelet coefficients.

As illustrated in Figure 3.8, a three-level WPT generates a total of eight sub-bands, and each sub-band covers one eighth of the frequency information successively. The simulated signal decomposed by discrete wavelet decomposition is also employed in Figure 3.9, which shows the decomposition process of a WPT. Different from wavelet transform, WPT analyses both the approximation part and the detail part of the signal.

3.3.6 Empirical Mode Decomposition

The EMD method introduced by Huang *et al.* [11] is a relatively new approach to signal analysis. It is developed from simple assumptions: (i) the signal is an integration of intrinsic components of oscillations, (ii) every linear or non-linear mode has at

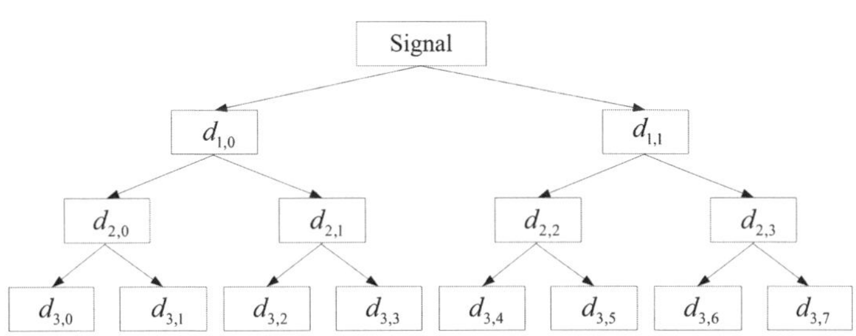

Figure 3.8 Illustration of wavelet packet transforms

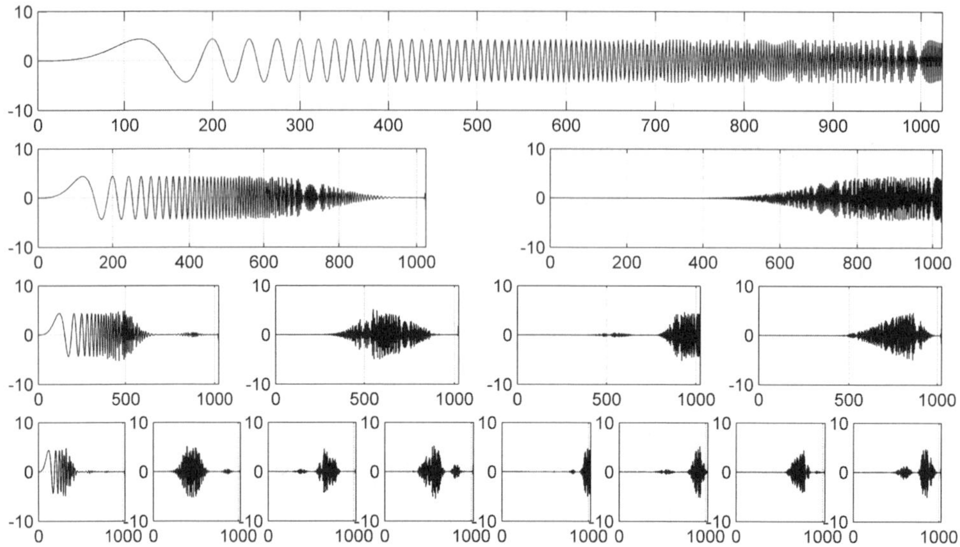

Figure 3.9 Example of wavelet packet transforms

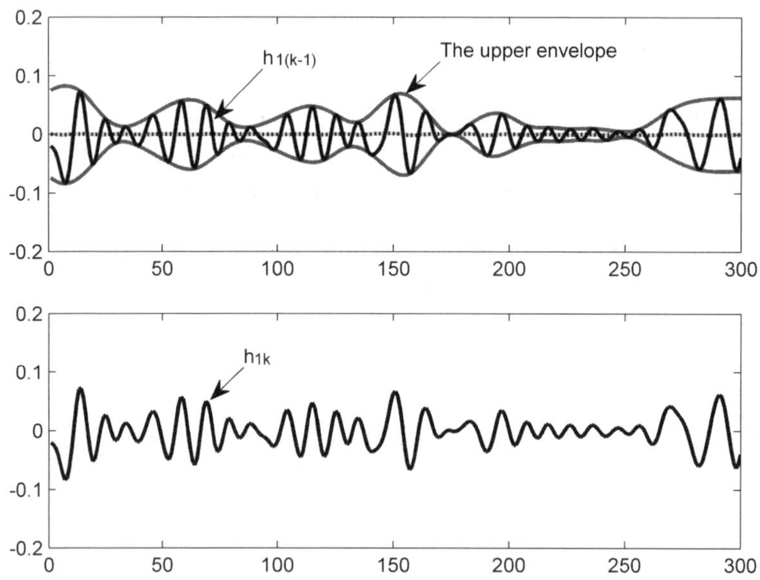

Figure 3.10 Sifting process of EMD

least one maximum and one minimum, (iii) if there is no extrema in the signal, then differentiation of the inflection point can reveal the extrema, and (iv) the signal is characterized by a time series between successive extrema. As shown in Figure 3.10, each signal is decomposed into a finite number of IMFs through a sifting process, and each IMF is examined to evaluate if it satisfies the following [15]:

1. In the whole dataset, the number of extrema and the number of zero-crossings must be equal or only have a difference of one.
2. At any point, the mean value between the local maxima envelope and the local minima envelope must be equal to zero.

An IMF represents a simple oscillatory mode as a counterpart to the simple harmonic function. With the definition, any signal $x(t)$ can be decomposed as follows:

Step 1: Identify all local extrema, and then connect all local maxima by a cubic spine line, forming the upper envelope.

Step 2: Repeat the procedure for local minima to produce the lower envelope. The upper and lower envelopes should cover all the data between them.

Step 3: Calculate the mean value of the upper and lower envelopes, $m_1(t)$, and the difference between the signal $x(t)$ and $m_1(t)$ is the first proto-mode $h_1(t)$,

$$h_1(t) = x(t) - m_1(t) \tag{3.30}$$

Ideally, if $h_1(t)$ satisfies the definition of IMF, $h_1(t)$ is the first empirical mode.

Step 4: If $h_1(t)$ is not an IMF, replace the original signal with $h_1(t)$ and repeat steps 1, 2, and 3, then calculate the proto-mode $h_{11}(t)$,

$$h_{11}(t) = h_1(t) - m_{11}(t) \tag{3.31}$$

where, $m_{11}(t)$ is the mean value of the upper envelope and the lower envelope. After repeating the sifting process k times, the approximate local envelope symmetry condition is satisfied, and $h_{1k}(t)$ becomes an IMF, that is

$$h_{1k}(t) = h_{1(k-1)}(t) - m_{1k}(t) \tag{3.32}$$

And the decomposed empirical mode can be designated as

$$c_1 = h_{1k}(t) \tag{3.33}$$

The approximate local envelope symmetry condition in the sifting process is called the stopping criterion, the most widely used type is given by limiting the size of the SD, the normalized squared difference between two successive sifting operations defined as,

$$\mathrm{SD} = \sum_{t=0}^{n} \frac{|h_{k-1}(t) - h_k(t)|^2}{h^2{}_{k-1}(t)} \tag{3.34}$$

where, n is the number of the sample point.

Step 5: Separating the first IMF from the $x(t)$,

$$r_1(t) = x(t) - c_1(t) \tag{3.35}$$

This residual $r_1(t)$ is then treated as new data and subjected to the same sifting process as described above to obtain an IMF of lower frequency. The procedure can be repeatedly applied to all subsequent iterations, and then n-IMFs of signal $x(t)$ can be obtained,

$$\begin{cases} r_2(t) = r_1(t) - c_2(t) \\ r_3(t) = r_2(t) - c_3(t) \\ \quad \cdots \\ r_n(t) = r_{n-1}(t) - c_n(t) \end{cases} \tag{3.36}$$

The decomposition process finally stops when the residue $r_n(t)$ becomes a monotonic function or a function with only one extremum from which no more IMF can be extracted. Then the original data $x(t)$ can be represented as,

$$x(t) = \sum_{i=1}^{n} c_i(t) + r_n(t) \tag{3.37}$$

Thus, the signal is decomposed into n-empirical modes, and a residue $r_n(t)$ which is a monotonic function or a function with only one extremum. Empirical modes $c_1(t),\ c_2(t), \cdots, c_n(t)$ include different frequency bands ranging from high to low, and they change with the variation of the investigated signal $x(t)$, while $r_n(t)$ represents the central tendency of signal $x(t)$. Therefore, the physical meanings hidden in non-linear and non-stationary signals can be revealed perfectly through an automatic sifting process.

The simulated signal is used to demonstrate the properties of the HHT method, which consists of three sinusoidal components as well as Gaussian noise [37] and is described as:

$$y(t) = 0.5 \sin\left(\frac{2\pi}{200}t\right) + 0.6 \cos\left(\frac{2\pi}{25}t\right) + \cos\left(\frac{2\pi}{50}t\right) \tag{3.38}$$

For the sake of clarity, the three sinusoidal modes with frequency of 0.04, 0.02, and 0.005 Hz were named the first order IMF, the second order IMF, and the third order IMF. As shown in Figure 3.11, the simulated signal was decomposed into three IMFs and a residue component. The corresponding time–frequency spectrum is shown in Figure 3.12, which clearly shows three components in the investigated signal, although the first order IMF and the second order IMF had slight fluctuation at the end of the signal.

In order to make a comparison study of wavelet decomposition and the EMD method in terms of estimating investigated modes the simulated signal was decomposed into 16 sub-modes with carefully selected wavelet parameters. As shown in Figure 3.13, the first IMF, second IMF, and third IMF were effectively detected based on wavelet decomposition. However, two problems occurred in the process, (i) selection of the

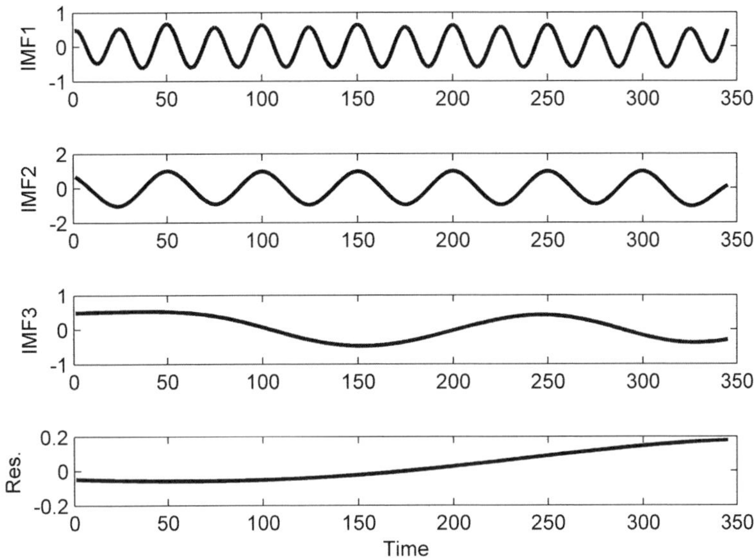

Figure 3.11 Signal decomposed by EMD

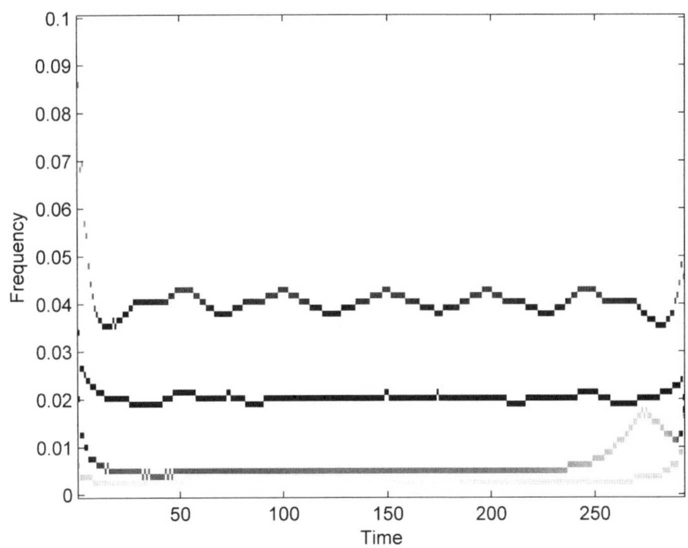

Figure 3.12 Signal analyses by HHT method

three target modes from the decomposed 16 modes; (ii) the difficulty of estimating target modes when wavelet parameters such as the decomposition level are not appropriate. The proposed method is a self-adaptive method without parameter selection and, as shown in Figure 3.14, the EMD method decomposed the signal into three modes and the corresponding frequency modes matched well with the investigated modes.

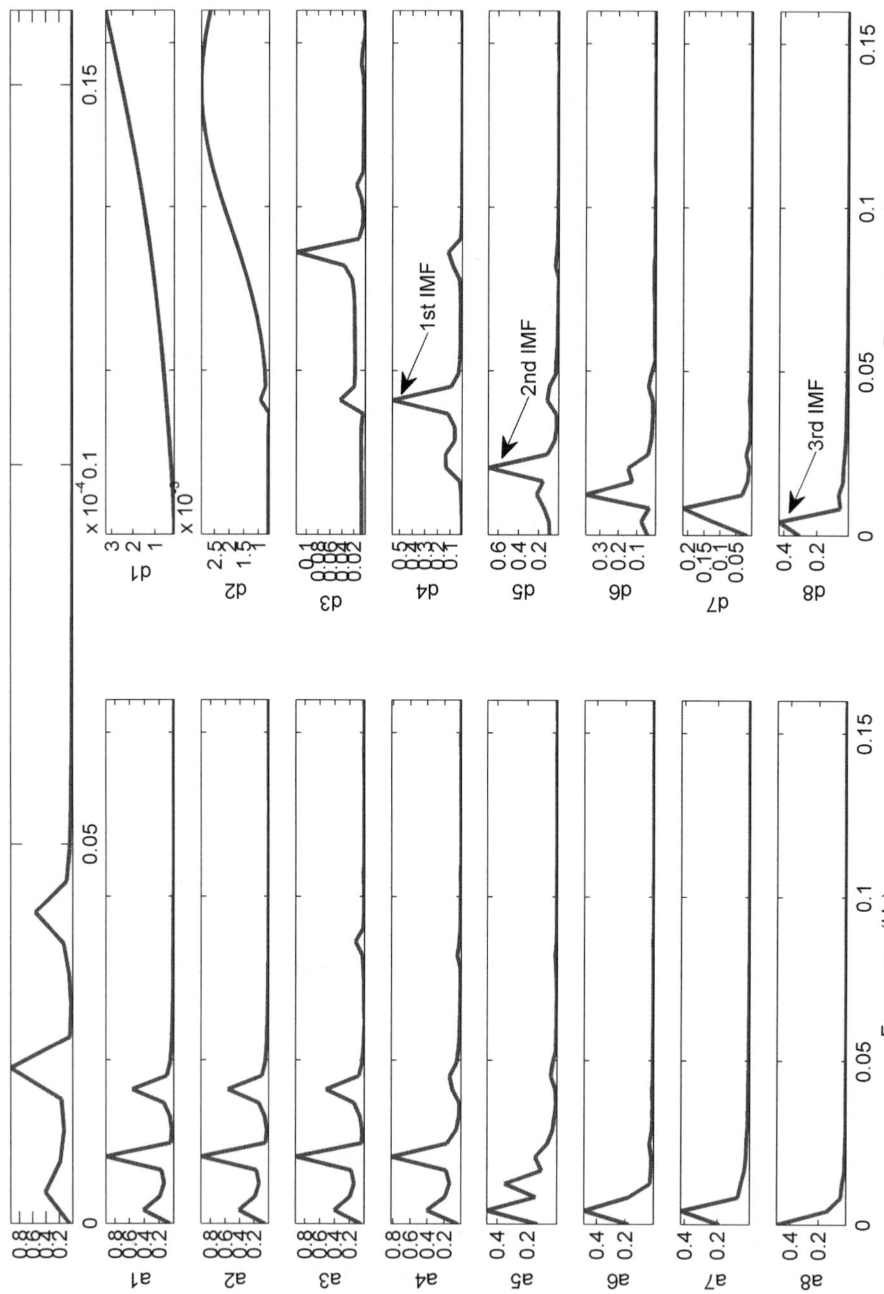

Figure 3.13 IMFs analysis in frequency-domain based on wavelet analysis

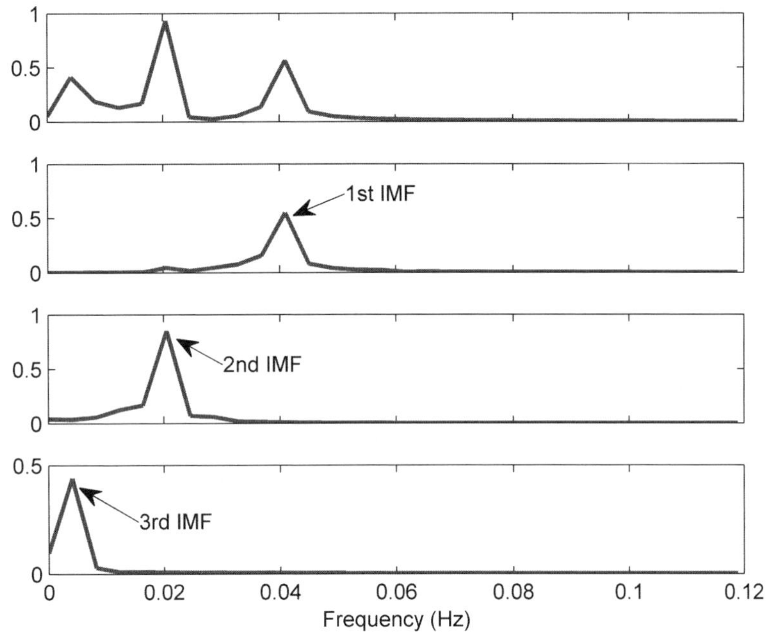

Figure 3.14 IMFs analysis in frequency-domain based on EMD

3.3.7 Improved Empirical Mode Decomposition

As discussed in Section 3.3.6, the EMD method is demonstrated to be an effective method for representing the characteristics of a signal, and has the advantage of needing no parameter selection. Nevertheless, the classical HHT suffers from end effects and redundant IMFs associated with EMD processes. Large swings occur in the interpolation fitting process, which eventually propagate inward and corrupt the whole data span [38].

Many schemes have been proposed in the literature for the purpose of alleviating the end effects and removing redundant IMFs. Rilling *et al.* [39] used a data flipping (mirror) technique by adding two extreme points on each side of the signal to furnish a complete periodic cycle of the waveform to suppress the end effect. Xun and Yan [40] applied artificial neural networks (ANNs) to extend each side of the signal and then performed the EMD method. Cheng *et al.* [41] proposed an improved HHT method based on the support vector regression machine (SVR). Roy and Doherty [42] introduced raised cosine interpolation to improve the classical EMD method. However, to date, improved EMD methods have the following shortcomings. First, these methods employ prediction approaches to improve the classical EMD method by extending each side of the signal, while signal extension methods such as the SVR machine, ANNs, auto-regressive moving average (ARMA), and mirror extension methods cannot completely eliminate boundary distortion. Also prediction errors will propagate during the sifting process and corrupt all IMFs. Secondly, signals of mechanical failures in the initial state often have small amplitude and with low signal-to-noise ratio, while signal extension based EMD methods are verified through analyzing a pure signal, and do not take a weak signal with low signal-to-noise ratio into consideration. Thirdly, the extension part of each side of the signal is empirical and cannot reflect real features of the original weak signal. In this section we propose a weak signal detection scheme based on an improved EMD method and wavelet analysis [43], which considers iterative errors of the sifting process and a correlation relationship between each IMF and the original signal.

3.3.7.1 The Solution of End Effects

The EMD is accomplished through an iterative algorithm called a sifting process, which employs cubic spline to interpolate upper envelopes between the local maxima, and lower envelopes between the local minima. However, the lack of enough extrema at both ends of the signal results in end effects during the spline-curve fitting

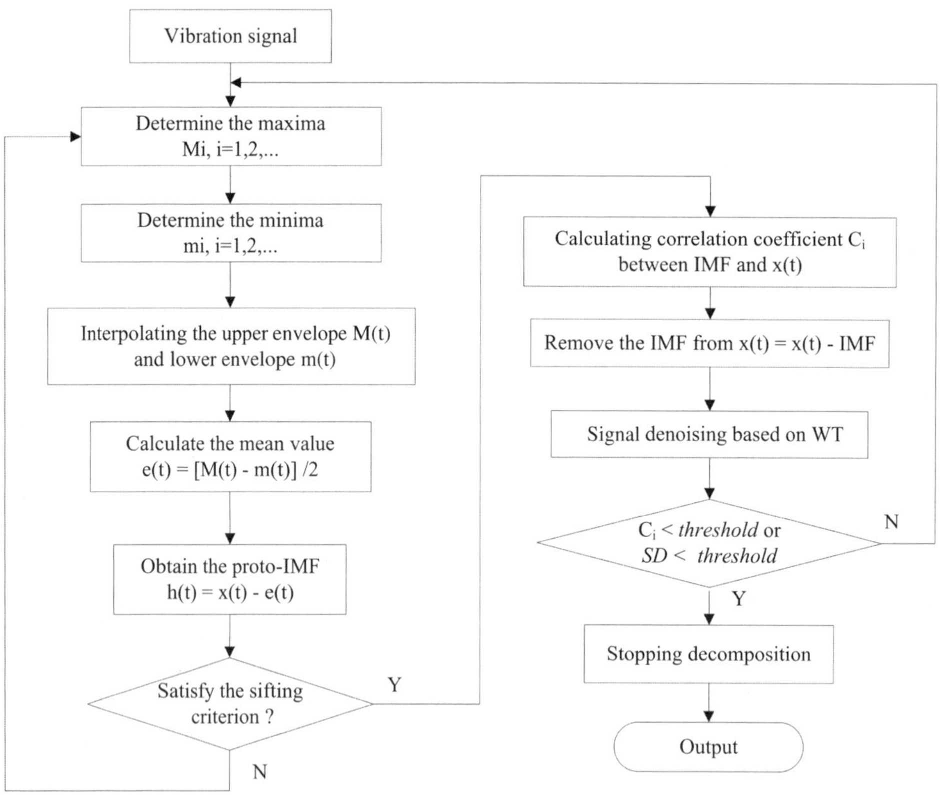

Figure 3.15 Flowchart of the proposed method

process, and the fitting error propagates inward during each iteration process and distorts each IMF with complex frequency components. In order to reduce the effect of noise signal and fitting error on each IMF, wavelet denoising is performed during the sifting process.

A flowchart of the proposed wavelet analysis embedded EMD method is shown in Figure 3.15, and the operation procedures are summarized as follows [43]:

Step 1: Compute IMF_i from the original signal $x(t)$ through the iteration process, where $i = 1,\ 2,\ 3,\ \ldots$ is the index of IMFs.

Step 2: Transform IMF_i into the wavelet domain through Equation 3.39, where $W_{j,k}$ is the kth wavelet coefficient at the jth level, $j, k \in Z$ andnd $\psi_{j,k}(t)$ is the commonly supported orthogonal wavelet functions (*coiflets*, *daublets,* and *symmlets*) [44].

$$W_{j,k} = \int_{-\infty}^{+\infty} \text{IMF}_i(t)\, \psi_{j,k}(t)\, \text{d}t \tag{3.39}$$

Step 3: Estimate the noise variance at each level and compute the denoising threshold T.

Step 4: Estimate new wavelet coefficients $W_{j,k}$ by threshold

$$d_t(W_{j,k}) = \text{sgn}(W_{j,k})(|W_{j,k}| - T)_+.$$

where T, computed above, is a positive real threshold.

Step 5: Reconstruct IMF_i' from the denoised detail coefficients and approximate coefficients through the inverse wavelet transform.

Step 6: Subtract IMF_i' from $x(t)$ and obtain the residual signal $r_i(t)$.

$$r_i(t) = x(t) - \text{IMF}_i'(t) \tag{3.40}$$

Step 7: Replace $x(t)$ with the residual signal $r_i(t)$ and return to *Step* 1, repeat the iteration process until the residual signal becomes a monotonic function or a function with only one extremum.

As shown in Figure 3.16, in order to make a comparative study of the improved EMD method proposed in this section with four existing signal extension based EMD methods, time series forecasting methods such as mirror extension [39], ANNs [40], the SVR machine [41], and ARMA [45] methods were used to extend both ends of the original signal. Signal extension using these four methods is presented first and then we will discuss the proposed method. As illustrated in Figure 3.17, the maximum point appears every 25 points, and it represents the periodicity of the signal, which was used as the extension length of the original signal.

Here, we employed a greedy search algorithm to find the optimal parameters of the ARMA model, the ANN model, and the SVR model. The order of the ARMA model was estimated based on the AIC (Akaike information criterion) method and the optimized order was 58 (see Figure 3.18). A radial basis kernel function was used

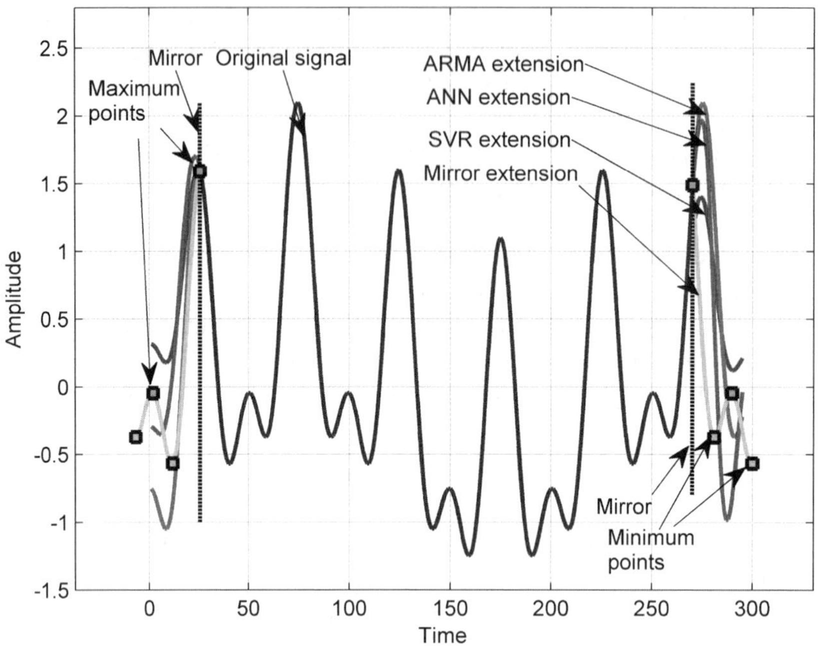

Figure 3.16 The original pure signal extension based on forecasting methods

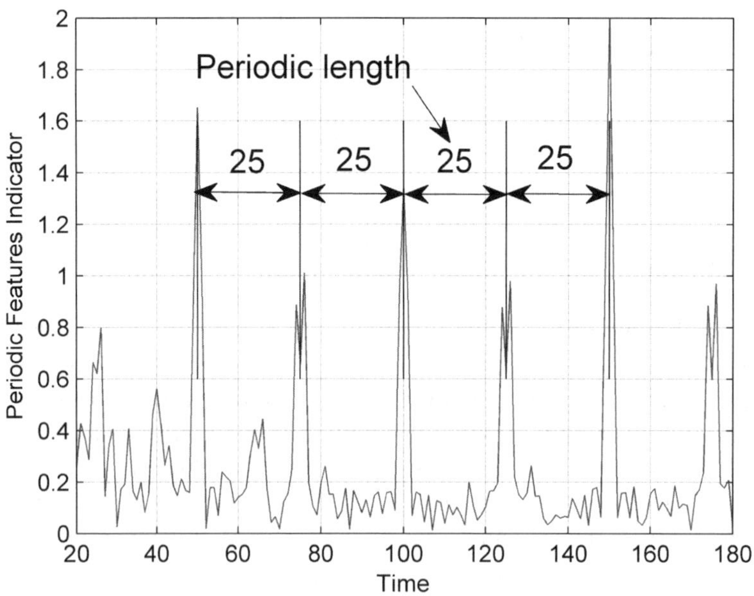

Figure 3.17 Periodic characteristic detecting

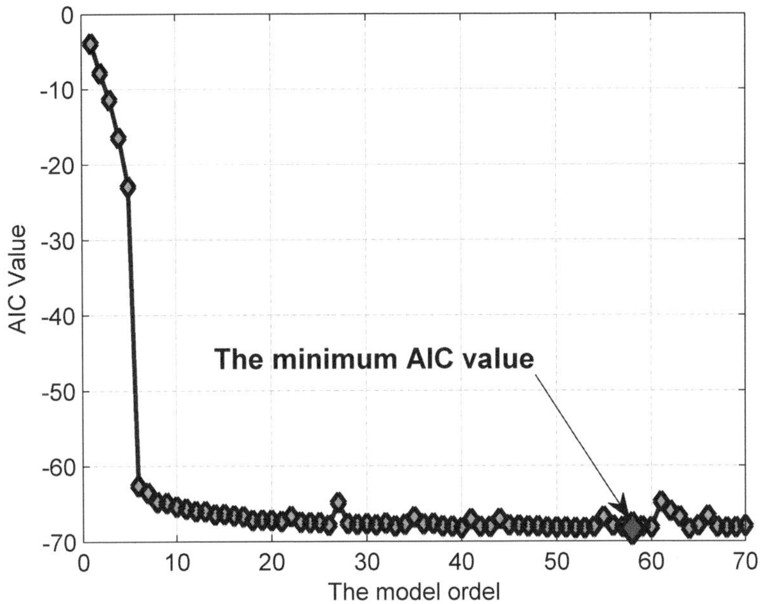

Figure 3.18 ARMA model training

in the SVR model and the cross validation method was used to find the optimal model. Shown in Figure 3.19, for the optimal SVR model, the polynomial parameter and cost parameter were estimated as 0.002 and 8, respectively. And the optimal ANN model reached the training target when the number of iterations was 361 (see Figure 3.20).

It can be seen in Figure 3.21a that the original pure signal was decomposed into four IMFs through the classical EMD method, and end effects occurred at both ends of the second order IMF, also the third order IMF has a large deviation from the ideal mode with 0.005 Hz frequency. Prediction errors of the investigated forecasting methods resulted in end effects and redundant IMFs during the sifting process (see Figure 3.21b–e). Although forecasting-based EMD methods can effectively improve the second order IMF, they caused low-frequency redundant IMFs. It can be found from comparative results that the wavelet analysis embedded EMD method was superior to that based on time series forecasting in dealing with the end effects of the HHT. As shown in Figure 3.21f, the proposed wavelet analysis embedded EMD method effectively improved the second order IMF and the third order IMF, and also removed the redundant IMFs.

3.3.7.2 The Improved Stopping Criterion

The widely used stopping criterion is given by limiting the size of the SD between two successive sifting operations. To evaluate the amplitude of the mean and the corresponding mode, Rilling *et al.* [39] proposed a novel stopping criterion based on two

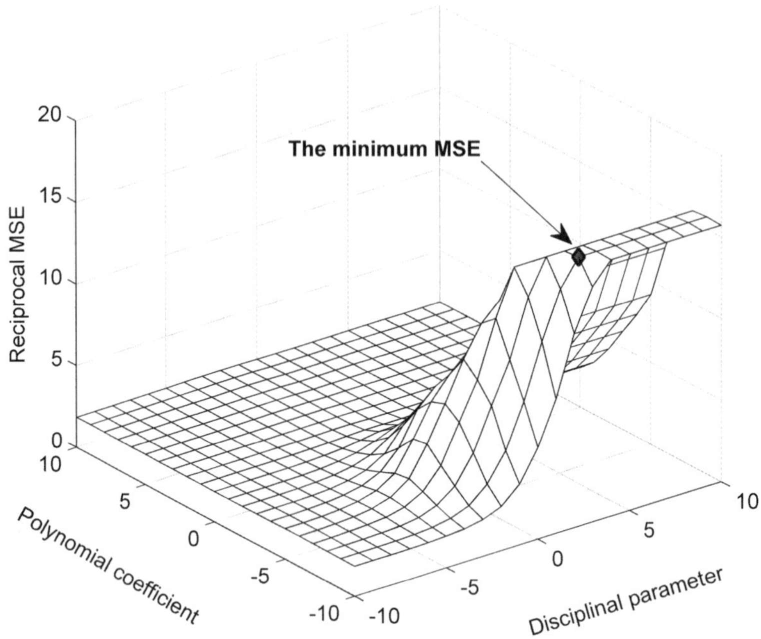

Figure 3.19 SVR model training

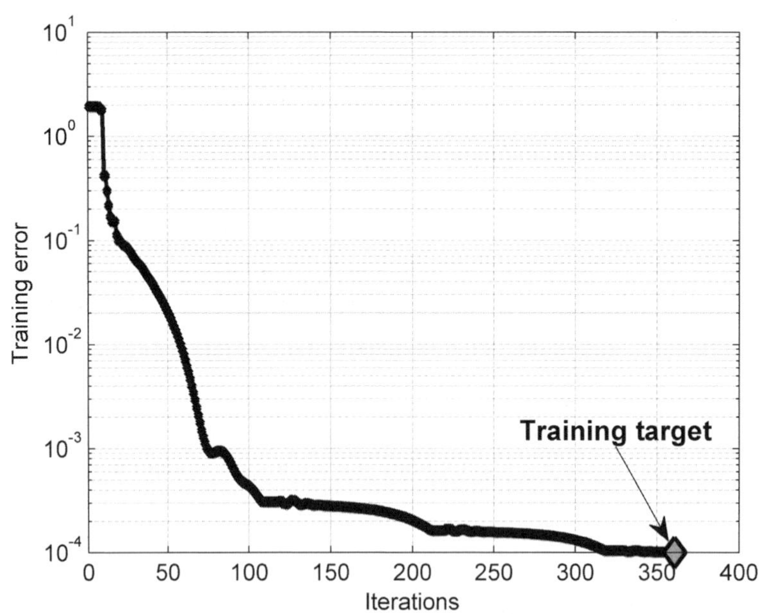

Figure 3.20 Iteration process of ANN model

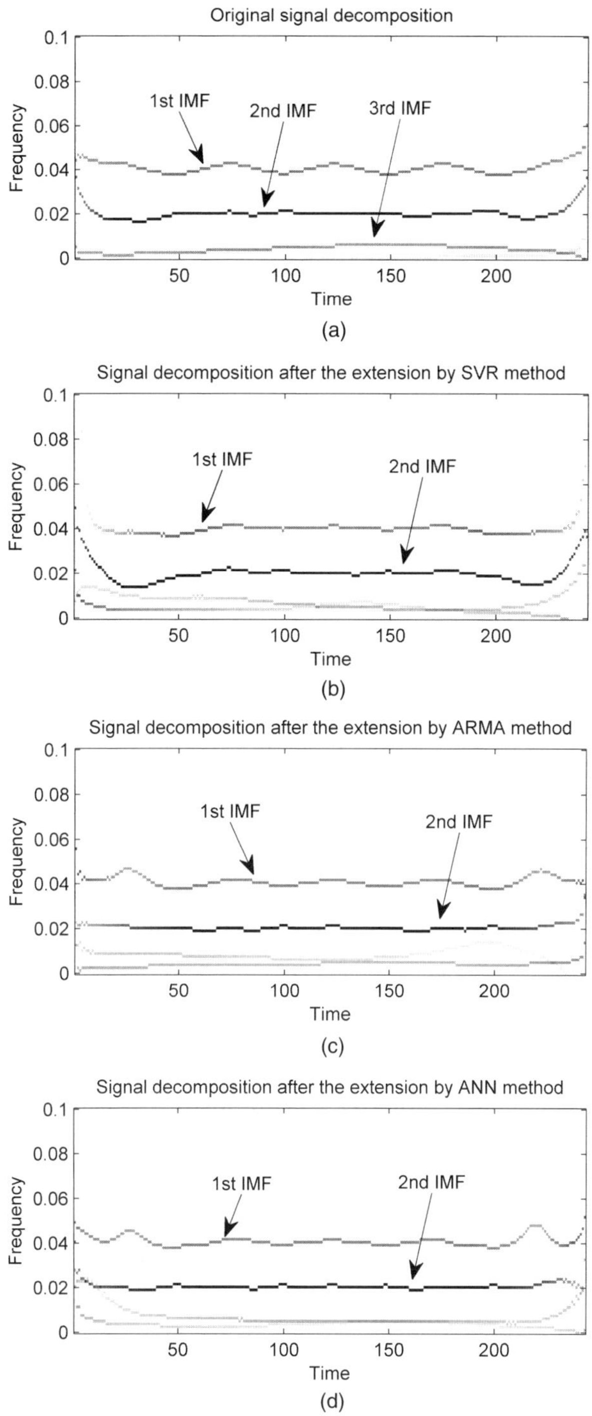

Figure 3.21 (a) Classical EMD, (b) SVR extension-based EMD, (c) ARMA extension-based EMD, (d) ANN extension-based EMD, (e) mirror extension-based EMD, and (f) the proposed improved EMD

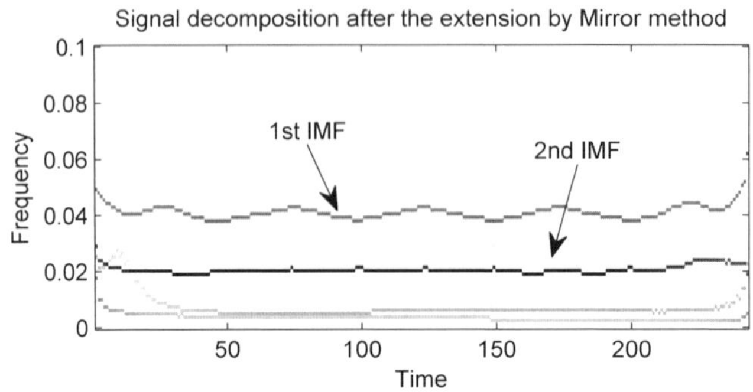

(e)

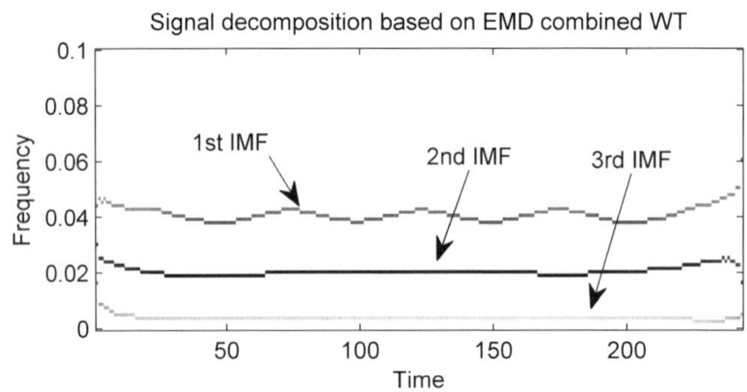

(f)

Figure 3.21 (*continued*)

thresholds, aiming to guarantee globally small fluctuations in the mean while taking locally large excursions into account. The evaluation function is described as,

$$\sigma(t) = \left| \frac{e_{\max}(t) + e_{\min}(t)}{e_{\max}(t) - e_{\min}(t)} \right| \tag{3.41}$$

where, $e_{\max}(t)$ is the upper envelope and $e_{\min}(t)$ is the lower envelope of the signal.

The sifting process iterates until $\sigma(t) < \theta_1$ for the prescribed fraction $(1 - \alpha)$ of the total duration, while $\sigma(t) < \theta_2$ for the remaining fraction. Typically, parameters can be set as $\alpha \approx 0.05$, $\theta_1 \approx 0.05$, and $\theta_2 \approx 10\theta_1$.

As discussed in Section 3.3.6, the EMD process is not established through rigorous mathematical deducing, and the sifting process will generate residual signal. The continuous decomposition of the residual signal leads to drawbacks similar to those mentioned previously (over-iteration leads to over-decomposition). The proposed solution effectively removes redundant IMFs based on the new stopping criterion, which considers the correlation coefficient between each decomposed IMF $c(t)$ and the investigated signal $x(t)$. The IMF is regarded as a redundant IMF when the correlation coefficient C between the IMF and the investigated signals or the SD is smaller than the pre-set threshold. Then the sifting process stops and the decomposed IMFs as well as the residual signal were obtained. The evaluation function can be described as,

$$\text{cross\_coef}_k = \frac{\sum (c_k(t) - \overline{c_k(t)})(x(t) - \overline{x(t)})}{\sqrt{\sum (c_k(t) - \overline{c_k(t)})^2}\sqrt{\sum (x(t) - \overline{x(t)})^2}} \tag{3.42}$$

where, $c_k(t)$ is the kth IMF, $\overline{c_k(t)}$ is the mean value, and θ_{coef} can be set from 0 to 0.1 [43].

To illustrate the capability of the proposed solution for removing undesired IMFs and to make a comparative study of Huang's stopping criterion [12] and Rilling's stopping criterion, we used the same example that was presented in Rilling's work [39], which is a sum of two sinusoidal frequency modulation components and one Gaussian wave packet (see Figure 3.25). The decomposition performed by Huang's stopping criterion was given in 10 IMFs, as shown in Figure 3.22, and the decomposition performed by Rilling's stopping criterion was given in nine IMFs, plotted in Figure 3.23. The comparative study performed by the proposed solution was given in three IMFs, as shown in Figure 3.24. The Hilbert spectrum of the decomposed IMFs based on the proposed stopping criterion is shown in Figure 3.25. As can be seen, the decomposed IMFs can extract true modes from the investigated signal.

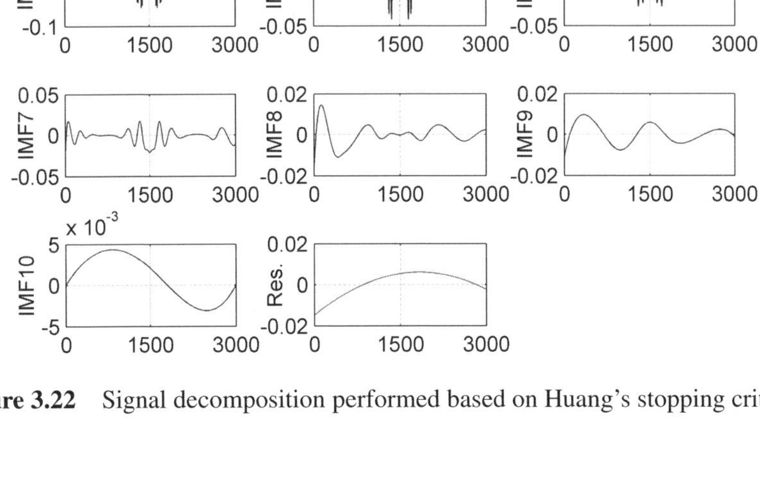

Figure 3.22 Signal decomposition performed based on Huang's stopping criterion

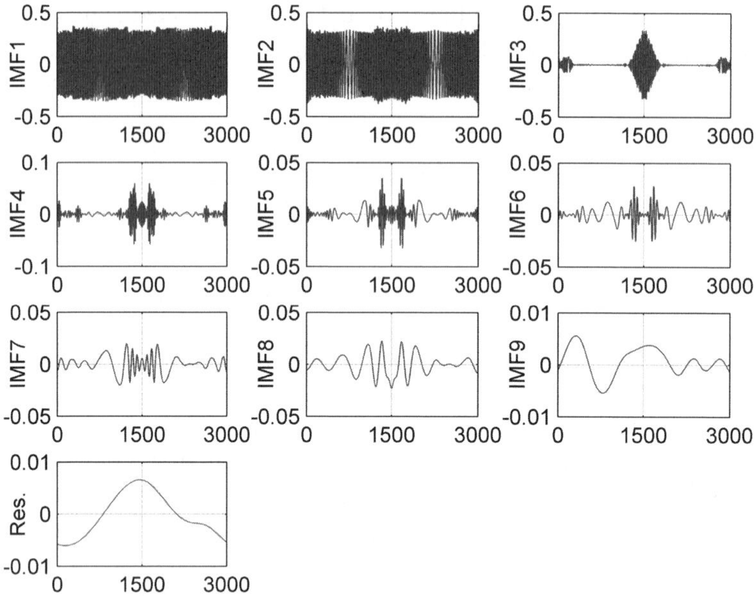

Figure 3.23 Signal decomposition performed based on Rilling's stopping criterion

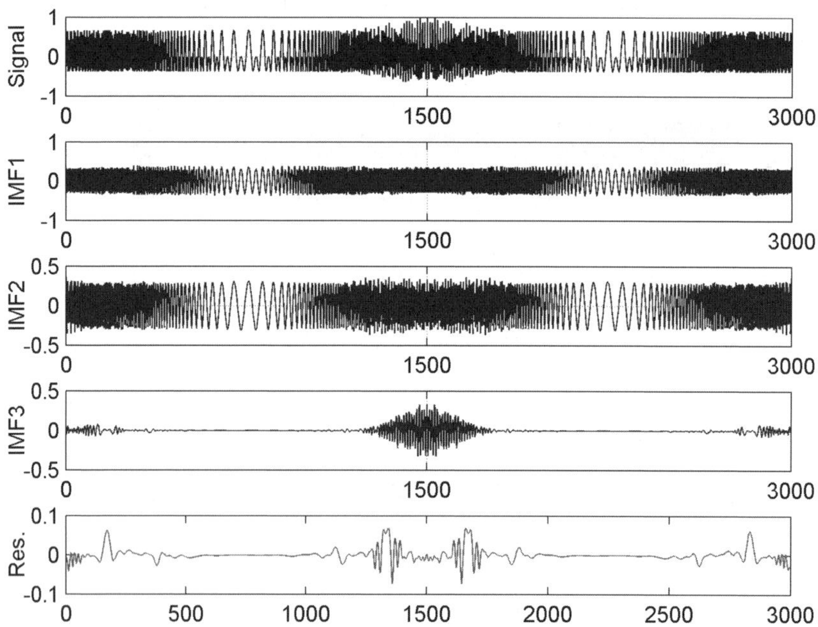

Figure 3.24 Signal decomposition performed based on the proposed stopping criterion

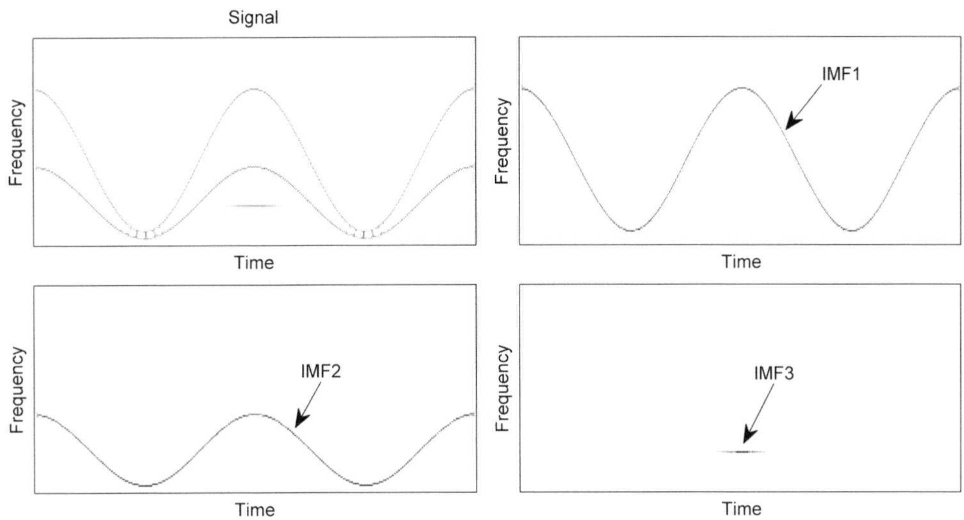

Figure 3.25 Hilbert spectrum analysis of the proposed stopping criterion

3.4 Real-Time Image Feature Extraction

3.4.1 Image Capture System

In mechanical components, the major cause of failure is usually internal to the device. The analyst cannot examine the part without first decapping it. Decapsulation of electrical and mechanical components tends to destroy or move the cause of failure, making the job of the analyst more frustrating and difficult to find the cause of failure of the device.

Radiography is a proven technique for the evaluation of electrical and mechanical components. However, several controlling factors must be taken into consideration [46, 47]. These factors are:

1. Exposure time
2. Position of subject
3. Material of subject
4. Type of film
5. Shielding
6. Interpretation of radiograph
7. X-ray source size
8. Subject to film distance.

Analysis of images from a radiographic process is widely used to examine internal structures of large and small objects. This process is the same in any medical, aircraft, and electronic industry. It consists of placing an X-ray sensitive material, such as film,

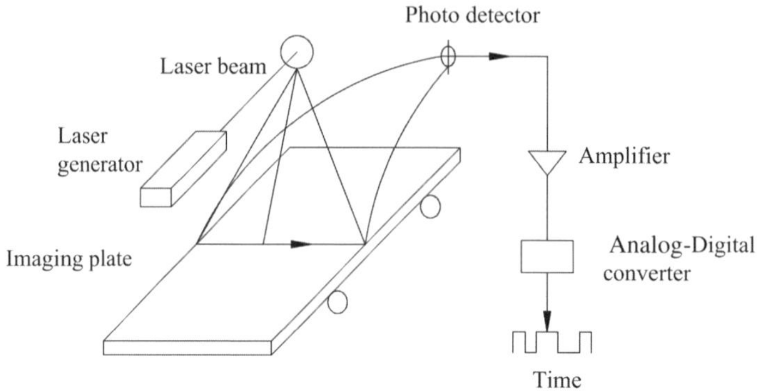

Figure 3.26 Method of reading imaging plate

on one side of an object, exposing the opposite side of the object to a source of X-ray radiation for a specific period of time. The resultant shadow cast by the X-ray beam projects an image of the internal structure of the object. This image is projected onto a recording device (usually film) and can then be used to assess the internal condition of the part [47].

An imaging plate device (IP) is a detector of radioactive rays. The imaging plate is coated with a two-dimensional, high density, thin layer of a special fluorescent material that emits light when irradiated with radioactive rays. As shown in Figure 3.26, as well as the IP the detection system consists of a device to read the IP, an image processing device to process the image which is read, a film image recording device, a CRT image display and a photo-disc image filing device. The IP data reading, after X-ray irradiation, is performed by scanning the surface of the IP with a laser beam.

From the irradiated IP photo-radiation in proportion to the quantity of X-rays is obtained. This photo signal is transformed to an electronic signal through a photo-detector and a photo-electronic amplifier, and changed to a digital signal by an analog to digital converter. Then the widely used method, euphony processing, can be applied to analyze the image data. Euphony shows the grade of brightness and the euphony value of IP equipment is 1024 [47]. In euphony processing, the density level of the image (gray level), that is, the euphony value, will be processed by characteristic functions.

3.4.2 Image Feature Extraction

3.4.2.1 Histogram Features

The histogram of an image is a plot of the gray level values or the intensity values of a color channel versus the number of pixels at that value. When considering an object as an image or sub-image, the nature of the image can be partly described by the

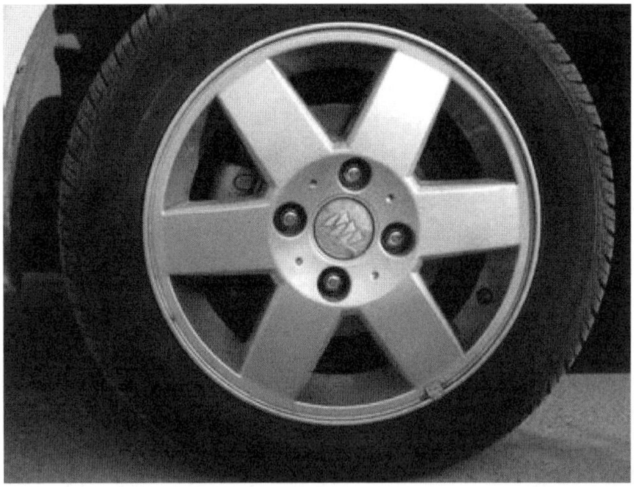

Figure 3.27 Original tire image

shape of the histogram provided. For example, a histogram skewed toward the high end implies a bright image, an image with a very narrow histogram shape implies low contrast, and a histogram with two major peaks (bimodal) implies an object that is of a different color to that of the background [48, 49].

The histogram can be regarded as a model of the probability distribution of the intensity levels. These statistical features provide information about the characteristics of the intensity level distribution for the image. The histogram probability can be described as,

$$P(g) = \frac{N(g)}{M} \tag{3.43}$$

where M is the number of pixels in the image (if the entire image is under consideration then $M = N^2$ for an $N \times N$ image) and $N(g)$ is the number of pixels at gray level g. As with any probability distribution all the values for $P(g)$ are less than or equal to 1, and the sum of all the $P(g)$ values is equal to 1. Figure 3.27 shows the original tire image, and the corresponding histogram features are shown in Figure 3.28, it can be seen that pixel values from 0 to 120 have a large count, which shows well that most of the original image is black in color.

3.4.2.2 Color Moments

The first color moment of the ith color component ($i = 1, 2, 3$) is defined by [50],

$$\text{CM}_i^1 = \frac{1}{N}\sum_{j=1}^{N} p_{i,j} \tag{3.44}$$

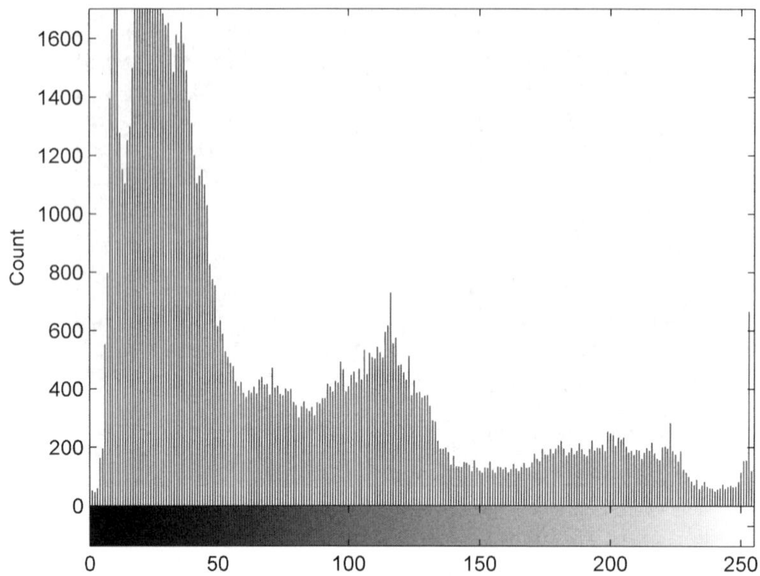

Figure 3.28 Histogram of the tire image

where $p_{i,j}$ is the color value of the ith color component of the jth image pixel and N is the total number of pixels in the image. The hth moment, $h = 2, 3, \ldots,$ of the ith color component is then defined as

$$\mathrm{CM}_i^h = \left(\frac{1}{N}\sum_{j=1}^{N}\left(p_{i,j} - \mathrm{CM}_i^1\right)\right)^{1/h} \tag{3.45}$$

3.4.2.3 Color Coherence Vectors

Color coherence vectors consist of two histograms: one of coherent and one of non-coherent pixels. Pixels are considered to be coherent if they are part of a continuous uniformly colored area and the size of this area exceeds some threshold τ, where τ is usually defined as 1% of the overall area of an image. The L_1 norm is used to obtain the distance metric between two color coherence vectors [51],

$$d_{\mathrm{CCV}}(I_1, I_2) = \sum_{k=1}^{N}\left[\left|H_1^c(k) - H_2^c(k)\right| + \left|H_1^s(k) - H_2^s(k)\right|\right] \tag{3.46}$$

where H_i^c and $H_i^s(k)$, $(i = 1, 2)$ are the histograms of coherent and non-coherent (scattered) pixels, respectively. In our implementation we first blurred the image using a 3×3 averaging filter and used $8 \times 8 \times 8$ RGB bins for representing the histograms.

3.4.2.4 Canny Edge Histogram

Canny proposed a new approach to edge detection that is optimal for step edges contaminated by white noise. The optimality of the detector is related to three criteria [52, 53].

1. The detection criterion expresses the fact that important edges should not be missed and that there should be no spurious responses.
2. The localization criterion says that the distance between the actual and located position of the edge should be minimal.
3. The one response criterion minimizes multiple responses to a single edge.

The model was based on a step edge corrupted by additive white Gaussian noise. The algorithm consists of the following steps [54]:

Step 1: Smoothing the input image by a Gaussian mask. The output smoothed image is denoted as $I(x, y)$.
Step 2: Calculating the horizontal gradient and vertical gradient at each pixel location by convolving the image $I(x, y)$ with partial derivatives of a 2D Gaussian function.
Step 3: Computing the gradient magnitude and direction at each pixel location.
Step 4: Applying non-maximum suppression (NMS) to thin edges.
Step 5: Computing the hysteresis high and low thresholds based on the histogram of the magnitudes of the gradients of the entire image.
Step 6: Performing a hysteresis threshold to determine the edge map.

The discussed Canny edge detection method is verified by analyzing the image presented in Figure 3.29, it can be seen that the edge of the tire is clearly detected (see Figure 3.27).

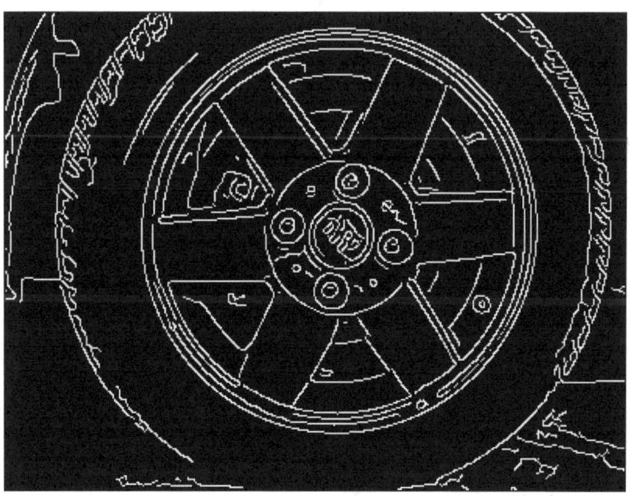

Figure 3.29 Canny edge detection of the tire image

3.5 Fusion or Integration Technologies

Data fusion is an information processing procedure, which can combine data from multiple information sources and related information from associated databases, to achieve improved accuracies and more specific inferences than can be achieved by the use of a single source alone. Data fusion involves data acquisition, data pre-processing, feature extraction, fusion computation, and fusion results output [55]. Here, we will discuss two widely used fusion methods, Dempster–Shafer evidence fusion and the fuzzy measure technique.

3.5.1 Dempster–Shafer Inference

The Dempster–Shafer theory is based on two non-additive evidential measures: belief and plausibility, which can be estimated from basic probability assignment [56].

Let $\{x_i\}_{i=1,2,\ldots,n}$ be a finite set X, called a frame of discernment. The power set composed of all possible subsets of X is 2^X. The hypotheses (classes) in X are assumed to be mutually exclusive and exhaustive [57]. The function $m : 2^X \to [0,1]$ is called a mass function if $\sum_{i=1}^{n} m(x_i) = 1$ and $m(\phi) = 0$.

A subset $\{A_i\}_{i=1,2,\ldots,P}$ with nonzero mass is called a focal element, expressed as $\{(A_i, m(A_i))|A_i \in X,\ \ m(A_i) > 0\}$. The value of $m(A_i)$ represents the degree of evidential support with which certain specific elements of X belong to the exact set A, not to subsets of A. In other words, it corresponds to the weight of evidence in favor of exactly and fully. Two types of focal elements exist: singletons and compound sets. This represents a major difference from the Bayesian probabilistic approach, which assigns probabilities to singletons only. Some common evidential measures are belief and plausibility, as defined in the following,

$$\text{Belief} : \text{Bel}(A) = \sum_{B \subseteq A} m(B) \tag{3.47}$$

$$\text{Plausibility} : \text{Pl}(A) = \sum_{A \cap B \neq \emptyset} m(B), \quad Pl(\emptyset) \neq 0 \tag{3.48}$$

where, the subset $B \subseteq X$ and subset $A \subseteq X$.

From the above definitions, the relationships $\text{Bel}(A) \leq \text{Pl}(A)$ and $\text{Pl}(A) = 1 - \text{Bel}(\overline{A})$ hold, where, $\overline{A} = 1 - A$ is the complement set of A. The Dempster–Shafer evidence theory provides an explicit measure of ignorance about a focal element A and its complement $\overline{A}$ as a belief interval: $[\text{Bel}(A),\ \ \text{Pl}(A)]$.

If the focal elements (sets of nonzero mass): $(A_1, A_2, \ldots, A_P)$, are closed intervals [56, 58]: $([a_1, b_1],\ [a_2, b_2], \ldots, [a_P, b_P])$, then a Dempster–Shafer structure is defined as a collection of pairs formed by an interval and an associated mass $\{(A_1, m_1),\ (A_2, m_2), \ldots, (A_P, m_P)\} = \{([a_1, b_1],\ [a_2, b_2], \ldots, [a_P, b_P])\}$, where, $a_i \leq b_i$ for all i, $b_i \neq b_j$ if $a_i = a_j$, and $\sum m_i = 1$.

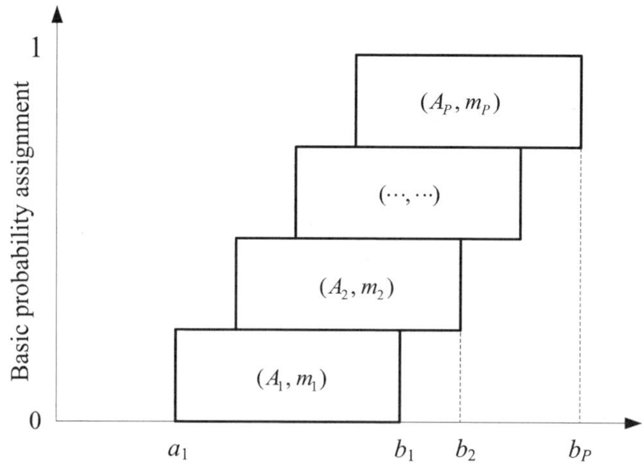

Figure 3.30 Dempster–Shafer structure

Graphically, each of these pairs can be represented as a rectangle whose base corresponds to the interval $[a_i, b_i]$ located on the horizontal axis and whose height, on the ordinate axis, is equal to the mass associated. The probabilistic interpretation was generalized [59] for a Dempster–Shafer structure: the cumulative plausibility and belief functions are recognized as the bounds of an area containing an associated distribution function. As shown in Figure 3.30 [56], based on these cumulative plausibility and belief functions, it is possible to make a Dempster–Shafer structure by drawing horizontal lines from each corner of the cumulative functions to the other bound. This process describes a collection of rectangles of various heights and locations [60].

3.5.2 Fuzzy Integral Fusion

A set function $g : P(Y) \to [0, 1]$ is called a fuzzy measure on condition that the following conditions are satisfied [61, 62]:

1. $g(\phi) = 0, \quad g(Y) = 1$
2. $g(A) \leq g(B)$, if $A \subset B$ and $A,\ B \in P(Y)$

Based on the definition, g_λ-fuzzy measure comes with an additional property:

$$g(A \cup B) = g(A) + g(B) + \lambda g(A)g(B) \tag{3.49}$$

For all $A,\ B \subset Y$ and $A \cap B = \emptyset$, and for some $\lambda > -1$.

Because of the boundary condition $g(Y) = 1$, λ is determined by solving the following polynomial equation:

$$\lambda + 1 = \prod_{i=1}^{n} (1 + \lambda g^i) \tag{3.50}$$

Let $g : Y \rightarrow [0, 1]$ be a fuzzy subset of Y and use the notation $A_i = \{y_i, y_{i+1}, \ldots, y_n\}$. For g being a g_λ-fuzzy measure, the values of $g(A_i)$, $1 < i \leq n$ can be determined recursively as

$$g(A_1) = g(\{y_1\}) = g^1 \tag{3.51}$$

$$g(A_i) = g^i + g(A_{i-1}) + \lambda g^i g(A_{i-1}) \tag{3.52}$$

Thus, a g_λ-fuzzy measure is completely determined by its densities, and the Choquet fuzzy integral [63] was proposed in the following form,

$$\int_Y h(y) \circ g(\cdot)\ \mathrm{d}y = \sum_{i=1}^{n} [h(y_i) - h(y_{i+1})] g(A_i) \tag{3.53}$$

where, $h(y_{n+1}) = 0$, the values of $h(\cdot)$ are ordered in decreasing sequence, that is $h(y_1) \geq h(y_2) \geq \cdots h(y_n)$.

3.6 Statistical Pattern Recognition and Data Mining

In the procedure of signal processing, pattern recognition is a crucial step that provides the final decision based on the extracted information. In previous sections, we have discussed the signal pre-processing techniques for outlier detecting (Section 3.2.2) and signal detrending (Section 3.2.3), signal processing approaches for statistical feature extraction (Section 3.3), as well as signal fusion or integration methods (Section 3.5). However, mapping the extracted high dimensional features with the desired patterns is a really challenging task. In this section, the widely used statistical pattern recognition and data mining techniques, Bayesian inference, ANNs, and SVM are discussed in detail.

3.6.1 Bayesian Decision Theory

The BN has been proved to be a powerful knowledge representation and reasoning algorithm under conditions of uncertainty. Domain specific knowledge can be incorporated in the network structure, and a complicated joint probability distribution can be reduced to a set of conditionally independent relationships that are easier to characterize. A BN $B = (S,\ \theta)$ is a directed acyclic graph (DAG), where $S = (N,\ A)$ represents the network structure consisting of nodes and arcs, N, known as the set of all the nodes in a BN structure represents the domain variables $X_1, \ldots, X_n$, and each arc $a \in A$ between the nodes describes a probabilistic dependence among the variables, quantified using the conditional probability distribution. For each node X_i, the set of parameters θ contains a single parameter $\theta_{X_i|\pi_i} = P(X_i|\pi_i)$ that encodes the corresponding conditional probabilities, where π_i denotes the set of direct parents of X_i, and the joint probability distribution can be expressed as

$$P(X_1, \ldots, X_n) = \prod_{i=1}^{n} P(X_i|\pi_i) = \prod_{i=1}^{n} \theta_{X_i|\pi_i} \tag{3.54}$$

The construction of a BN consists of two sub-problems, namely the structure learning and parameter estimation. The process of learning the structure of a BN is to find the DAG that best reflects all interdependence relations between variables. Two popular approaches to perform structure learning have been introduced in the literature in the last two decades, one is the scoring function, and the other is the search algorithm. Commonly used scoring functions are the log-likelihood, the minimal description length (MDL) score, and the Bayesian score. The log-likelihood function is the log of the likelihood function which increases linearly with the data length, the higher scoring networks are those with high correlation between the nodes and their parents. When adding a node to the networks the log-likelihood always increases, thus the network structure with maximum likelihood is often complexly connected, this is the deficiency of the log-likelihood method. The MDL scoring algorithm has a synthetic consideration both on likelihood function and computing complexity, and uses the MDL as the objective function, the BN with the least MDL score is said to model the underlying distribution in the best possible way [64]. The Bayesian score function is another widely used approach. The Bayesian score function captures the full Bayesian posterior probability and, consequently, the prior over graphs need to be specified. Compared with scoring functions, search algorithms are more popular, mainly because they search the highest scoring graph using different heuristic methods, the problem of finding the highest-scoring network structure by using scoring functions is NP-hard, while heuristic searches can run indefinitely and stop at any time to reveal the highest scoring graph. Researchers have proposed many heuristic search methods, such as K2 hill climbing (HC) and Markov chain Monte Carlo (MCMC) algorithms.

After establishing the BN structure, the next step is to perform parameter estimation and compute the conditional probability $P(X_i|\pi_i)$ for each variable X_i. There are two types of parameter estimation, depending on whether all the variables are complete or not. If the variable set is incomplete, the expectation maximization (EM) algorithm is widely used, or else, as in the case mentioned in this chapter, maximum likelihood estimation is more practical. Generally, parameters can be estimated from the observed data, let θ_{ijk} denote the conditional probability that a variable x_i has the value v_{ik}, for some k from 1 to r_i, given the parents of x_i, represented by π_i and instantiated as w_{ij}, then $\theta_{ijk} = P(X_i = v_{ik}|\pi_i = w_{ij})$ is termed a network conditional probability. The simplest form of parameter estimation is based on frequency counts shown as

$$\theta^f_{ijk} = \frac{n(X_i, \pi_i)}{n(X_i)} \tag{3.55}$$

Bayesian inference is followed by the procedure of BN learning, which is defined as the process of computing posterior distribution of the target variable. BN is one of the most computationally efficient algorithms for machine learning, document classification, and data mining [65]. So far a number of Bayesian classifiers have been proposed, such as the naive Bayesian classifier (NBC), tree augmented naive Bayes (TAN), and Bayesian network augmented naive Bayes (BAN) and general Bayesian network (GBN), among which NBC is the most widely used and the simplest. In spite

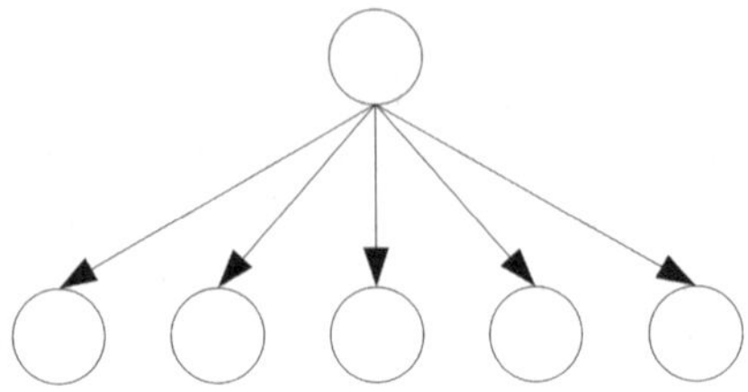

Figure 3.31 The structure of NBC

of its simplicity, the NBC can perform surprisingly well in many domains compared with other alternatives such as decision trees and ANNs, especially when variables are not significantly correlated with each other and the number of variables is relatively few. As shown in Figure 3.31, the graphical structure of the BN representing the NBC encodes the assumption that there is only one edge from the class node to each attribute node and each attribute is conditionally independent of the other attributes given the class.

Since NBC has a fixed structure, BN learning simply involves the estimation of parameters according to the procedure shown as Equation 3.55, where π_i is equivalent to the class node ω_i. Then a new case $\{X_1 = x_1, \ldots, X_n = x_n\}$ is classified by computing the posterior probability of each class according to the Bayesian theorem,

$$P(\omega_i|X_1 = x_1, \ldots, X_n = x_n) = \frac{P(X_1 = x_1, \ldots, X_n = x_n|\omega_i)P(\omega_i)}{P(X_1 = x_1, \ldots, X_n = x_n)} \tag{3.56}$$

The Naive Bayesian approach tries to get around the problem by a simplifying assumption regarding the relationship between features, thus it employs the class conditional independence assumption between the features. Hence, the above numerator becomes,

$$P(X_1 = x_1, \ldots, X_n = x_n|\omega_i) = \prod_{i=1}^{n} P(X_i = x_i|\omega_i) \tag{3.57}$$

3.6.2 Artificial Neural Networks

A feed forward back-propagation (BP) network is one of the most popular techniques in the field of ANNs. The architecture of a three layer feed forward ANN is illustrated in Figure 3.32. The source nodes in the input layer of the network supply the respective elements of the activation pattern or input vector, which constitute the input signals applied to the neurons in the hidden layer. The output signals of the hidden layer are used as inputs to the output layer. The output signals of the neurons in the output layer of the network constitute the overall response of the network to the activation patterns applied by the input layer neurons [66].

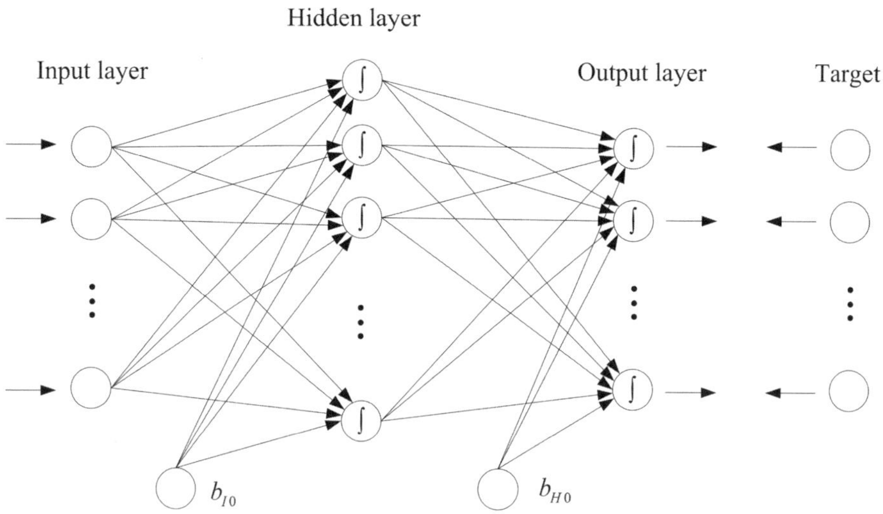

Figure 3.32 Schematic diagram of the BP algorithm in a multilayer neural network

The BP algorithm consists of two passes – forward pass and backward pass. With n input neurons, m hidden neurons, and p output neurons, the training process of the BP network can be described as follows.

1. *Feed forward pass*

The input vector $X = (x_0, x_1, \ldots, x_n)$ with x_0 being the bias b_{I0}, the outputs of all hidden layer nodes can be calculated as,

$$net_j = \sum_{i=0}^{n} w_{i,j}x_i \quad (i = 0, 1, \ldots, n;\ j = 1, 2, \ldots, m) \tag{3.58}$$

$$z_j = f_H(net_j) \qquad (j = 1, 2, \ldots, m) \tag{3.59}$$

where net_j is the activation value of the jth node, $w_{i,j}$ is the connection weight from input node i to the hidden node j, z_j is the corresponding output of the jth node in the hidden layer, and f_H is called the activation function of a node.

The outputs of all output layer neurons can be calculated as,

$$o_k = f_o\left(\sum_{j-0}^{m} w_{j,k}z_j\right) \qquad (j = 0, 1, \ldots, m;\ k = 1, 2, \ldots, p) \tag{3.60}$$

where f_o is the activation function, $w_{j,k}$ is the connection weight from hidden node j to output node k, z_j is the corresponding out of the jth node in the hidden layer with z_0 being the bias b_{H0}. All the connection weights and bias values are assigned with random values initially, and then modified according to the results of the BP training process.

The global error E is generated based on the output obtained o_k and the desired output T_k,

$$E = \frac{1}{2}\sum_{k=1}^{p}(T_k - o_k)^2 \tag{3.61}$$

2. *Backward pass*

According to the calculated error, changes in the weights are made. An output layer weight is updated as,

$$\Delta w_{j,k} = \frac{\partial E}{\partial w_{j,k}} \tag{3.62}$$

Similarly, changes in the synaptic weights of the hidden layer can be evaluated. As this process of weight change is iterative so a learning rule is to be applied to make the process smooth. The gradient descent learning rule is widely used. Using a modified gradient descent learning rule with momentum [67],

$$w_{j,k}(t+1) = w_{j,k}(t) - \eta\Delta w_{j,k} + \alpha w_{j,k}(t-1) \tag{3.63}$$

where η and α are introduced to make the learning process smooth and to ensure that the weight changes take place in the same direction.

The illustration shown in Figure 3.33 is the classification of simulation data with three patterns by the BP algorithm. The hidden layer is set with a sigmoid function, and the training error is 0.001. As shown in Figure 3.34, the training error has a decreasing trend and reaches the training target when the iteration is 28.

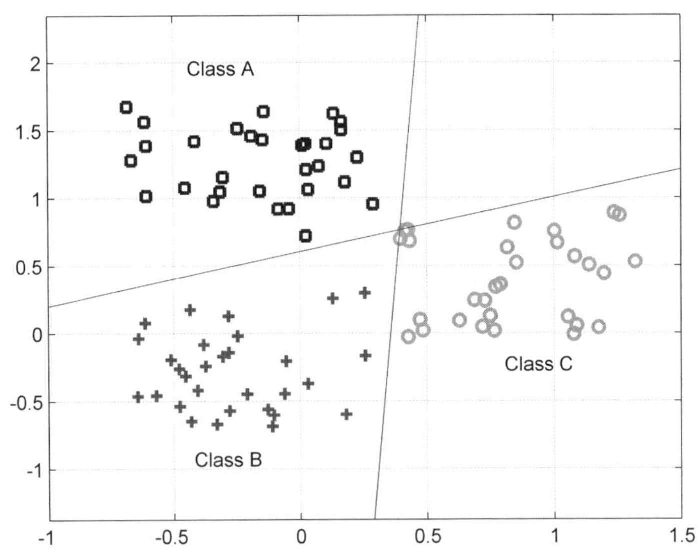

Figure 3.33 Pattern classifications by the BP algorithm

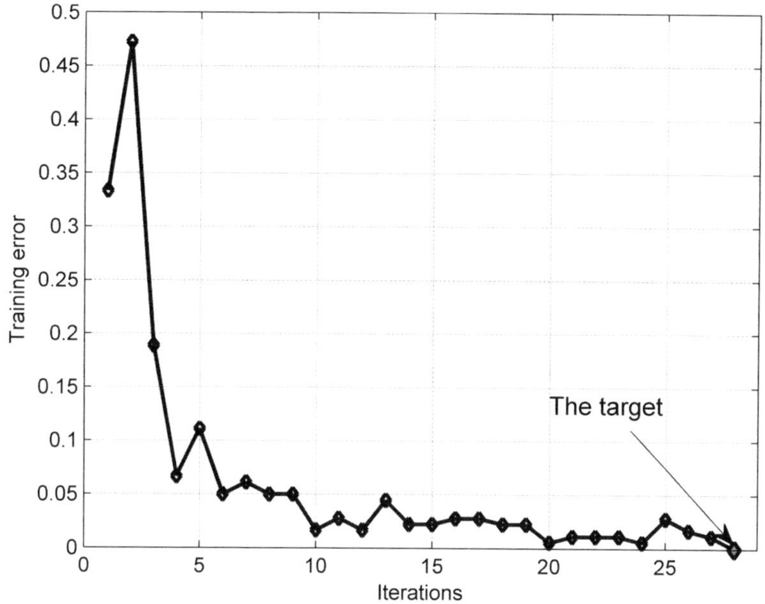

Figure 3.34 Training process of ANN

3.6.3 Support Vector Machine

3.6.3.1 Fundamentals of the Support Vector Machine

SVMs have become one of the most popular approaches to learning from examples with many potential applications in science and engineering in the last few years. The key concept of SVMs, which were originally first developed for binary classification problems, is the use of hyperplanes to define decision boundaries separating data points of different classes. SVMs are able to handle both simple, linear, classification tasks, as well as more complex and non-linear classification problems. The idea behind SVMs is to map the original data points from the input space to a high-dimensional feature space such that the classification problem becomes simpler in the features pace [68].

The basic principle of SVMs can be illustrated in a two-dimensional way as shown in Figure 3.35, the classification of a set of data with class A− and class A+, the SVM algorithm tries to place a boundary between the two classes and orients it in such way that the margin is maximized, the nearest data points are used to define the margin and are known as support vectors.

Considering the training data $\{x_i, y_i\}_{i=1}^{n}$ with d-dimensional input vectors x_i and the class labels $y_i \in \{-1, +1\}$, suppose there exists a hyperplane which separates the positive from the negative examples. The point x_i that lies on the hyperplane must satisfy $w \cdot x_i + b = 0$, where the weight w is a row vector and b is a bias. Thus, the input data

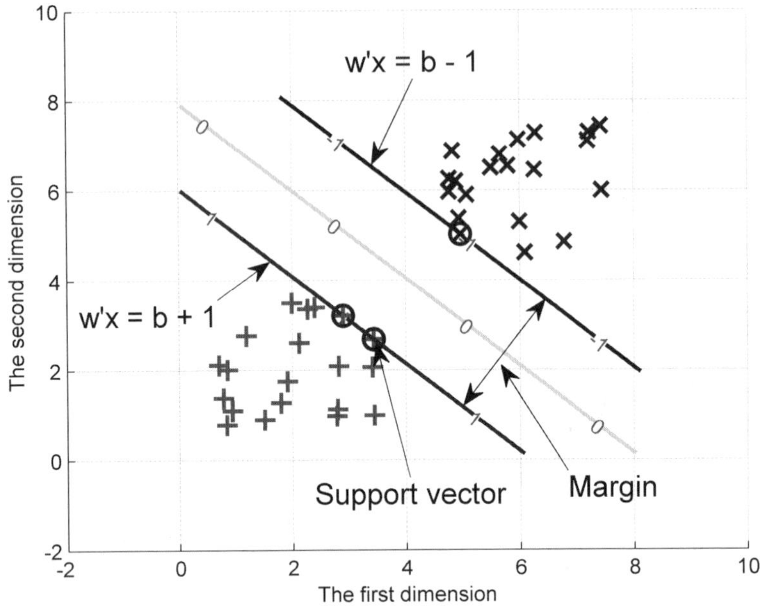

Figure 3.35 Classification of two classes using SVM

can be classified through the following constraints,

$$\begin{cases} w \cdot x_i + b \geq +1 & \text{for } y_i = +1 \\ w \cdot x_i + b \leq -1 & \text{for } y_i = -1 \end{cases} \tag{3.64}$$

The optimal hyperplane can be obtained as a solution to the following constrained optimization problem [69],

$$\text{Minimize} \frac{1}{2}\|w\|^2 \tag{3.65}$$

$$\text{Subject to } y_i[w \cdot x_i + b] - 1 \geq 0, \quad i = 1, 2, \cdots, l \tag{3.66}$$

The above formulation plays perfectly when the data are linearly separable. However, the investigated data in most real-life situations are overlapping, therefore, the soft variable ξ_i is adopted which allows toleration of a restricted number of misclassifications around the margin, and the soft constrained condition can be written as

$$y_i[w \cdot x_i + b] - 1 + \xi_i \geq 0, \quad i = 1, 2, \cdots, l \tag{3.67}$$

In order to determine model parameters for SVMs, either the original primal problem or its dual counterpart are taken as the starting point. Primal and dual problems are defined in the sequel. Applying the structure risk minimization principle to the dichotomous classification case, the so-called primal problem in Equation 3.68 subject to the constraints given in Equation 3.69, needs to be solved in praxis. The first term accounts for the VC dimension of the learning machine. The second term is an upper bound on the number of misclassifications making use of the slack variables.

$$\text{Minimize } \frac{1}{2}\|w\|^2 + C\sum_{i=1}^{l} \xi_i \tag{3.68}$$

$$\text{Subject to } y_i[w \cdot x_i + b] - 1 + \xi_i \geq 0, \quad \xi_i \geq 0, \quad i = 1, 2, \cdots, l \tag{3.69}$$

where, C is the disciplinal parameter introduced to define the trade-off between the large margin and misclassification error.

Alternatively, the equivalent optimization problem, the so-called dual problem, needs to be solved, whose solution in the dichotomous classification case is the solution of Equation 3.70 subject to Equation 3.71. For the constrained optimization problem, Lagrange multipliers α_i are introduced, and this form evolves among others, by replacing $w = \sum_{i=1}^{m} \alpha_i y_i x_i$, $\alpha_i \neq 0$ only for the support vectors x_i, $i = 1, 2, \ldots, m$.

$$\text{Minimize } L(w, b, \alpha) = \sum_{i=1}^{m} \alpha_i - \frac{1}{2}\sum_{i,j=1}^{m} \alpha_i \alpha_j y_i y_j \varphi(x_i) \cdot \varphi(x_j) \tag{3.70}$$

$$\text{Subject to } 0 \leq \alpha_i \leq C, \qquad \sum_{i=1}^{m} \alpha_i y_i = 0 \tag{3.71}$$

Methods to solve the corresponding optimization problem to SVM learning include sequential minimal optimization (SMO) and derivatives [70] decomposition methods [71], and methods to solve the least-squares SVM formulations [72]. When the following parameters were determined, the bias b, the number of support vectors m, the support vectors x_i, and associated y_i values, $i = 1, 2, \ldots, m$, as well as the Lagrange multipliers α_i, the SVM classifier in the following form was determined,

$$f(x) = \text{sign}\left(\sum_{i,j=1}^{l} \alpha_i y_i K\left(x_j, x_i\right) + b\right) \tag{3.72}$$

where the kernel function $K(\cdot\ ,\ \cdot)$ is positive definite, $K(x_i, x_j) = \varphi(x_i)^{\mathrm{T}}\varphi(x_j)$. The typical examples of kernel function are polynomial kernel, radial basis function (RBF) kernel, linear kernel, and sigmoid kernel [73],

- *Linear function*: $K(x_i, x_j) = {x_i}^T x_j$
- *Polynomial function*: $K(x_i, x_j) = (\gamma \cdot {x_i}^{\mathrm{T}} x_j + c_0)^d$
- *Radial basis function*: $K(x_i, x_j) = \exp(-\|x_i - x_j\|^2/2\gamma^2)$, $\gamma > 0$
- *Sigmoid kernel function*: $K(x_i, x_j) = \tanh(\gamma \cdot {x_i}^{\mathrm{T}} x_j + c_0)$

where, d is the index of the polynomial function, γ is the width parameter of the kernel-function, and c_0 is the bias.

The solution to the convex quadratic programing problem is global and unique when a positive definite kernel is used and the employing of a kernel function enables SVMs to work in a high dimensional feature space and solve complex and non-linear classification problems.

3.6.3.2 Experimental and Application

The experimental set-up and schematic diagram are shown in Figure 3.36 [74], the test rig consists of a three-phase induction motor (left), a torque transducer (center), a dynamometer (right), and control electronics. Faults of size 7, 14, and 21 mils (1mil = 0.001 inches) were introduced into the drive-end bearings (6205-2RSJEMSKF) using electro-discharge machining (EDM). Then the faulted bearings were reinstalled into the test motor and vibration data were recorded for motor loads of 0–3 hp (four motor speeds range from 1720 to 1797 rpm).

An accelerometer with a band width up to 5000 Hz and a 1 V/g output is mounted on the motor housing at the 12 o'clock position at the drive-end of the motor to acquire the vibration signals from the bearing. The data collection system consists of a high band width amplifier particularly designed for vibration signals and a data recorder with

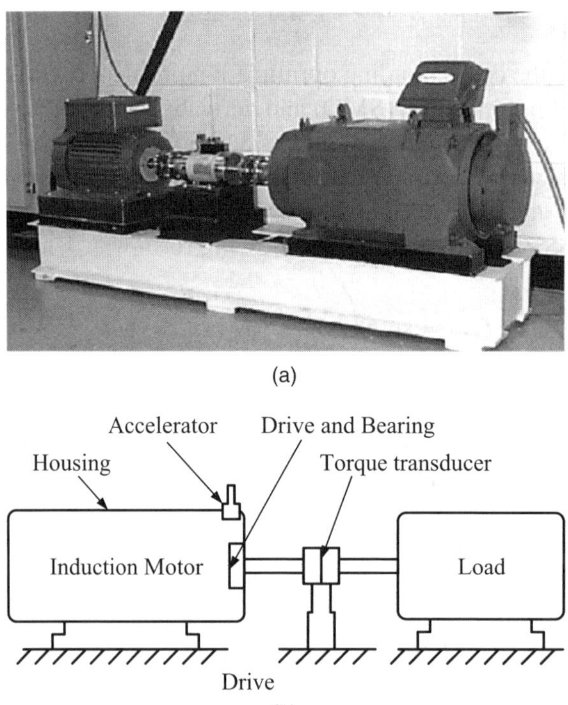

Figure 3.36 (a) Experimental set-up and (b) schematic diagram of the test rig

Table 3.1 Bearings information (size: inches)

Derive end bearing: 6205-2RSJEMSKF, deep groove ball bearing				
Inside diameter	Outside diameter	Thickness	Ball diameter	Pitch diameter
0.9843	2.0472	0.5906	0.3126	1.537

Table 3.2 Fault bearing data description

Fault diameter (mil)	Motor load (hp)	Motor speed (rpm)	Inner race	Ball	Outer race (center)
7	0	1797	IR007_0	B007_0	OR007@6_0
7	1	1772	IR007_1	B007_1	OR007@6_1
7	2	1750	IR007_2	B007_2	OR007@6_2
7	3	1730	IR007_3	B007_3	OR007@6_3
14	0	1797	IR0014_0	B0014_0	OR0014@6_0
14	1	1772	IR0014_1	B0014_1	OR0014@6_1
14	2	1750	IR0014_2	B0014_2	OR0014@6_2
14	3	1730	IR0014_3	B0014_3	OR0014@6_3
21	0	1797	IR0021_0	B0021_0	OR0021@6_0
21	1	1772	IR0021_1	B0021_1	OR0021@6_1
21	2	1750	IR0021_2	B0021_2	OR0021@6_2
21	3	1730	IR0021_3	B0021_3	OR0021@6_3

a sampling frequency of 12 000 Hz per channel. The data recorder is equipped with low-pass filters at the input stage for anti-aliasing. On the other hand, the frequency content of interest in the vibration signals of the system under study did not exceed 5000 Hz, for which the sampling rate is ample. Drive end bearings specifications and the collected fault bearing data description are listed in Tables 3.1 and 3.2 [75].

The method that consisted of EMD and SVM was applied to identify nine kinds of failure of a rolling bearing, the raw signal of bearing failures was collected from the test bed. The pre-processed data were decomposed by EMD, and a series of IMFs was obtained. As shown in Figure 3.37, the inner fault sample was decomposed into 12 IMFs, it can be clearly seen that the amplitude of the last 4 IMFs was so small that they were generally considered as undesired IMFs, which resulted from envelope fitting errors and lack of sampling points at both ends of the signal. A screening process was employed to select the vital IMFs from the decomposed IMFs [40]. Cross-correlation coefficients between each IMF and the original signal were calculated and the IMF was regarded as an undesired mode when the calculated coefficient was less than the threshold, which was defined as the absolute value of a ratio of the maximal correlation coefficient to a factor

$$\lambda = |\max(\mu_1)|/\eta \tag{3.73}$$

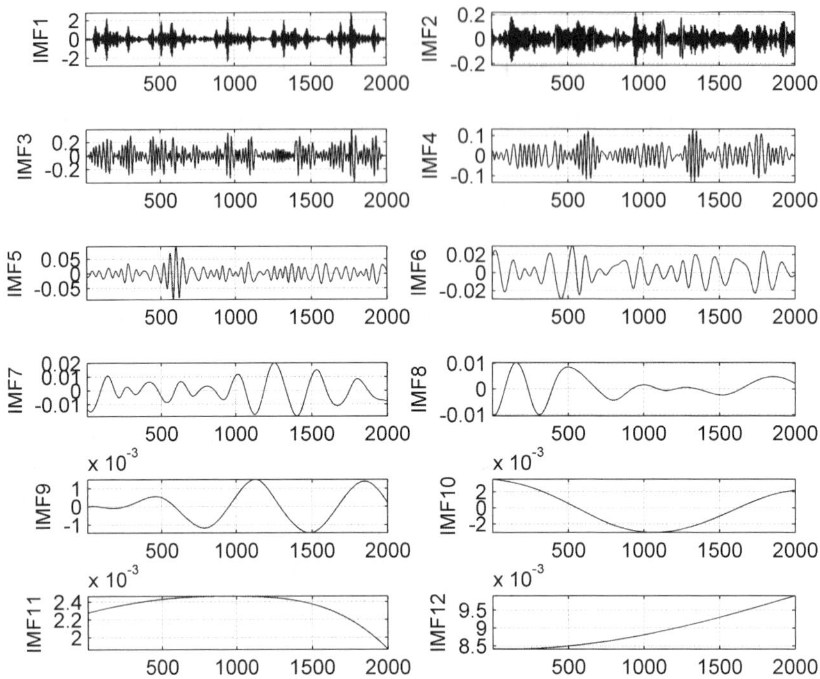

Figure 3.37 Inner fault signal decomposed based on EMD

Table 3.3 Cross-correlation coefficients between IMFs and the original signal

IMF	IMF1	IMF2	IMF3	IMF4	IMF5	IMF6	IMF7	IMF8
Cross-correlation coefficient	0.8656	0.3618	0.2538	0.1300	0.0323	0.0337	0.0071	0.0021
IMF	IMF9	IMF10	IMF11	IMF12				
Cross-correlation coefficient	0.0022	0.0052	0.0093	0.0486				

where, μ_1 is the obtained cross-correlation coefficient and η is an optional parameter.

Typically, the optional parameter can be estimated as $\eta = 4$, and the threshold can be calculated as $\lambda = 0.2164$ [76]. Then, as shown in Table 3.3, IMF1, IMF2, and IMF3 were selected, which had larger coefficients than the threshold and were employed to mine bearing failure information.

As discussed previously, statistical analysis of vibration signals in the time-domain and frequency-domain is able to yield different primary and secondary statistical parameters to characterize the shape of the vibration data. In the experiment, statistical features which were extracted from the raw vibration signals were selected as the basis to classify different bearing faults.

Fault features such as RMS value, peak factor, kurtosis, and margin factor were extracted from the obtained IMFs, which were regarded as input vectors in the SVM

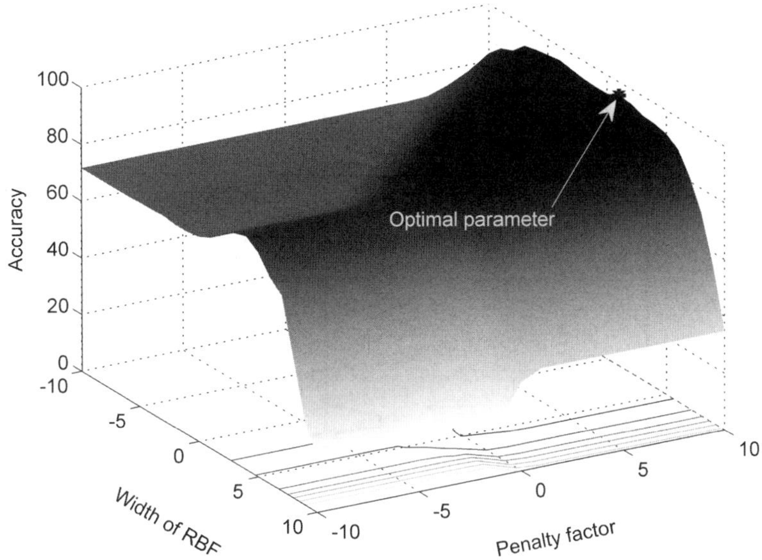

Figure 3.38 Relationship between training accuracy and related parameters

classification process. Identification of nine kinds of bearing faults was conducted based on SVM, the widely used RBF was selected as the kernel function. A greedy searching algorithm was used to find the optimal parameters of the SVM model. As shown in Figure 3.38, when the penalty factor is $C = 2^{10}$ and the width is $\gamma = 2$, the training model of the SVM researched the best classification accuracy. Then, the optimal model was used to classify nine kinds of bearing failures. As shown in Figure 3.39, all kinds of bearing faults can be identified with minimal accuracy of 80%. The left three sub-figures represented the classification accuracy of early bearing failures, the 7 mil fault diameters in three components of the bearing were identified effectively with a very high accuracy, even when the training samples were in short supply. Especially, in the initial stage of bearing failure, the classification accuracy can achieve 95% with small training samples. Experimental results demonstrated that the presented technique gave a very good solution for fault identification of mechanical equipment.

3.7 Advanced Technology for Feature Extraction

As a commonly used technology for parts classification in industry, group technology (GT) is employed according to certain principles of the system, which results in convenient information management and parts processing [77].

However, GT has not been introduced to the field of signal processing. This section presented a GT-based feature extraction methodology, as a simple and effective technology of information management, which provides a useful analytical tool for feature extraction and selection of non-stationary signals.

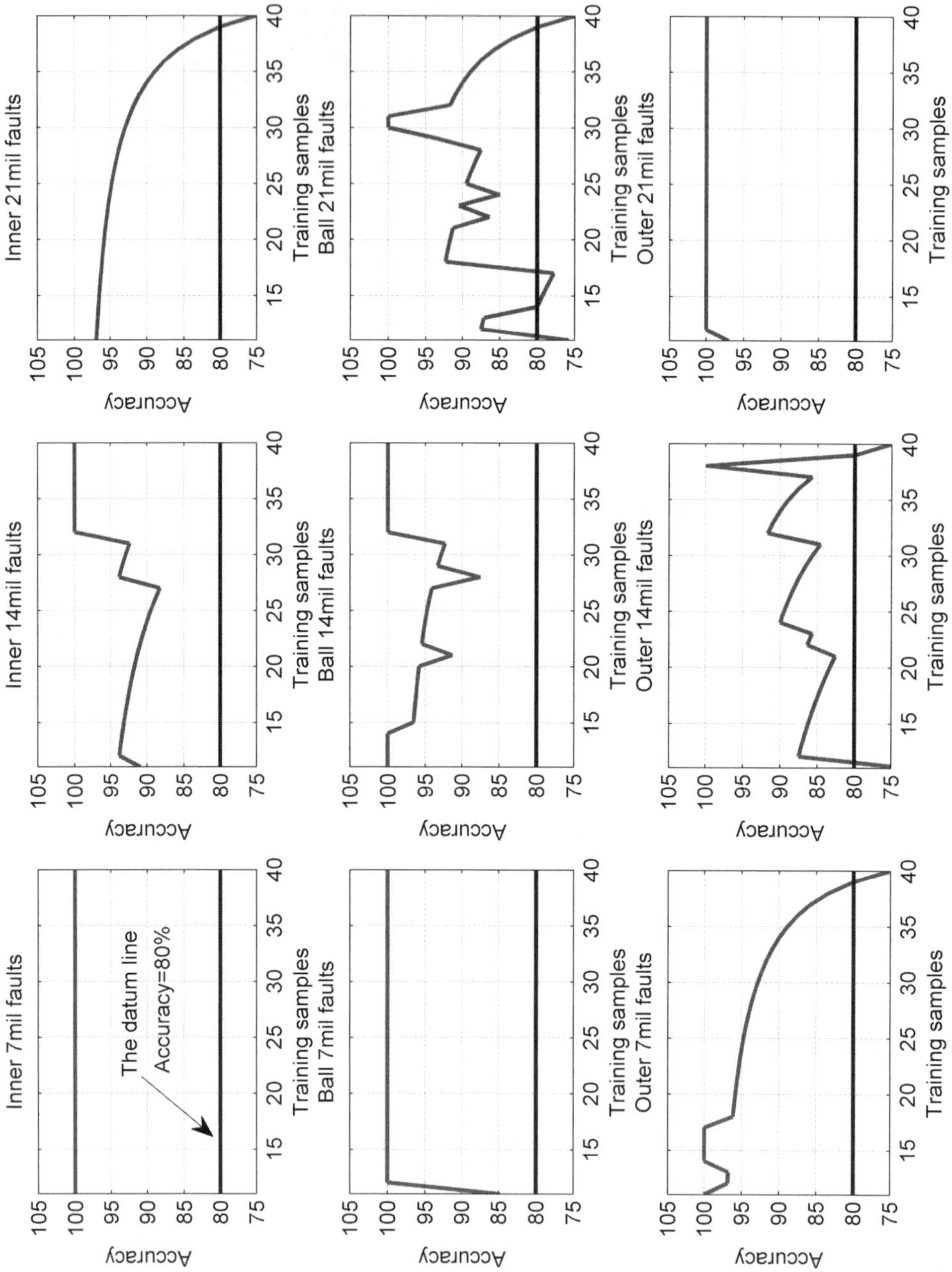

Figure 3.39 Bearing faults identification based on SVM

3.7.1 Group Technology

3.7.1.1 A Brief Introduction to GT

The mechanism of GT is grouping according to certain criteria by making use of similarities between objectives, in order to deal with objectives in the same group by identical methods, and eventually improve system efficiency [77, 78]. As the functionality of grouping similar elements, GT provides a strong theoretical support for analyzing interrelationships among information and reducing dimensions of information.

3.7.1.2 Theory of GT

The essence of GT is a measurement set, which is constructed by correlation functions defined by corresponding measurement. Set analytical methods, as well as other relevant theories, are employed to group certain related samples into entirely non-overlap groups. Namely, making use of proper mathematical methods, collectivity I will be absolutely disassembled where

$$I = S_1 \cup S_2 \ldots \cup S_n \; S_1,\ S_2,\ S_n \text{ are subsets of } I; \tag{3.74}$$

$$S_i \cap S_j = \Phi, \quad i, j \in \{1, 2, \ \ldots \ n\}, \quad i \neq j \tag{3.75}$$

$$S_i \neq \Phi, \quad i, j \in \{1, 2, \ \ldots \ n\} \tag{3.76}$$

In GT, all the samples have to exist in the form of vectors, and all vectors have the same length. Norms are used to calculate generalized distances between samples in different normalized spaces. The most popular way to measure the similarity of different sample points is to calculate Euclidean distances between samples in the m-dimensional Euclidean space [79], which is the most common measurement in practical application.

$$\|P_i - P_j\|_2 = \sqrt{\sum [(P_i(m) - P_j(m))]^2} \tag{3.77}$$

However, there is a problem when the form of two vectors is identical but proportional in value, the distance between the two vectors will be relatively large. Therefore, generalized distance does not reflect the similarity of form.

The generalized cosine of the vectors provides us with an appropriate tool. Samples will be placed in the m-dimensional linear space, thus each vector is made up of samples and the origin has a definite direction. Each can be expressed as vector $A\angle\Phi$, where A is the vector of the length, angle Φ stands for the direction. It can be proved that the vectors with the same direction have the same form, no matter what the length of the vectors is. Therefore, the inconvenience caused by the change of length can be avoided by using the generalized cosine of two vectors as a measure of similarity. The samples compose a similarity measure set. The generalized cosine of two vectors is defined as [79]:

$$\cos(p_i, p_j) = \sum_m \frac{p_i \times p_j}{\|p_i\|_2 \bullet \|p_j\|_2,} \quad i, j \in \{1, 2, \ \ldots \ n\} \tag{3.78}$$

$$\cos(p_i, p_j) \to 0 \tag{3.79}$$

when the two vectors are almost entirely dissimilar;

$$\cos(p_i, p_j) = 1 \tag{3.80}$$

when the two vectors are completely similar.

Obviously, the generalized cosine can be employed as a similarity measure in GT. This measure is determinate and monotonic. Any similarity can be quantified as a fixed value with a generalized cosine, which provides a convenient basis for forthcoming grouping.

3.7.1.3 Algorithm of Group Technology

For the sample set **I,** the similarities of samples can be valued through calculating the generalized cosine. Then group all the elements. The traditional approach is:

1. Array the samples $p_1, p_2 \ldots p_n$ according to the order, obtain an m-dimensional sample set with n elements contained.
2. Start from the first elements, take p_1 as the core, and calculate the generalized cosine of p_1 with other elements to obtain: $\{\cos(p_1, p_2), \cos(p_1, p_3) \cdots \cos(p_1, p_n)\}$
3. Choose a suitable threshold e, p_j would be elected if $\cos(p_1, p_j) \geq e$; similarly, we can finally obtain a set S_1 with the core of p_1 and all other elements meet the requirements;
4. Form set $I_1 = I\text{-}S_1$, obtain set S_2 by repeating the above steps;
5. Repeat the above steps, obtain $I = S_1 \cup S_2 \ldots \cup S_n$.

The procedure of traditional GT is shown in Figure 3.40.

The traditional grouping algorithm presented above is straightforward where reduplication would never happen in the grouping process. However, there is an inherent shortage that results in the limitation of grouping quality since the core point is selected arbitrarily.

3.7.2 Improved Algorithm of Group Technology

We put forward an optimal-core determination algorithm for GT. The optimal core satisfies the following conditions (see Figure 3.41):

1. The optimal core is in the densest location of the set.
2. The similarity of any samples in the set with an optimal core is less than the preset threshold.
3. Samples can be completely grouped without overlap.

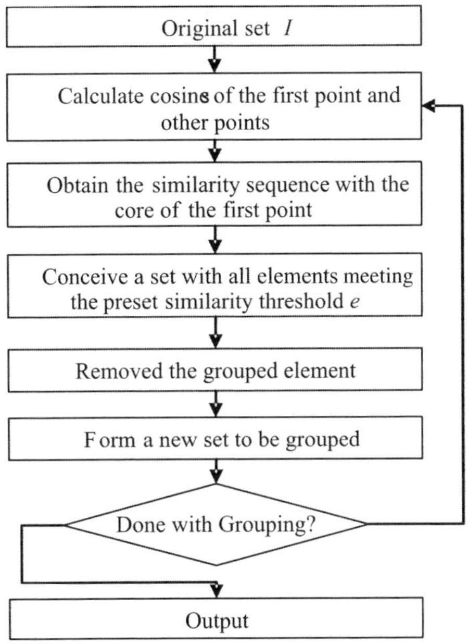

Figure 3.40 Traditional group algorithm

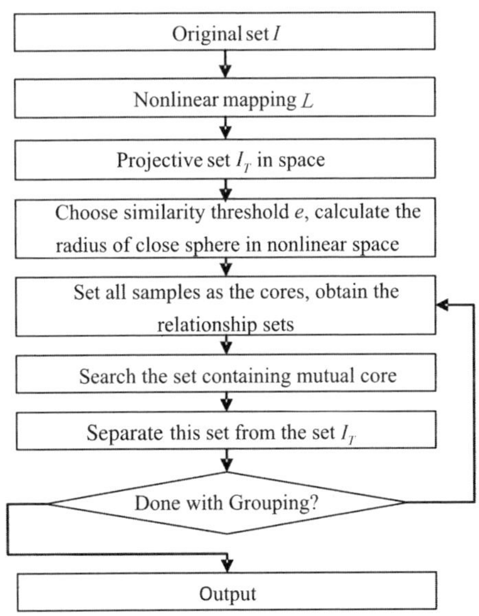

Figure 3.41 Improved group algorithm

As it is necessary to identify the point in the densest position, the point in a group which has greatest number of points is selected. The procedures of the improved algorithm are as follows:

1. Array the sample points $p_1, p_2 \dots p_n$ according to the order, obtain an m-dimensional point set with n elements contained.
2. Set $p_1, p_2 \dots p_n$ as the core, respectively, calculate the generalized cosine of these samples with others, then obtain: $\{\cos(p_1,p_2), \cos(p_1,p_3) \dots \cos(p_1,p_n)\}$
3. Choose a suitable threshold e, $P_{\rm j}$ would be elected if $\cos(p_1, p_j) \geq e$; similarly, we can finally obtain sets as $S_1, S_2 \dots\dots S_{\rm n}$ with the cores $p_1, p_2 \dots p_n$, and all other elements will meet the requirements;
4. Select the set containing the most elements from $S_1, S_2 \dots\dots S_n$ as a group G_1
5. Form set $I_1 = I\text{-}S_1$, obtain set S_2 by repeating the above steps;
6. Repeat the above steps, obtain $I = S_1 \cup S_2 \dots \cup S_n$.

The advantage of this algorithm is that, for each sample set, we are able to find the optimal core sample, and completely group without any overlap. In addition, the effect of grouping can be controlled by a pre-set threshold to ensure the quality of grouping. However, the calculation quantity is much greater than that of the original algorithm, and the computational speed is relatively slow since it is required to identify the optimal core in each iteration.

3.7.3 Numerical Simulation of Improved Group Algorithm

As GT has the property of grouping similar elements, it can certainly be used in pattern recognition.

The experimental data are generated from the following four categories:

1. $y = 1 + rand$
2. $y = x^2/40 + rand$
3. $y = e^{-x} + rand$
4. $y = \sin(x) + rand$.

Here, *rand* is the uniform random noise in [0, 0.3].

Each category of simulation data has 3 sample vectors sized (1×10), a total of 12 vectors are generated for simulation. In order to classify samples belonging to the same category, the GT-based methodology presented in Section 3.7.1 is applied. The threshold of the generalized cosine is set as 0.95. The final results of group sets are shown in Figure 3.42.

Obviously, the samples from the same category are grouped together accurately.

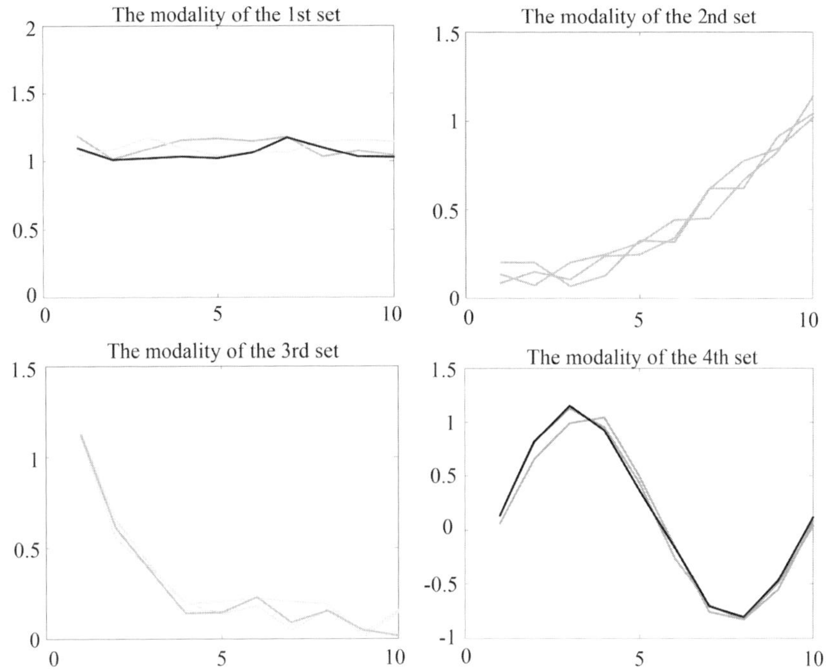

Figure 3.42 Group technology for similar modality recognition

3.7.4 Group Technology for Feature Extraction

3.7.4.1 The Introduction of a Traditional Feature Extraction Method for Extraction of Wavelet Packet Energy

In this context, GT is introduced to reduce redundant information as a feature selection methodology. Currently, wavelet packet decomposition has become a typical and widely used feature extraction method for non-stationary signals. It is deemed that the extracted features should cover the majority of the information of the original signals, consequently greater frequency band energies are selected according to a preset threshold. Therefore, the procedure of feature selection is interpreted as selecting the first several bands' energies sorted in a declining order until the threshold is satisfied (for example, 85% of total), see Figure 3.43.

This method has two inherent problems:

1. In order to obtain high frequency resolution, wavelet packet decomposition of more layers is required, which results in a geometric increase in the number of decomposition bands. Obviously, traditional methods of energy proportion based truncation

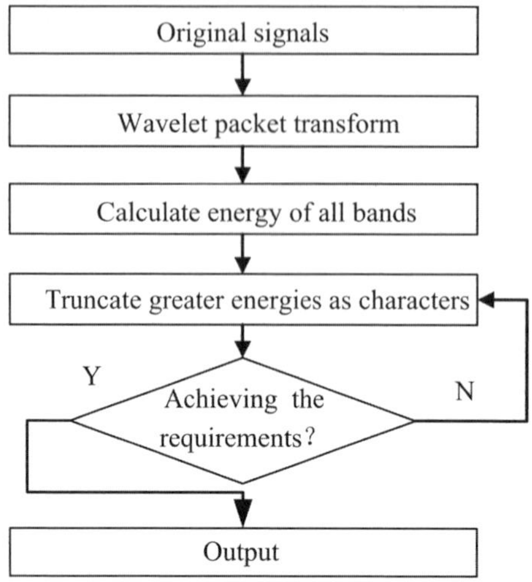

Figure 3.43 Traditional feature extraction method of non-stationary signals

inevitably result in eigenvector dimension oversize, which makes feature fusion difficult.

2. Non-stationary signals, especially vibration signals, have internally syntonic characteristics, each resonance is caused by a bunch of factors instead of a single one. Traditional methods could not provide deep insight into the internal factors. For some frequency components, a syntonic and linear relationship is apparent because of the emergence of resonance. As the relationship is not considered by the traditional method, eigenvectors of the signal contain greater redundancy but short of ultimate simplification of the information.

3.7.4.2 Group Technology Based Feature Extraction Method

In fact, for the first problem mentioned in Section 3.7.4.1, it is not feasible to reduce the eigenvector dimensions by decreasing the number of decomposition layers which would result because the final result is at the cost of sacrificing frequency resolution. For the second problem, the crux is to mine information hidden in signals, and eventually classify them. Therefore, there is a feasible way of analyzing the entire or sampled data set to obtain resonant relationships among signals.

GT is such an approach, which can extract similar relationships among information, hence simplifying it. The procedure for the GT-based feature extraction method is shown in Figure 3.44.

3.7.5 Application

3.7.5.1 Description of Experiment and Data

The experimental data is a one-dimensional vibration signal acquired in an accelerated degradation experiment on cutting tools. The experiment and the corresponding data set are described below:

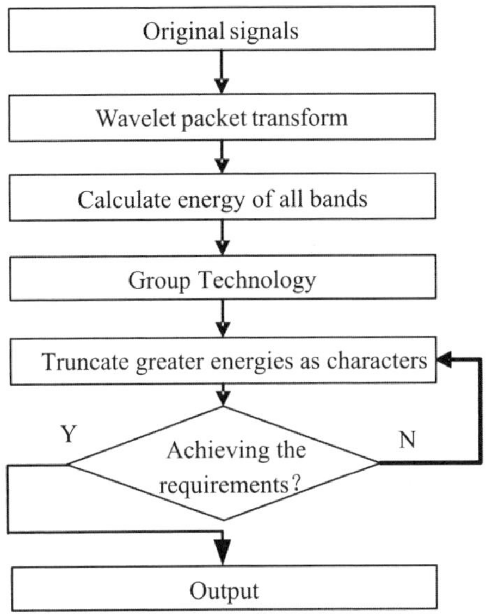

Figure 3.44 Feature extraction method based on GT

Experiments were conducted on an FADAL machining center
Data set:

drilling_data: 1024 × 194 × 10

The accelerometer is mounted on a spindle to acquire a vertical vibration signal. Ten sets of full life-cycle samples of the cutting tool are measured from brand-new to worn-out, each life-cycle has a total of 194 samples/holes with 1024 data points.

Experimental parameters:

Feed rate	9.8 ipm
V	1200 rpm
Sampling rate	15 kHz
Filter (lowpass)	6 kHz
Depth of hole	0.5 in.

3.7.5.2 Data Processing

In this case, wavelet packet decomposition is employed to extract features from vibration signals, the number of decomposition layers is six, correspondingly, an energy matrix of 194 × 64 is obtained based on the entire data set, where row number represents the number of the sample and each column refers to the wavelet energy vector for each sample.

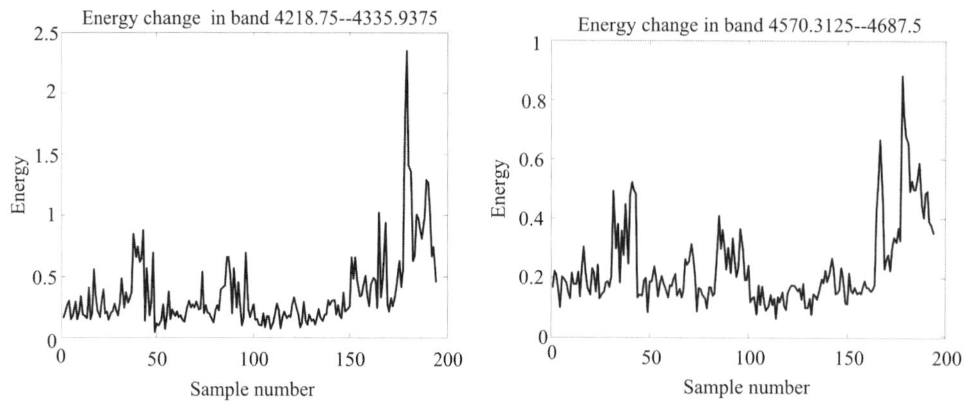

Figure 3.45 Energies in different bands

As for the signals acquired from practical applications, the relationships among frequencies are dependent on resonance, which reflects hidden characteristics of the system, and is worthy of investigation. Figure 3.45 illustrates the energies in terms of the number of samples, when more and more samples/holes were machined, the degradation process emerged which is represented by the increment in the value of the energies.

Obviously, the energies in different frequency bands have a similar trend of changes, which illustrates that there are resonant relations in different bands, and identification of these interrelated bands is conducive to reducing redundant information.

3.7.5.3 Experiment Results

Some of the results achieved by applying the GT-based feature selection methodology are demonstrated in Figure 3.46 where the generalized cosine threshold is pre-set at 0.9. Eventually, the dimension of the feature matrix was reduced to 11×194 from 64×194, namely, a significant amount of information is compressed. As a result, 11 clusters were achieved as $\{6, 7, 8, 9, 10, 11, 12, 13, 14, 15, 16, 19, 21, 22, 23, 24, 27, 28, 29, 30, 31, 32, 35, 39, 41, 51\}$, $\{37, 38, 40, 45, 46, 48\}$, $\{17, 18, 20, 49, 50\}$, $\{25, 42, 43, 44\}$, $\{2, 3, 4\}$, $\{34, 36\}$, $\{1\}$, $\{5\}$, $\{26\}$, $\{33\}$, $\{47\}$, respectively.

GT can not only access the system attributes by excavating the implicit relationships hidden in signals, but also make the information able to be dealt with intuitively by simplifying and compression.

3.7.5.4 Prognostics

The wavelet packet-band energies of the entire life-cycle of the other nine cutting tools were processed following the same procedures presented above, a three-dimensional

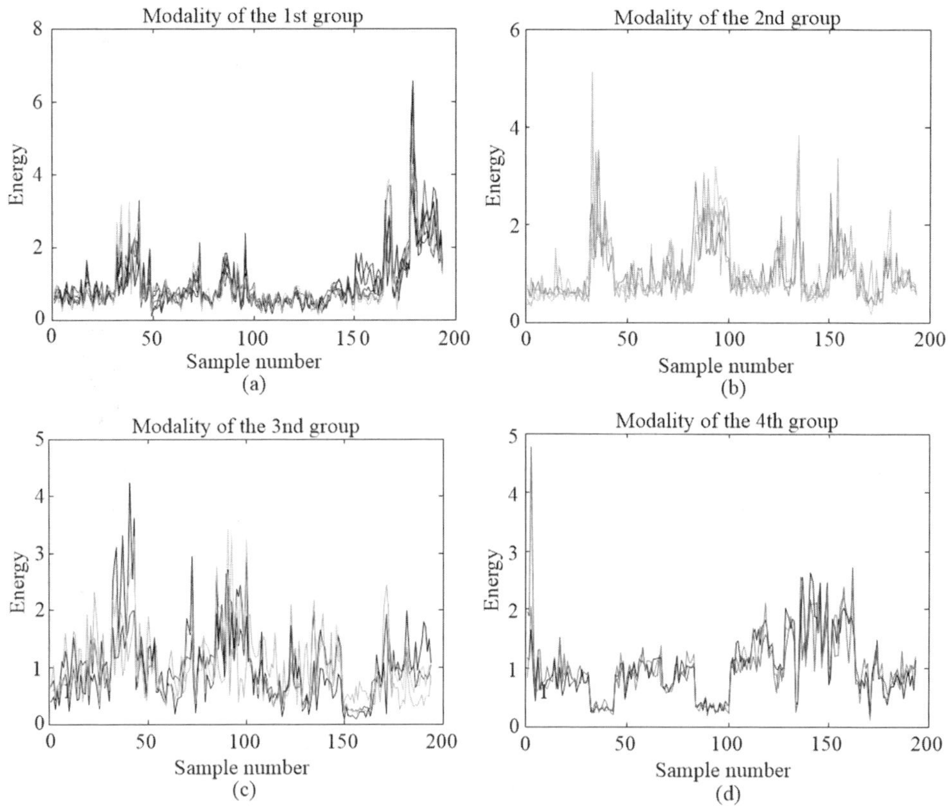

Figure 3.46 The patterns of the first four clusters (a–d) obtained by GT for superfluous information reduction

matrix was obtained which represents the feature vectors of the acquired drilling data, with size $11 \times 194 \times 10$.

In order to validate and demonstrate the effectiveness of the proposed GT-based feature extraction methodology, four data sets were constructed, which represent four phases of degradation severity from brand new to worn out:

1. Group the feature vectors for the 11th to the 20th holes as the first set to represent the brand new condition.
2. Group the feature vectors for the 51st to the 60th holes as the second set to represent an OK condition.
3. Group the feature vectors for the 101st to the 110th holes as the third set to represent a moderate wear condition;
4. Group the feature vectors for the 151st to the 160th holes as the last set to represent worn out condition;

Table 3.4 Classification results using SVM

SVM No.	1	2	3
Total number of support vectors	80	63	39
Error ratio of classification for the training set	0	0	0
Error ratio of classification for the validation set (%)	20	17.3	0

Eventually a feature matrix was set up using data from the four sets, with size 11 × 400. The first 100 columns stand for the feature vectors of the brand new condition; the 101st to the 200th columns stand for the feature vectors of an OK condition, the 201st to the 300th columns stand for the feature vectors of a moderate wear condition; and the last 100 columns stand for the worn out condition.

The above matrix constitutes the data sources for feature fusion and prognostics. Herein, half the data from each set is used for training and the other is used for validation.

SVM was employed for feature fusion and prognostic purposes. In this case, three SVMs were obtained after training, where a Gaussian kernel function was applied with a basic width of 1.1. The results by validating the trained SVMs using the other half of the data are given in Table 3.4.

These results indicate that GT for feature extraction can implement large-scale compression of the information, while ensuring group information with a similar pattern and distinguishing information with different patterns. The classification results of the first two sets are reasonable, since the data sets used here represent degradation severities, instead of sets of different failures, there are overlaps between "brand new" and "OK" conditions.

References

1. Žvokelj, M., Zupan, S. and Prebil, I. (2011) Non-linear multivariate and multiscale monitoring and signal denoising strategy using Kernel Principal Component Analysis combined with Ensemble Empirical Mode Decomposition method. *Mechanical Systems and Signal Processing*, **25** (7), 2631–2653.
2. Bozchalooi, I.S. and Liang, M. (2007) A smoothness index-guided approach to wavelet parameter selection in signal de-noising and fault detection. *Journal of Sound and Vibration*, **308** (1–2), 246–267.
3. Liu, B. (2005) Selection of wavelet packet basis for rotating machinery fault diagnosis. *Journal of Sound and Vibration*, **284** (3-5), 567–582.
4. Hadad, K., Pourahmadi, M. and Majidi-Maraghi, H. (2011) Fault diagnosis and classification based on wavelet transform and neural network. *Progress in Nuclear Energy*, **53** (1), 41–47.
5. Kankar, P.K., Sharma, S.C. and Harsha, S.P. (2011) Fault diagnosis of ball bearings using continuous wavelet transform. *Applied Soft Computing*, **11** (2), 2300–2312.

6. Purushotham, V., Narayanan, S. and Prasad, S.A.N. (2005) Multi-fault diagnosis of rolling bearing elements using wavelet analysis and hidden Markov model based fault recognition. *NDT & E International*, **38** (8), 654–664.
7. Saravanan, N. and Ramachandran, K.I. (2010) Incipient gear box fault diagnosis using discrete wavelet transform (DWT) for feature extraction and classification using artificial neural network (ANN). *Expert Systems with Applications*, **37** (6), 4168–4181.
8. Mohammed, O.A., Abed, N.Y. and Ganu, S. (2006) Modeling and characterization of induction motor internal faults using finite-element and discrete wavelet transforms. *IEEE Transactions on Magnetics*, **42** (10), 3434–3436.
9. Rajagopalan, S., Aller, J.M., Restrepo, J.A. *et al.* (2007) Analytic wavelet ridge based detection of dynamic eccentricity in Brushless Direct Current (BLDC) motors functioning under dynamic operating conditions. *IEEE Transactions on Industrial Electronics*, **54** (3), 1410–1419.
10. Zanardelli, W.G., Strangas, E.G. and Aviyente, S. (2007) Identification of intermittent electrical and mechanical faults in permanent-magnet AC drives based on time-frequency analysis. *IEEE Transactions on Industry Applications*, **43** (4), 971–980.
11. Huang, N.E., Shen, Z. and Long, S.R. (1998) The Empirical mode decomposition and the Hilbert spectrum for nonlinear and non-stationary time series analysis. *Proceedings of the Royal Society of London, Series A*, **454**, 903–995.
12. Huang, N.E. and Wu, Z. (2008) A review on Hilbert-Huang transform: method and its applications to geophysical studies. *Reviews of Geophysics*, **46** (2), RG2006.
13. Ong, K.C.G., Wang, Z. and Maalej, M. (2008) Adaptive magnitude spectrum algorithm for Hilbert-Huang transform based frequency identification. *Engineering Structures*, **30** (1), 33–41.
14. Peng, Z.K., Tse, P.W. and Chu, F.L. (2005) A comparison study of improved Hilbert-Huang transform and wavelet transform: application to fault diagnosis for rolling bearing. *Mechanical Systems and Signal Processing*, **19** (5), 974–988.
15. Cheng, J., Yu, D., Tang, J. *et al.* (2008) Application of frequency family separation method based upon EMD and local Hilbert energy spectrum method to gear fault diagnosis. *Mechanism and Machine Theory*, **43** (6), 712–723.
16. Widodo, A. and Yang, B.S. (2007) Support vector machine in machine condition monitoring and fault diagnosis. *Mechanical Systems and Signal Processing*, **21** (6), 2560–2574.
17. Mandal, S., Ghoshal, S.P., Kar, R. *et al.* (2012) Design of optimal linear phase FIR high pass filter using craziness based particle swarm optimization technique. *Journal of King Saud University - Computer and Information Sciences*, **24** (1), 83–92.
18. Komsta, Ł. (2009) A comparative study on several algorithms for denoising of thin layer densitograms. *Analytica Chimica Acta*, **641** (1–2), 52–58.
19. Litwin, L. (2000) FIR and IIR digital filters. *IEEE Potentials*, **19** (4), 28–31.
20. Kidambi, S.S. (1997) Computationally efficient weighted least-squares design of FIR filters satisfying prescribed magnitude and phase specifications. *Signal Processing*, **60** (1), 127–130.
21. Marple, S.L. Jr., (1987) *Digital Spectral Analysis with Applications*, Prentice-Hall, Inc., Englewood Cliffs, NJ.
22. Hodge, V. and Austin, J. (2004) A survey of outlier detection methodologies. *Artificial Intelligence Review*, **22** (2), 85–126.
23. Todeschini, R., Ballabio, D., Consonni, V. *et al.* (2013) Locally centred Mahalanobis distance: a new distance measure with salient features towards outlier detection. *Analytica Chimica Acta*, **787**, 1–9.
24. Park, S., Inman, D.J. and Yun, C.-B. (2008) An outlier analysis of MFC-based impedance sensing data for wireless structural health monitoring of railroad tracks. *Engineering Structures*, **30** (10), 2792–2799.

25. Bashan, A., Bartsch, R., Kantelhardt, J.W. *et al.* (2008) Comparison of detrending methods for fluctuation analysis. *Physica A: Statistical Mechanics and its Applications*, **387** (21), 5080–5090.
26. Pouzols, F.M. and Lendasse, A. (2010) Effect of different detrending approaches on computational intelligence models of time series. The 2010 International Joint Conference on Neural Networks (IJCNN), July 18–23, 2010.
27. Shafqat, K., Pal, S.K. and Kyriacou, P.A. (2007) Evaluation of two detrending techniques for application in Heart Rate Variability. 29th Annual International Conference of the IEEE Engineering in Medicine and Biology Society, 2007. EMBS 2007, pp. 267–270.
28. van Ommen, J.R., Sasic, S., van der Schaaf, J. *et al.* (2011) Time-series analysis of pressure fluctuations in gas–solid fluidized beds – A review. *International Journal of Multiphase Flow*, **37** (5), 403–428.
29. Lei, Y., Zuo, M.J., He, Z. *et al.* (2010) A multidimensional hybrid intelligent method for gear fault diagnosis. *Expert Systems with Applications*, **37** (2), 1419–1430.
30. Yuan, J. and Liu, X. (2013) Semi-supervised learning and condition fusion for fault diagnosis. *Mechanical Systems and Signal Processing*, **38** (2), 615–627.
31. Decker, H.J. (2003) Effects on Diagnostic Parameters After Removing Additional Synchronous Gear Meshes. Technical Report NASA/TM – 2003-212312, ARL–TR–2933, NASA, April 2003.
32. Oswald, F.B. (2004) Mechanical Components Branch Test Facilities and Capabilities. Technical Report NASA/TM – 2004-212722, NASA, January 2004.
33. Perko, M., Fajfar, I., Tuma, T., *et al.* (1998) Fast Fourier transform computation using a digital CNN simulator. 1998 Fifth IEEE International Workshop on Cellular Neural Networks and Their Applications Proceedings, pp. 230–235.
34. Lei, Y., He, Z., Zi, Y. *et al.* (2007) Fault diagnosis of rotating machinery based on multiple ANFIS combination with GAs. *Mechanical Systems and Signal Processing*, **21** (5), 2280–2294.
35. Leung, A.K.-M., Chau, F.-T. and Gao, J.-B. (1998) A review on applications of wavelet transform techniques in chemical analysis: 1989–1997. *Chemometrics and Intelligent Laboratory Systems*, **43** (1–2), 165–184.
36. Yan, R., Gao, R.X. and Chen, X. (2014) Wavelets for fault diagnosis of rotary machines: a review with applications. *Signal Processing*, **96** (Pt. A), 1–15.
37. Li, L., Li, M. and Lu, Y. (2010) Improved EMD algorithm and its application to striation distance measurement. *Journal of Applied Sciences - Electronics and Information Engineering*, **28** (1), 32–37.
38. Feldman, M. (2011) Hilbert transform in vibration analysis. *Mechanical Systems and Signal Processing*, **25** (3), 735–802.
39. Rilling, G., Flandrin, P., and Gonçalvès, P. (2003) On empirical mode decomposition and its algorithms. Proceedings of IEEE EURASIP Workshop on Nonlinear Signal and Image Processing NSIP, Grado, Italy, June, 2003.
40. Xun, J. and Yan, S. (2008) A revised Hilbert-Huang transformation based on the neural networks and its application in vibration signal analysis of a deployable structure. *Mechanical Systems and Signal Processing*, **22** (7), 1705–1723.
41. Cheng, J., Yu, D. and Yang, Y. (2007) Application of support vector regression machines to the processing of end effects of Hilbert-Huang transform. *Mechanical Systems and Signal Processing*, **21** (3), 1197–1211.
42. Roy, A. and Doherty, J.F. (2010) Improved signal analysis performance at low sampling rates using raised cosine empirical mode decomposition. *Electronics Letters*, **46** (2), 176–177.
43. Yan, J. and Lu, L. (2014) Improved Hilbert–Huang transform based weak signal detection methodology and its application on incipient fault diagnosis and ECG signal analysis. *Signal Processing*, **98**, 74–87.
44. Daubechies, I. (1996) Where do wavelets come from? A personal point of view. *Proceedings of the IEEE*, **84** (4), 510–513.

45. Hu, J. and Yang, S. (2007) AR model prediction-based EMD method and its application to data extension. *Journal of Vibration, Measurement & Diagnosis*, **27** (2), 116–120.
46. Jones, L. (1982) X-ray radiographic techniques in failure analysis. 20th Annual Reliability Physics Symposium, 1982, pp. 152–155.
47. Nakano, S., Tsubaki, T. and Yoneda, Y. (2000) External diagnosis of power transmission and distribution equipment using X-ray image processing. *IEEE Transactions on Power Delivery*, **15** (2), 575–579.
48. Sergyan, S. (2008) Color histogram features based image classification in content-based image retrieval systems. 6th International Symposium on Applied Machine Intelligence and Informatics, 2008. SAMI 2008, pp. 221–224.
49. Ju, H. and Kai-Kuang, M. (2002) Fuzzy color histogram and its use in color image retrieval. *IEEE Transactions on Image Processing*, **11** (8), 944–952.
50. Shih, J.L. and Chen, L.H. (2002) Colour image retrieval based on primitives of colour moments. *IEEE Proceedings - Vision, Image and Signal Processing*, **149** (6), 370–376.
51. Schaefer, G. and Stich, M. (2004) UCID: an uncompressed color image database. Proceedings of SPIE, Storage and Retrieval Methods and Applications for Multimedia, San Jose, CA, pp. 472–480.
52. Wenhao, H. and Kui, Y. (2008) An improved Canny edge detector and its realization on FPGA. 7th World Congress on Intelligent Control and Automation, 2008. WCICA 2008, pp. 6561–6564.
53. Canny, J. (1986) A computational approach to edge detection. *IEEE Transactions on Pattern Analysis and Machine Intelligence*, **PAMI-8** (6), 679–698.
54. Qian, X., Chakrabarti, C., and Karam, L.J. (2011) A distributed Canny edge detector and its implementation on FPGA. Digital Signal Processing Workshop and IEEE Signal Processing Education Workshop (DSP/SPE), 2011 IEEE, pp. 500–505.
55. Jiang, S.-F., Fu, D.-B., Hu, C.-M. *et al.* (2011) Damage identification of concrete-filled steel tubular arch bridge using data fusion based on information allocation theory. *Procedia Engineering*, **15**, 1705–1710.
56. Talavera, A., Aguasca, R., Galván, B. *et al.* (2013) Application of Dempster–Shafer theory for the quantification and propagation of the uncertainty caused by the use of AIS data. *Reliability Engineering and System Safety*, **111**, 95–105.
57. Basir, O., Karray, F. and Hongwei, Z. (2005) Connectionist-based Dempster-Shafer evidential reasoning for data fusion. *IEEE Transactions on Neural Networks*, **16** (6), 1513–1530.
58. Sadiq, R. and Rodriguez, M.J. (2005) Interpreting drinking water quality in the distribution system using Dempster–Shafer theory of evidence. *Chemosphere*, **59** (2), 177–188.
59. Yager, R.R. (1986) Arithmetic and other operations on Dempster-Shafer structures. *International Journal of Man-Machine Studies*, **25** (4), 357–366.
60. Ferson, S. and Hajagos, J.G. (2004) Arithmetic with uncertain numbers: rigorous and (often) best possible answers. *Reliability Engineering and System Safety*, **85** (1–3), 135–152.
61. Fu, H., Yang, Y.-K., Ma, K. *et al.* (2011) A novel fuzzy sensor fusion algorithm. *Journal of Coal Science and Engineering (China)*, **17** (4), 457–460.
62. Kwak, K.-C. and Pedrycz, W. (2005) Face recognition: a study in information fusion using fuzzy integral. *Pattern Recognition Letters*, **26** (6), 719–733.
63. Murofushi, T. and Sugeno, M. (1989) An interpretation of fuzzy measures and the Choquet integral as an integral with respect to a fuzzy measure. *Fuzzy Sets and Systems*, **29** (2), 201–227.
64. Ouali, A., Ramdane Cherif, A. and Krebs, M.-O. (2006) Data mining based Bayesian networks for best classification. *Computational Statistics & Data Analysis*, **51** (2), 1278–1292.
65. Porwal, A., Carranza, E.J.M. and Hale, M. (2006) Bayesian network classifiers for mineral potential mapping. *Computers & Geosciences*, **32** (1), 1–16.
66. Li, G. and Shi, J. (2010) On comparing three artificial neural networks for wind speed forecasting. *Applied Energy*, **87** (7), 2313–2320.
67. Kankar, P.K., Sharma, S.C. and Harsha, S.P. (2011) Fault diagnosis of ball bearings using machine learning methods. *Expert Systems with Applications*, **38** (3), 1876–1886.

68. Akay, M.F. and Abaslkeles, I. (2010) Predicting the performance measures of an optical distributed shared memory multiprocessor by using support vector regression. *Expert Systems with Applications*, **37** (9), 6293–6301.
69. Vapnik, V.N. (2000) *The Nature of Statistical Learning Theory*, Springer, New York.
70. Flake, G. and Lawrence, S. (2002) Efficient SVM regression training with SMO. *Machine Learning*, **46** (1–3), 271–290.
71. Keerthi, S.S. and Shevade, S.K. (2003) SMO algorithm for least-squares SVM formulations. *Neural Computation*, **15** (2), 487–507.
72. Suykens, J.A.K., De Brabanter, J., Lukas, L. *et al.* (2002) Weighted least squares support vector machines: robustness and sparse approximation. *Neurocomputing*, **48** (1–4), 85–105.
73. Luts, J., Ojeda, F., Van de Plas, R. *et al.* (2010) A tutorial on support vector machine-based methods for classification problems in chemometrics. *Analytica Chimica Acta*, **665** (2), 129–145.
74. Case Western Reserve University, Bearing Data Center http://csegroups.case.edu/bearingdatacenter /home (accessed 2nd July 2014).
75. Liu, H., Liu, C. and Huang, Y. (2011) Adaptive feature extraction using sparse coding for machinery fault diagnosis. *Mechanical Systems and Signal Processing*, **25** (2), 558–574.
76. Yan, J. and Lu, L. (2011) Incipient bearing fault diagnosis based on improved Hilbert-Huang transform and support vector machine. *Applied Mechanics and Materials*, **80-81**, 875–879.
77. Group Technology Research Group (1987) *Principle and Application of Group Technology*, Publishing House of Harbin Institute of Technology, Harbin, pp. 1–10, 40-68.
78. Xu, X. and Cai, J. (2004) *Group Technology*, Machinery Industry Press, Beijing.
79. Andrew, R.W. (2004) *Statistical Pattern Recognition*, Publishing House of Electronics Industry, Beijing.

4

Health Monitoring and Prognosis

4.1 Health Monitoring as a Concept

The word *health* comes first from the field of health care and is used mainly to describe the state of a biological organism. The word *monitoring* means observing and checking the progress or quality of something (in this case health) over a period of time.

Over the past decades there has been a growing interest in monitoring the ongoing "health" of products and systems. The aim of "health monitoring" in the engineering field is to find and predict the early signs of failure before total mechanical failure leads to a calamitous incident.

Health monitoring techniques have already been widely applied in industry. Generally, health monitoring is a process of monitoring the condition of machinery and processes by using advanced sensing and modern signal processing techniques. Here, health is a description of the performance of monitored objects which can be regarded as the extent of degradation or deviation from an expected normal condition. Sometimes health monitoring is also called health condition monitoring or condition monitoring in the literature.

As the foundation of diagnostics and prognostics, health monitoring aims to increase machinery availability and performance and reduce consequential damage and breakdown maintenance. An efficient condition monitoring scheme is capable of preventing unexpected machine failure, minimizing costly downtime, and reducing maintenance cost [1, 2]. With the development of technologies for sensing, recording, computing, and signal processing, health monitoring has been widely used in a number of diverse application areas such as tool-wear, power plants, gearboxes, rotating machines, and airplanes.

4.2 Degradation Indices

In the traditional understanding of human beings, it often seems that machines fail suddenly, but in fact machines usually go through a measureable process of degradation

Machinery Prognostics and Prognosis Oriented Maintenance Management, First Edition. Jihong Yan.

before they fail. Degradation indices are the selected indicators which can represent the evolution of degradation of the targeted system or critical components. The information obtained by the sensors is in the form of primary data or raw data, such as vibration data, temperature data, acoustic emission signals, pressure data, moisture data, weather data, or environment data. However, these data have not been effectively analyzed and it is difficult to use them in practice due to their enormous volume. The "data rich but information poor" phenomenon exists in various social sectors and fields, including marketing, business, management, education, psychology, and so on, as well as in the area of mechanical engineering, which calls for the implementation of a data mining technique in a mechanical system, or critical component condition monitoring, diagnosis, and prognosis process.

For slow-changing signals, we can obtain information on the trend of the change in the signals directly from the time domain waveform. As shown in Figure 4.1, weather temperature keeps steady from 11 pm to 4 am, and drops linearly after 3 pm.

For fast-changing signals, it is difficult to use the time domain waveform because of the tremendous size. So it is necessary to extract features related to the health state or performance of the machine or component and set up an appropriate degradation indicator based on these features. The features are usually in various domains such as the time, frequency, and wavelet domains, including root mean square (RMS) [3], kurtosis [4], crest factor, frequency features obtained from Fourier transform, wavelet or wavelet packet transform (WPT), empirical mode decomposition, independent component analysis, Hilbert transform, and so on. For a simple component/system, a single feature for a sensor can be used as the degradation index.

For instance, in Figure 4.2, 57 groups of experiments were carried out to simulate the imbalance fault of the rotor-ball bearing system, and each group of experiments has a different set of loadings. After using fast Fourier transform (FFT) on each group of data, we can see from the result that as the loading increased, the amplitude of each data set also increased, which means the FFT spectrum can be used as a degradation indicator for prediction of the rotor's remaining life prediction.

Sometimes, even for a simple system, a single feature of the signal is not sufficient for fault diagnosis and prognosis. So in this case, multiple features are needed in order to provide complementary information, this method is called feature fusion.

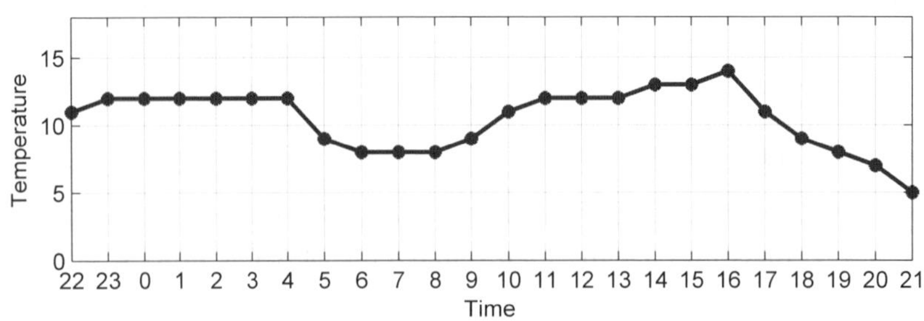

Figure 4.1 Temperature variation over 24 hours

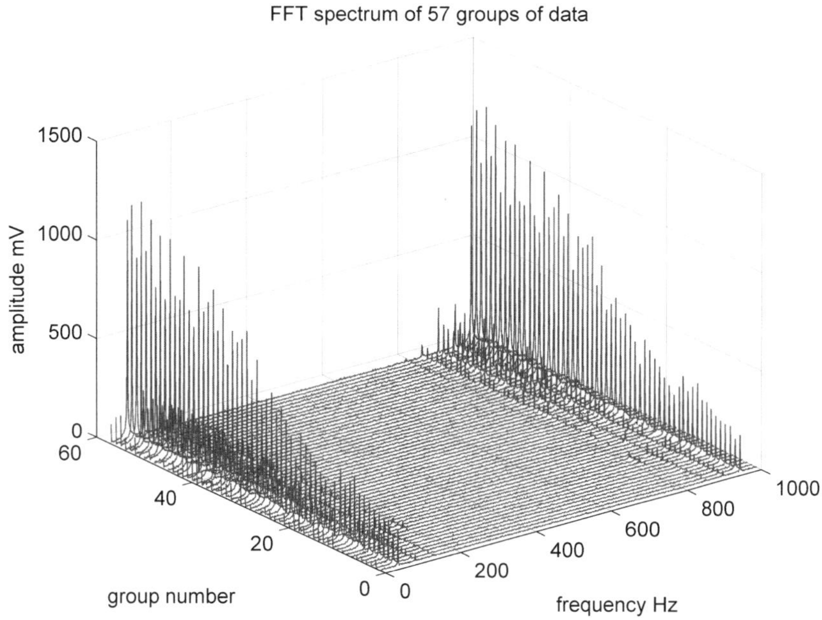

Figure 4.2 Rotor degradation signals

Combining the results obtained by more than one domain analysis method, the feature fusion technique presents a more accurate fault diagnosis and prognosis than can be achieved by any single feature analysis method.

Three stress signals of a turbine blade are shown in Figure 4.3: the maximum stress signal, the minimum stress signal, and the mean stress signal. From each single feature of the signal, we can only tell that the stress varies with time, but we cannot achieve any accurate fault diagnosis and prognosis, so we use feature fusion technology to carry out the performance evaluation, and the result is shown in Figure 4.4.

The feature fusion techniques are very popular in system monitoring for fault diagnostics and prognostics. However, the degradation indices generated by the feature fusion models lack physical meaning. How to assess the performance and get the degradation indicator in relation to the physical properties is a challenge in prognostics.

However, for a complex system, a single sensor is incapable of collecting sufficient data for accurate condition monitoring, fault diagnosis, and prognosis. So under these circumstances, multiple sensors are needed in order to provide complementary data in addition to the redundant information.

With the rapid development of computer science and advanced sensor technology, there has been an increasing trend toward using multiple sensors for condition monitoring, fault diagnosis, and prognosis. When multiple sensors are used, data collected from different sensors may contain different partial information about the same machine condition.

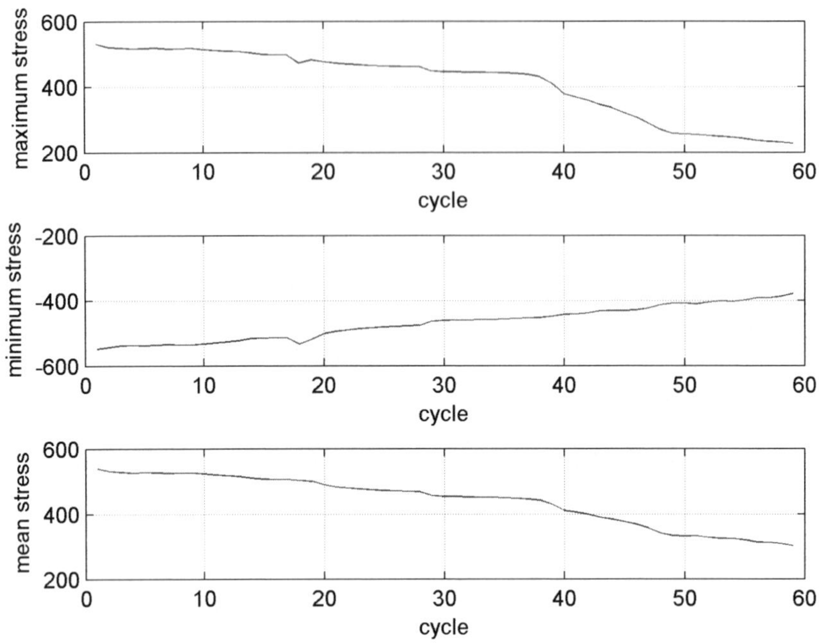

Figure 4.3 Three stress signals of turbine blades

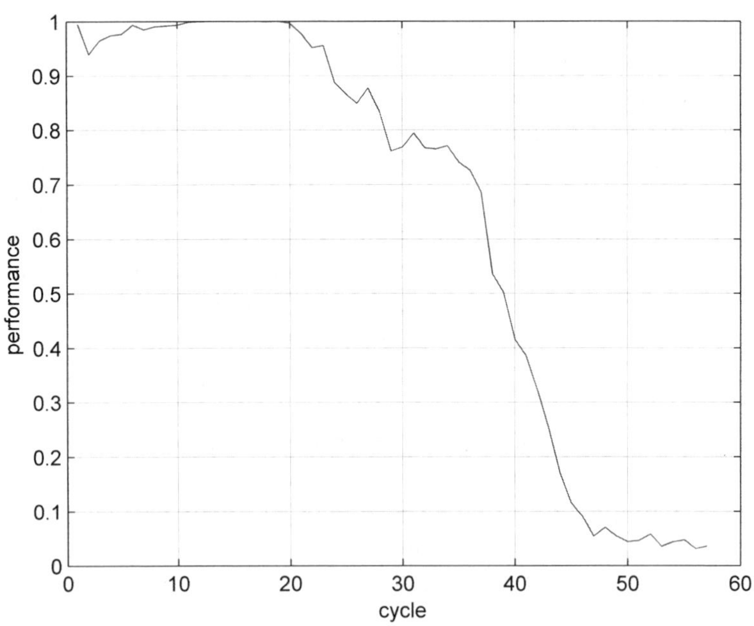

Figure 4.4 Turbine blade performance evaluation

Now the problem is how to combine all the partial information obtained from different sensors for more accurate machine diagnosis and prognosis. The solution to this problem is known as multi-sensor data fusion. Multi-sensor data fusion is an emerging technology applied to Department of Defense (DoD) areas, such as automated target recognition, battlefield surveillance, and guidance and control of autonomous vehicles, and to non-DoD applications such as monitoring of complex machinery, medical diagnosis, and smart buildings. Techniques for multi-sensor data fusion are drawn from a wide range of areas, including artificial intelligence, pattern recognition, statistical estimation, and others. There are many techniques for multi-sensor data fusion. They can be grouped into three main approaches: (i) data-level fusion, (ii) feature-level fusion, and (iii) decision-level fusion.

In Figure 4.5, there are four levels in the proposed fusion sketch which divides the data fusion into signal fusion and pixel fusion. At the signal level, the signals from each sensor are modeled as random variables to estimate the combined signal output. At the decision level, mono-source classification results are combined, based on the predefined degree of belief using some combination operators. There are broadly four types of pixel level fusion methods: statistical, fuzzy logic, Dempster–Shafer evidence theory, and neural networks. Feature level fusion is performed at an intermediate level based on the features detected. In fact, during the health monitoring process, how to fully use these features for performance assessment is an attractive topic for the worldwide research community. A good performance assessment method

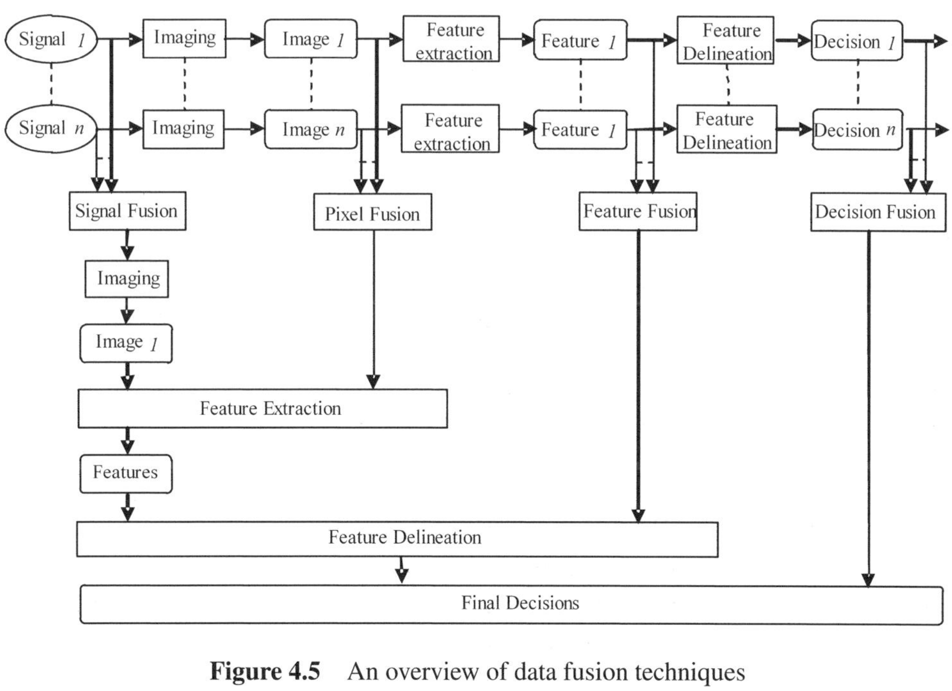

Figure 4.5 An overview of data fusion techniques

should take advantage of mutual information from multiple features for system degradation assessment [5]. The multi-sensor assessment component is realized through the feature-level, or decision-level sensor fusion, as defined by the Joint Directors of Laboratories standard of multi-sensor data fusion [6].

4.3 Real-Time Monitoring

With the rapid development of computer and advanced sensor technologies, real-time monitoring for prognostics and health management is becoming more affordable and feasible. In practice, the monitoring systems are various. For a simple system or component, for instance, a bearing monitoring system, the monitoring system could contain only several sensors (three for instance) and obtain a single feature from each sensor. While for a complex system, such as a wind turbine monitoring system, for which a few sensors are not capable of collecting sufficient data for condition monitoring and further diagnosis and prognosis, there could be a variety of sensors, such as air velocity transducers, temperature sensors, torque sensors, vibrating sensors, angle sensors, and so on. These sensors are needed in order to provide complementary data in addition to the redundant information. But, in essence, a real-time monitoring system usually consists of data acquisition (DAQ), data processing, and result displaying. DAQ will mainly focus on obtaining and collecting raw data which contains useful performance information from the critical machine or key component. In data processing the important part of the information will be extracted from the raw data collected in the previous procedure since it is difficult to use directly due to the large amount of noise, redundant information together with the useful information. Result displaying will show the analysis results on the control computer in an intelligible way so that the decision-maker can have a good understanding of the machine or component's operating condition.

4.3.1 Data Acquisition

DAQ is the process of measuring an electrical or physical phenomenon, such as voltage, current, temperature, pressure, or sound with a computer. As shown in Figure 4.6, the hardware of DAQ systems typically includes sensors, a signal conditioning device, an analog-to-digital (A/D) converter, a data transmission device, and a data recording circuit. The main techniques involved in the monitoring systems are introduced here.

4.3.1.1 Sensors

The measurement of a physical phenomenon, such as the temperature of a room, the intensity of a light source, or the force applied to an object, begins with a sensor.

A sensor, also called a transducer, is a converter that measures a physical quantity and converts it into a measurable electrical signal which can be read by an observer

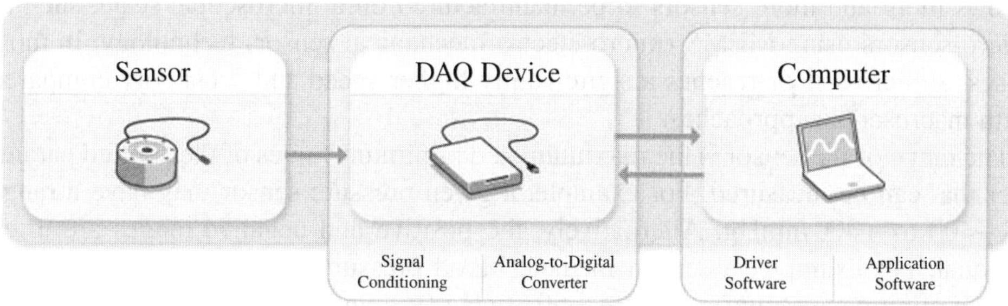

Figure 4.6 Data acquisition hardware system

or by a (mostly electronic) instrument. Depending on the type of sensor, its electrical output can be a voltage, current, resistance, or another electrical attribute that varies over time. Some sensors may require additional components and circuitry to produce properly a signal that can accurately and safely be read by a DAQ device.

For instance, a thermocouple converts temperature to an output voltage which can be read by a voltmeter. Depending on the types of the measurements, many different sensors have been created, such as vibration sensors, acoustic sensors, chemical sensors, current sensors, magnetic sensors, fluid velocity sensors, position sensors, optical sensors, force sensors, thermal sensors, and so on. For accuracy, most sensors are calibrated against known standards. Common sensors are listed in Table 4.1.

A sensor's sensitivity indicates how much the sensor's output changes when the measured quantity changes. For instance, if the mercury in a thermometer moves 1 cm when the temperature changes by 1 °C, the sensitivity is 1 cm/°C (it is basically the slope $\Delta y/\Delta x$ assuming a linear characteristic). Sensors that measure very small changes must have very high sensitivities. Sensors also have an impact on what they measure; for instance, a room temperature thermometer inserted into a hot cup of liquid cools the liquid while the liquid heats the thermometer. Sensors need to be designed to have a small effect on what is measured; making the sensor smaller often improves this and may introduce other advantages. Technological progress

Table 4.1 Common sensors

Sensor	Phenomenon
Thermocouple, RTD, thermistor	Temperature
Photo sensor	Light
Microphone	Sound
Strain gage, piezoelectric transducer	Force and pressure
Potentiometer, LVDT, optical encoder	Position and displacement
Accelerometer	Acceleration
pH electrode	pH

allows more and more sensors to be manufactured on a microscopic scale, such as micro-sensors using MEMS (micro-electro-mechanical sensor) technology. In most cases, a micro-sensor reaches a significantly higher speed and sensitivity compared with macroscopic approaches.

The range of the sensor is the maximum and minimum values of the applied parameter that can be measured. For example, a given pressure sensor may have a range of −400 to +400 mmHg. Alternatively, the positive and negative ranges are often unequal. For example, a certain medical blood pressure transducer is specified to have a minimum (vacuum) limit of −50 mmHg (y_{min} in Figure 4.7) and a maximum (pressure) limit of +450 mmHg (y_{max} in Figure 4.7). This specification is common, incidentally, and is one reason why doctors and nurses sometimes destroy blood pressure sensors when attempting to draw blood through an arterial line without being mindful of the position of the fluid stopcocks in the system. A small syringe can exert a tremendous vacuum on a closed system.

A sensor is also a device which responds to an input quantity by generating a functionally related output, usually in the form of an electrical or optical signal. A good sensor should be sensitive to the measured property only, insensitive to any other

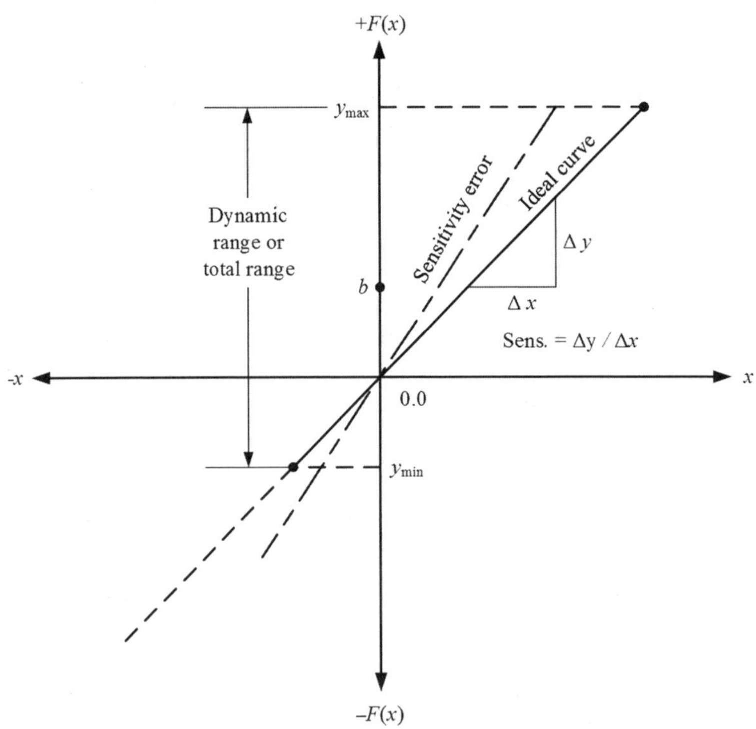

Figure 4.7 Ideal curve and sensitivity error

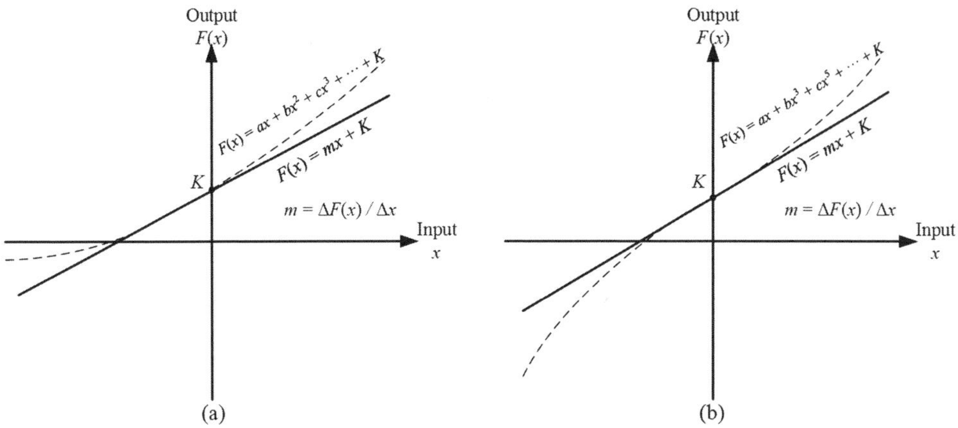

Figure 4.8 Output versus input signal curves showing (a) quadratic error and (b) cubic error

property likely to be encountered in its application, and should not influence the measured property. As shown in Figure 4.8, there may be two kinds of error: a quadratic error and a cubic error. Ideal sensors are designed to be linear or linear to some simple mathematical function of the measurement, typically logarithmic. The output of such a sensor is an analog signal and is linearly proportional to the value or simple function of the measured property. The sensitivity is then defined as the ratio between the output signal and the measured property. For example, if a sensor measures temperature and has a voltage output, the sensitivity is a constant with the unit (V/K); this sensor is linear because the ratio is constant at all points of measurement. For an analog sensor signal to be processed, or used in digital equipment, it needs to be converted to a digital signal, using an analog-to-digital converter (ADC).

4.3.1.2 Signal Conditioning Device

As listed in Table 4.2, many applications require environment or structural measurements, such as temperature and vibration, from sensors. These sensors, in turn, require signal conditioning before a DAQ device can effectively and accurately measure the signal. Key signal conditioning technologies provide distinct enhancements to both the performance and accuracy of DAQ systems.

1. *Amplification*

   Amplifiers increase the voltage level to better match the ADC range, thus increasing the measurement resolution and sensitivity. In addition, using external signal conditioners located closer to the signal source, or transducer, improves the measurement signal-to-noise ratio by magnifying the voltage level before it is affected by environmental noise.

Table 4.2 Signal conditioning is recommended for sensor measurements

	Amplification	Attenuation	Isolation	Filtering
Thermocouple	√		√	√
Thermistor	√		√	√
RTD	√		√	√
Strain gage	√		√	√
Load, pressure, torque (mV/V)	√		√	√
Load, pressure, torque (±5 V, ±10 V, 4–20 mA)	√		√	√
Accelerometer	√		√	√
Microphone	√		√	√
Proximity probe	√		√	√
LVDT/RVDT	√		√	√
High voltage		√	√	

	Excitation	Linearization	CJC	Bridge completion
Thermocouple		√	√	
Thermistor	√	√		
RTD	√	√		
Strain gage	√	√		√
Load, pressure, torque (mV/V)	√	√		
Load, pressure, torque (±5 V, ±10 V, 4–20 mA)	√	√		
Accelerometer	√	√		
Microphone	√	√		
Proximity probe	√	√		
LVDT/RVDT	√	√		
High voltage				

2. *Attenuation*

   Attenuation, the opposite of amplification, is necessary when voltages to be digitized are beyond the ADC range. This form of signal conditioning decreases the input signal amplitude so that the conditioned signal is within the ADC range. Attenuation is typically necessary when measuring voltages that are more than 10 V.

3. *Isolation*

   Isolated signal conditioning devices pass the signal from its source to the measurement device without a physical connection, by using transformer, optical, or capacitive coupling techniques. In addition to breaking ground loops, isolation blocks high-voltage surges and rejects high common-mode voltage, thus protecting both the operators and the expensive measuring equipment.

4. *Filtering*

   Filters reject unwanted noise within a certain frequency range. Often, lowpass filters are used to block out high-frequency noise in electrical measurements, such as 60 Hz power. Another common use for filtering is to prevent aliasing from high-frequency signals. This can be done by using an anti-aliasing filter to attenuate signals above the Nyquist frequency.
5. *Excitation*

   Excitation is required for many types of transducers. For example, strain gages, accelerometers, thermistors, and resistance temperature detectors (RTDs) require external voltage or current excitation. RTD and thermistor measurements are usually made with a current source that converts the variation in resistance to a measurable voltage. Accelerometers often have an integrated amplifier, which requires a current excitation provided by the measurement device. Strain gages, which are very-low-resistance devices, are used typically in a Wheatstone bridge configuration with a voltage excitation source.
6. *Linearization*

   Linearization is necessary when sensors produce voltage signals that are not linearly related to the physical measurement. Linearization is the process of interpreting the signal from the sensor and can be done either with signal conditioning or through software. Thermocouples are the classic example of a sensor that requires linearization.
7. *Cold-junction compensation*

   Cold-junction compensation (CJC) is a technology required for accurate thermocouple measurements. Thermocouples measure temperature as the difference in voltage between two dissimilar metals. Based on this concept, another voltage is generated at the connection between the thermocouple and the terminal of your DAQ device. CJC improves the measurement accuracy by providing the temperature at this junction and applying the appropriate correction.
8. *Bridge completion*

   Bridge completion is required for quarter- and half-bridge sensors to comprise a four resistor Wheatstone bridge. Strain gage signal conditioners typically provide half-bridge completion networks consisting of high-precision reference resistors. The completion resistors provide a fixed reference for detecting small voltage changes across the active resistor(s).

4.3.1.3 Analog-to-Digital Converter

Analog signals from sensors must be converted into digital before they are manipulated by digital equipment such as a computer. An analog-to-digital converter (abbreviated ADC, A/D, or A to D) is a device that converts a continuous physical quantity (usually voltage) to a digital number that represents the quantity's amplitude.

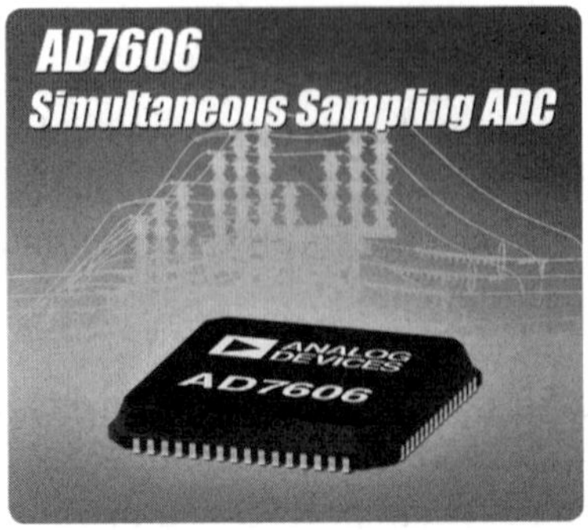

Figure 4.9 A/D converter

The conversion involves quantization of the input, it unavoidably generates a small amount of error. Instead of doing a single conversion, an ADC often performs the conversions ("samples" the input) periodically. The result is a sequence of digital values that have converted a continuous-time and continuous-amplitude analog signal to a discrete-time and discrete-amplitude digital signal.

An ADC (shown in Figure 4.9) is defined by its bandwidth (the range of frequencies it can measure) and its signal to noise ratio (how accurately it can measure a signal relative to the noise it introduces). The actual bandwidth of an ADC is characterized primarily by its sampling rate, and to a lesser extent by how it handles errors such as aliasing. The dynamic range of an ADC is influenced by many factors, including the resolution (the number of output levels it can quantize a signal to), linearity and accuracy (how well the quantization levels match the true analog signal) and jitter (small timing errors that introduce additional noise). The dynamic range of an ADC is often summarized in terms of its effective number of bits (ENOB), the number of bits of each measure it returns that are on average not noise. An ideal ADC has an ENOB equal to its resolution. ADCs are chosen to match the bandwidth and required signal to noise ratio of the signal to be quantized. If an ADC operates at a sampling rate greater than twice the bandwidth of the signal, then perfect reconstruction is possible given an ideal ADC and neglecting quantization error. The presence of quantization error limits the dynamic range of even an ideal ADC, however, if the dynamic range of the ADC exceeds that of the input signal, its effects may be neglected, resulting in an essentially perfect digital representation of the input signal.

An ADC may also provide an isolated measurement, such as an electronic device that converts an input analog voltage or current to a digital number proportional to the magnitude of the voltage or current. However, some non-electronic or only partially electronic devices, such as rotary encoders, can also be considered ADCs. The digital output may use different coding schemes. Typically, the digital output will be a two's complement binary number that is proportional to the input, but there are other possibilities. An encoder, for example, might output a Gray code. The inverse operation is performed by a digital-to-analog converter (DAC).

An ADC has several sources of errors. Quantization error and (assuming the ADC is intended to be linear) non-linearity are intrinsic to any analog-to-digital conversion. These errors are measured in a unit called the least significant bit (LSB). In the above example of an eight-bit ADC, an error of one LSB is 1/256 of the full signal range, or about 0.4%.

4.3.1.4 Data Transmission Device

Data transmission is the physical transfer of data (a digital bit stream) over a point-to-point or point-to-multipoint communication channel. Examples of such channels are copper wires, optical fibers, wireless communication channels, and storage media. The data are represented as an electromagnetic signal, such as an electrical voltage, radio wave, microwave, or infrared signal.

While analog transmission is the transfer of a continuously varying analog signal, digital communication is the transfer of discrete messages. The messages are either represented by a sequence of pulses by means of a line code (baseband transmission), or by a limited set of continuously varying wave forms (passband transmission), using a digital modulation method. The passband modulation and corresponding demodulation (also known as detection) is carried out by modem equipment. According to the most common definition of a digital signal, both baseband and passband signals representing bit-streams are considered as digital transmission, while an alternative definition only considers the baseband signal as digital, and passband transmission of digital data as a form of digital-to-analog conversion.

In real-time monitoring systems, the control computers are far from the targeted assets. The digital signals including the health state inside need to transmit from the on-site plant to the control computer. Usually, there are two ways to implement the data transmission: via the internet or wirelessly. Nowadays, the internet has been well constructed and is widely used in daily life and industry. It is very convenient to transmit data by the internet, especially when optical fibers are used so that the transmitting speed is much improved compared to using copper wires. However, in some places where the internet is not available or difficult to be constructed, wireless communication is a better choice. Wireless technologies have been under rapid development during recent years. The types of wireless technologies being developed range from simple IrDA that uses infrared light for short-range, point-to-point communications, to the wireless personal area network (WPAN) for short range, point-to multi-point communications, such as Bluetooth and ZigBee, to the mid-range, multi-hop wireless local area network (WLAN), to long-distance cellular phone systems, such as GSM/GPRS and CDMA. Figure 4.10 shows various kinds of modules and equipment for us to choose.

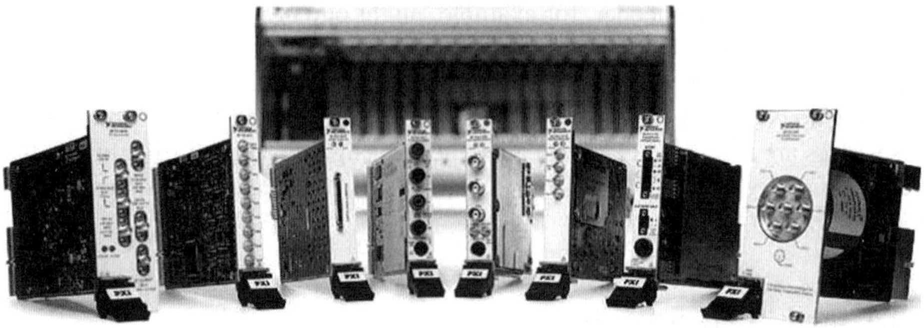

Figure 4.10 PXI DAQ equipment

4.3.1.5 Nyquist–Shannon Sampling Theorem

In the field of digital signal processing, the sampling theorem is a fundamental bridge between continuous signals (analog domain) and discrete signals (digital domain). Strictly speaking, it only applies to a class of mathematical functions whose Fourier transforms are zero outside of a finite region of frequencies. The analytical extension to actual signals, which can only approximate that condition, is provided by the discrete-time Fourier transform, a version of the Poisson summation formula.

Intuitively, we expect that when one reduces a continuous function to a discrete sequence (called samples) and interpolates back to a continuous function, the fidelity of the result depends on the density (or sample-rate) of the original samples. The sampling theorem introduces the concept of a sample-rate that is sufficient for perfect fidelity for the class of band-limited functions. It expresses the sample-rate in terms of the function's bandwidth. The theorem also leads to a formula for the mathematically ideal interpolation algorithm.

An important issue in sampling is the determination of the sampling frequency. We want to minimize the sampling frequency to reduce the data size, thereby lowering the computational complexity in data processing and the costs for data storage and transmission. However, we also want to avoid losing information contained in the signal, which may happen when the sampling frequency is too low. The Nyquist–Shannon theorem states:

If a function $x(t)$ contains no frequencies higher than B hertz, it is completely determined by giving its ordinates at a series of points spaced $1/(2B)$ seconds apart.

A sufficient sample-rate is therefore $2B$ samples/second, or anything larger. Conversely, for a given sample-rate, f_s, the band limit for perfect reconstruction is $B \leq f_s/2$. When the band limit is too high (or there is no band limit), the reconstruction exhibits imperfections known as aliasing. Modern statements of the theorem are sometimes careful to state explicitly that $x(t)$ must contain no sinusoidal component at exactly frequency B, or that B must be strictly less than 1/2 the sample rate. The two thresholds, $2B$ and $f_s/2$ are called the Nyquist rate and the Nyquist frequency, respectively. They are attributes of $x(t)$ and of the sampling equipment, respectively. The condition

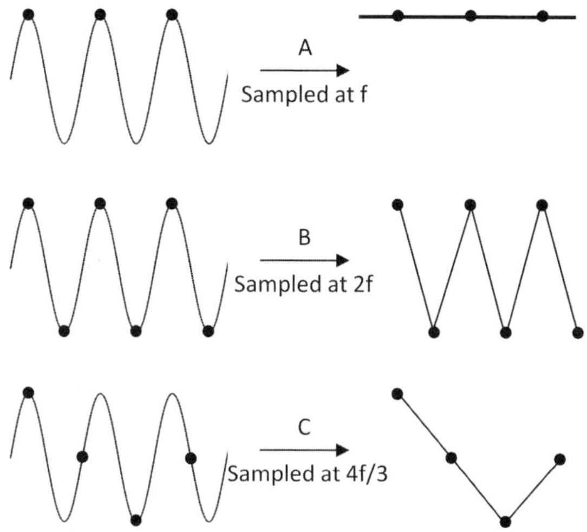

Figure 4.11 Effects of various sampling rates while sampling a signal

described by these inequalities is called the Nyquist criterion, or sometimes the *Raabe condition*. The theorem is also applicable to functions of other domains, such as space, in the case of a digitized image. The only change, in the case of other domains, is the units of measure applied to t, f_s, and B. It is shown in Figure 4.11 that, if we choose different sampling rates while sampling a signal, the results we get will be different.

In practice, however, it is often the case that the signal to be sampled contains frequency components higher than the Nyquist frequency. In such cases, one can still avoid aliasing by anti-aliasing low-pass filtering to remove all frequencies higher than the Nyquist frequency before sampling.

4.3.2 Data Processing Techniques

DAQ collects the original information from the monitored objects such as machines, structures. However, the amount of the original data is large, including noise, unimportant information, and important information. It is difficult to perform fault diagnostics and prognostics by directly utilizing the original signals since the useful information is hidden in them. Various signal processing methods have been developed for noise reduction, redundant information elimination, and to extract important information from the collected monitored monitoring data. Here we just give a brief introduction. Detailed description of the methods can be found in Chapter 2.

4.3.2.1 Time-Domain Analysis

This is the analysis of mathematical functions and physical signals with respect to time. As shown in Figure 4.12, a time-domain graph shows how a signal changes

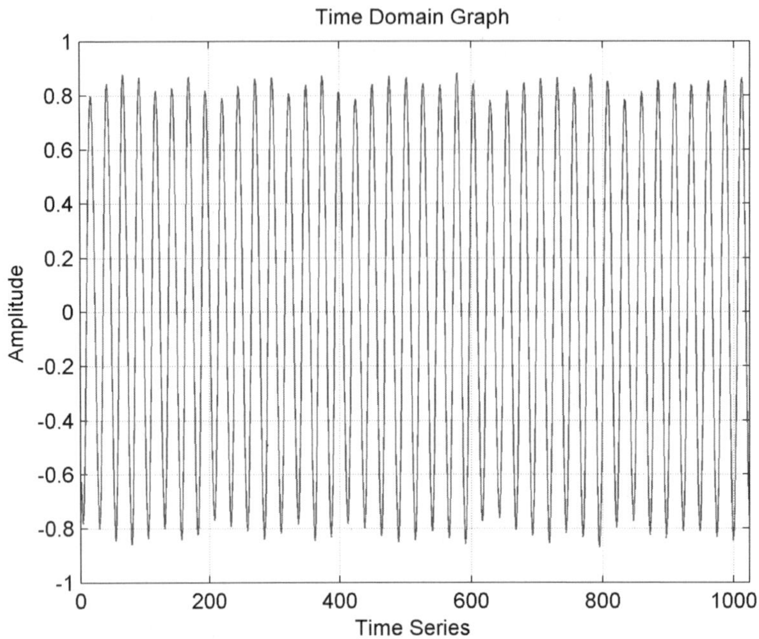

Figure 4.12 Time-domain waveform

with time. In the time domain, the signal or function's value is known for all real numbers, for the case of continuous time, or at various separate instants in the case of discrete time.

Statistical methods are used in time-domain analysis, which is directly based on the time waveform itself. Traditional time-domain analysis calculates characteristic features from time waveform signals as descriptive statistics.

One common application of statistical algorithms for the purposes of CM is to analyze the data signals from the various sensors in wavelet transforms (WTs). Common statistical measures such as RMS and peak amplitude are widely used for the diagnosis of failures. Other important statistical parameters are the maximum value, minimum value, means, peak to peak, interval, standard deviation, shape factor, crest factor, impulse factor, definite integral, energy ratio, skewness, kurtosis, and so on. These fault features are studied in the time domain.

4.3.2.2 Frequency-Domain Analysis

Frequency-domain analysis transforms the signal from the time domain to the frequency domain in order to study the fault information in the frequency domain. A particular frequency appears when there is a certain fault. The advantage of frequency-domain analysis over time-domain analysis is its ability to identify and isolate certain frequency components of interest.

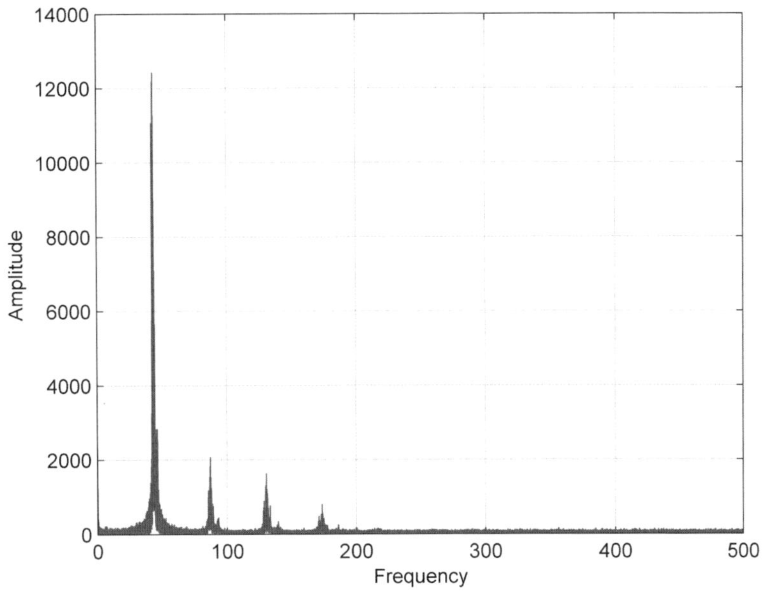

Figure 4.13 Fast Fourier transform

1. *FFT*
   FFT is one of the most widely used frequency spectrum analysis methods. The main idea is either to look at the whole spectrum or to look closely at certain frequency components of interest and thus extract features from the signal. An example of FFT is shown in Figure 4.13.
2. *Power spectrum*
   The most commonly used tool in spectrum analysis is the power spectrum. It is defined as $E[X(f)X^*(f)]$, where $X(f)$ is the Fourier transform of signal $x(t)$, E denotes expectation and * denotes the complex conjugate. Some useful auxiliary tools for spectrum analysis are graphical presentation of the spectrum, frequency filters, envelope analysis (also called amplitude demodulation), side band structure analysis, and so on. The Hilbert transform, which is a useful tool in envelope analysis, has also been used for machine condition monitoring, prognosis, fault detection, and diagnostics. An example of a power spectrum is shown in Figure 4.14.

4.3.2.3 Time–Frequency-Domain Analysis

The drawback of the frequency-domain analysis is it is not suitable for non-stationary signals, which are very common when machinery degradation or faults occur. Thus, time–frequency analysis, which investigates waveform signals in both the time and frequency domains, has been developed for non-stationary waveform signals.

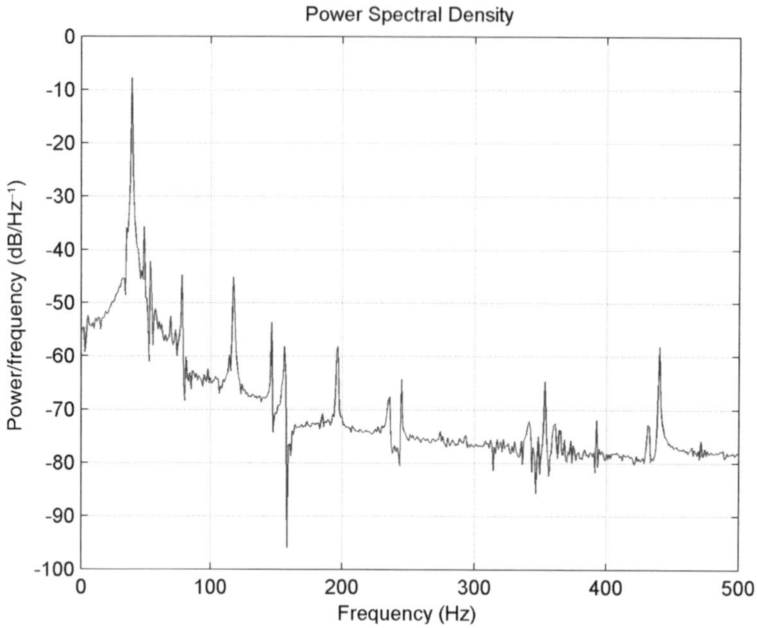

Figure 4.14 Power spectrum waveform

Traditional time–frequency analysis uses time–frequency distributions, which represent the energy or power of waveform signals in two-dimensional functions of both time and frequency to better reveal fault patterns for more accurate diagnostics.

1. *Short-Fourier transform*

   The short-time Fourier transform (STFT), or alternatively short-term Fourier transform, is a Fourier-related transform used to determine the sinusoidal frequency and phase content of local sections of a signal as it changes over time.

   The idea of STFT is to divide the whole waveform signal into segments with a short-time window and then apply a Fourier transform to each segment. The spectrogram has some limitation in time–frequency resolution due to signal segmentation. It can only be applied to non-stationary signals with slow change in their dynamics. An example of STFT is shown in Figure 4.15.
2. *Wavelet transform*

   Wavelet analysis is becoming a common tool for analyzing localized variations of power within a time series. By decomposing a time series into time–frequency space, one is able to determine both the dominant modes of variability and how those modes vary in time. The waveform is zooming and panning to match the input signal. In the last decade, WT has been widely applied in diverse fields of random signal processing. The transformation of a signal to another form using WT does not change the information content in the original signal. WT uses a multi-resolution technique where different frequencies are analyzed with different

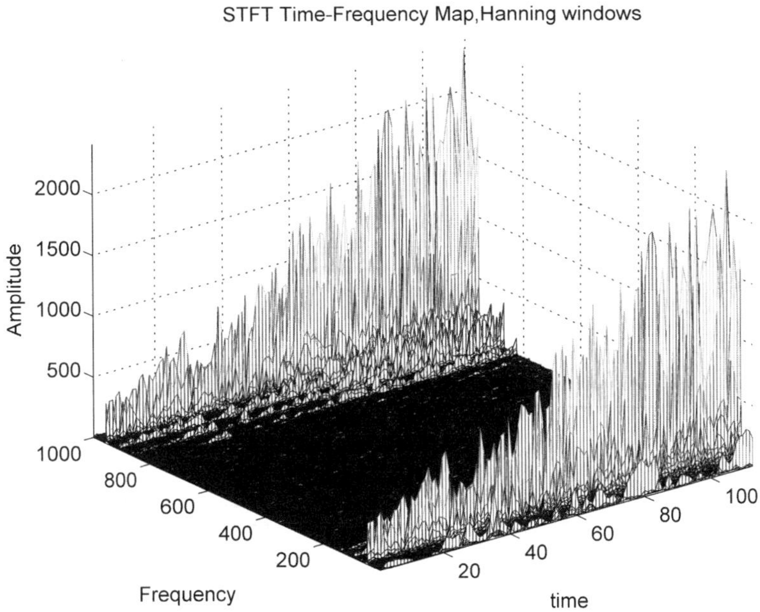

Figure 4.15 Short Fourier transform

resolutions in order to generate a time-frequency representation of the signal. Discrete wavelet transform (DWT) and WPT were derived from the WT family. Although DWT and WPT all decompose a signal into several bands representing low and high frequencies, they differ in the number of resultant bands. The details about DWT and WPT are introduced in the following sections.

One main advantage of WT is its ability to produce a high frequency resolution at low frequencies and a high time resolution at high frequencies for signals with long duration low frequencies and short duration high frequencies. Another advantage of WT is its ability to reduce noise in raw signals. Due to these advantages, WT has been successfully applied to waveform data analysis in condition monitoring, prognosis and fault diagnostics of gears, bearings, and other mechanical systems. An example of WT is shown in Figure 4.16.

3. *Discrete wavelet transform*

   In numerical analysis and functional analysis, a DWT is any WT for which the wavelets are discretely sampled. As with other WTs, a key advantage it has over Fourier transforms is temporal resolution: it captures both frequency and location information (location in time). DWT has been proven very efficient in signal analysis for many engineering applications.

4. *Wavelet package transform*

   Originally known as optimal sub-band tree structuring (SB-TS) also called wavelet packet decomposition (WPD) (sometimes known as just wavelet packets or sub-band tree) is a WT where the discrete-time (sampled) signal is passed through more filters than the DWT. An example of WPT is shown in Figure 4.17.

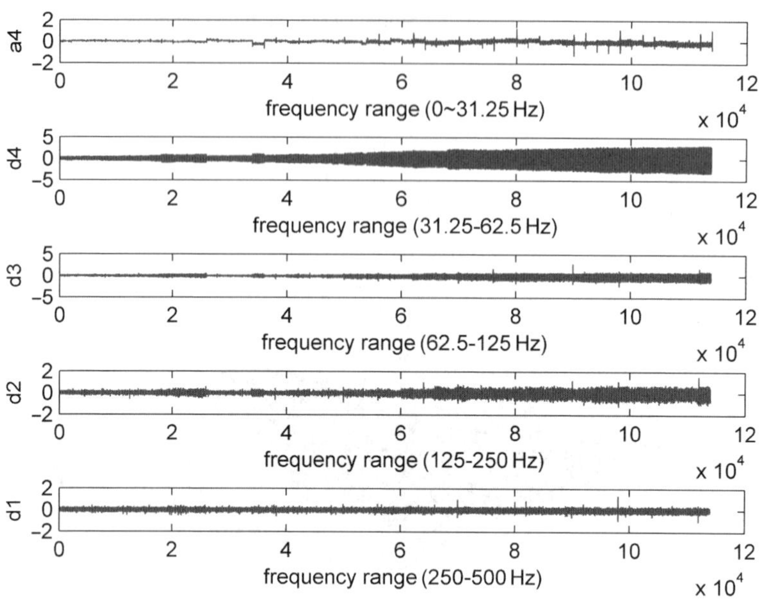

Figure 4.16 Wavelet transform

4.3.3 Example

The real-time monitoring system is widely applied in many fields, including bearings [7, 8], gear boxes [9, 10], wind turbines [11, 12], bridges and roads [13, 14], tool wear [9, 15, 16], aero-engines [17], and nuclear power plants [18, 19].

A monitoring system is developed to collect the critical data for an unbalanced rotor about the displacement and acceleration at a certain position. The structure of the rotor experiment platform is shown in Figure 4.18, and a schematic of the monitoring system can be seen in Figure 4.19.

The system is composed of front-end sensors, an amplifier filter circuit, an ADC circuit, a central processing unit (CPU), and a data center. When the rotor is running steadily, the sensing analog signals after amplification and noise reduction will be converted by the ADC into digital signals. These digital data will be distinguished by the CPU, and then the displacement and acceleration of the rotor is obtained and stored in the data center for further analysis.

1. *Sensors*

   In this system we will collect both acceleration and displacement data, so two different kinds of sensors are needed: an acceleration sensor and a displacement sensor.

   As shown in Figure 4.20, a PCB acceleration sensor can conduct acceleration monitoring with high sensitivity and fast response, because of the advantage of good installable performance, little influence on the structural properties, and the

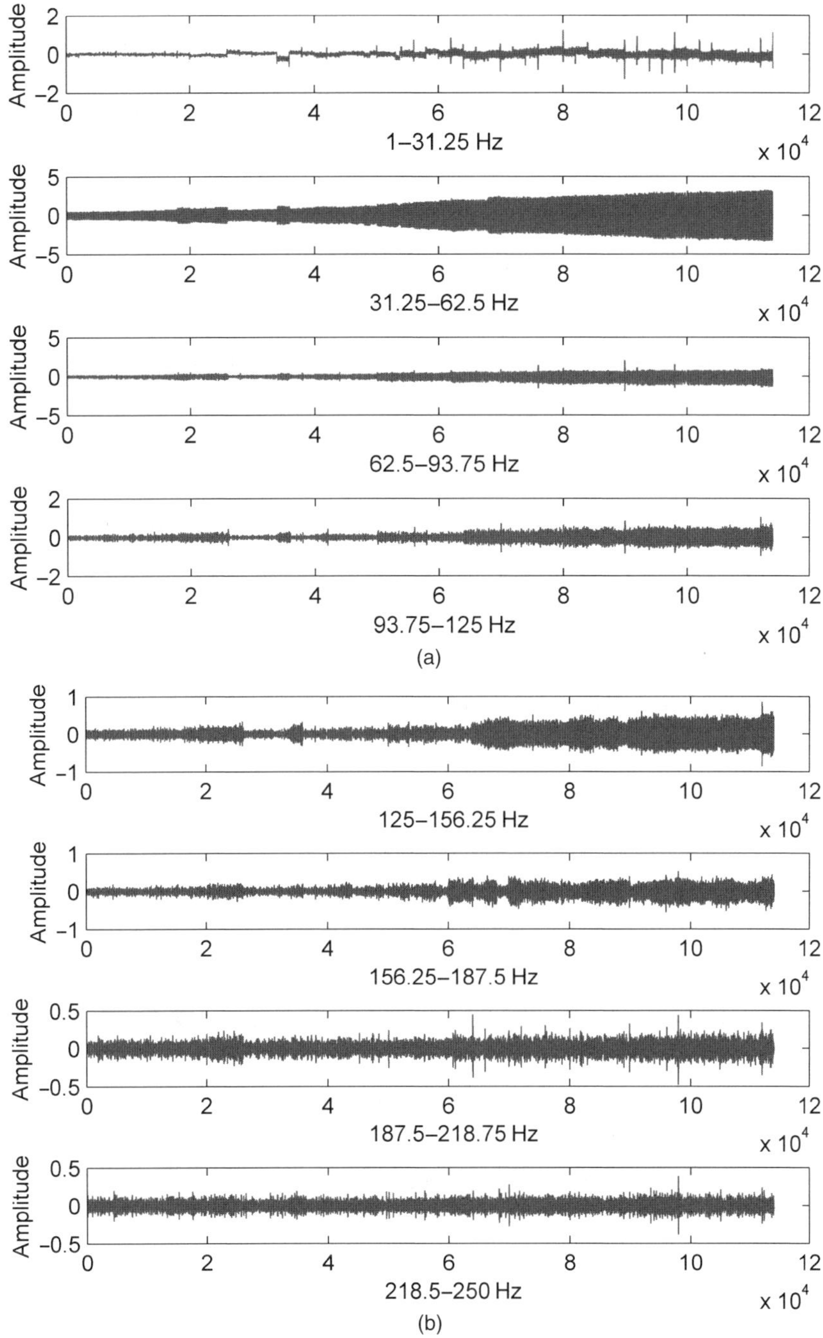

Figure 4.17 (a–d) Wavelet package transform

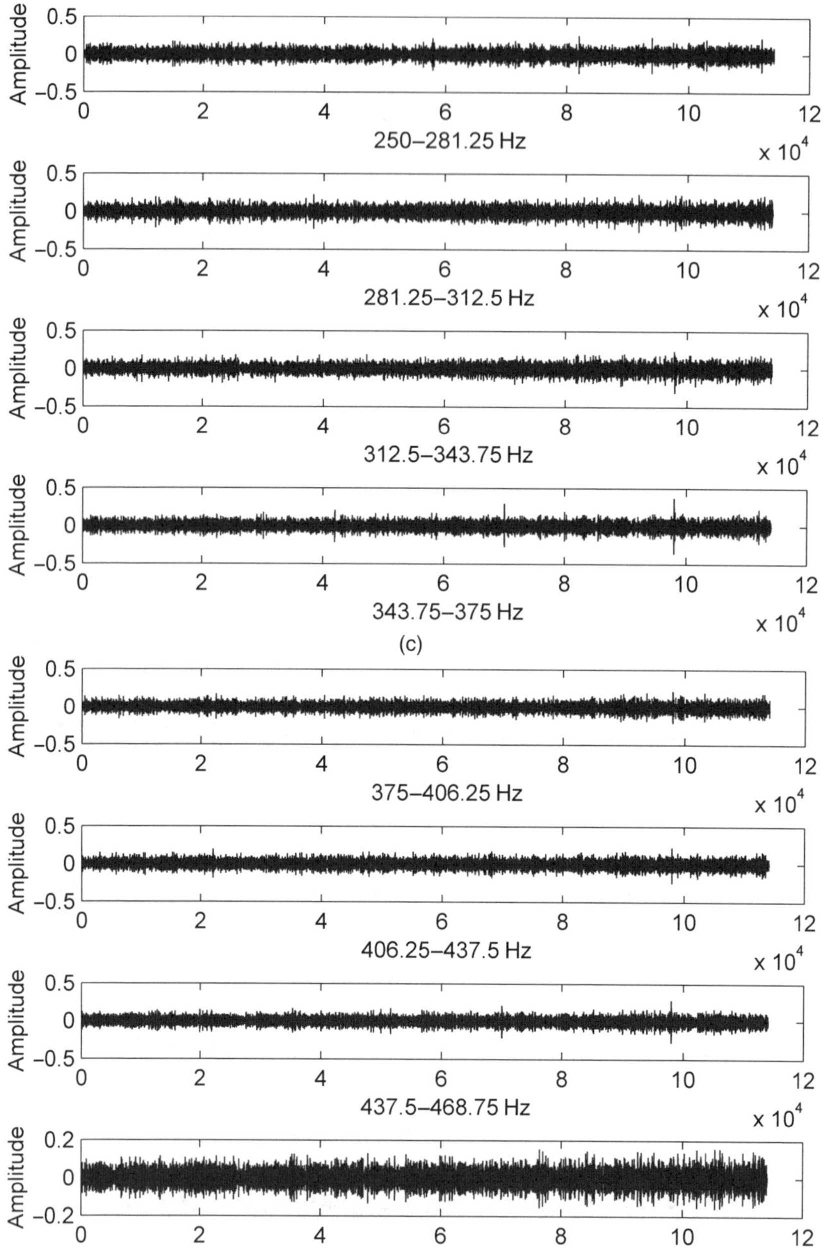

(d)

Figure 4.17 (*continued*)

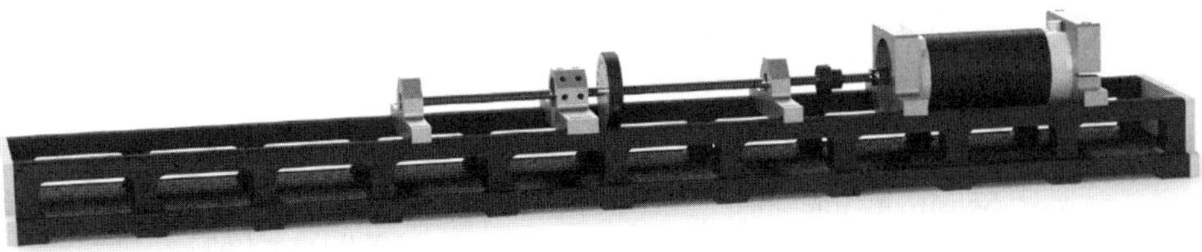

Figure 4.18 Rotor experiment platform

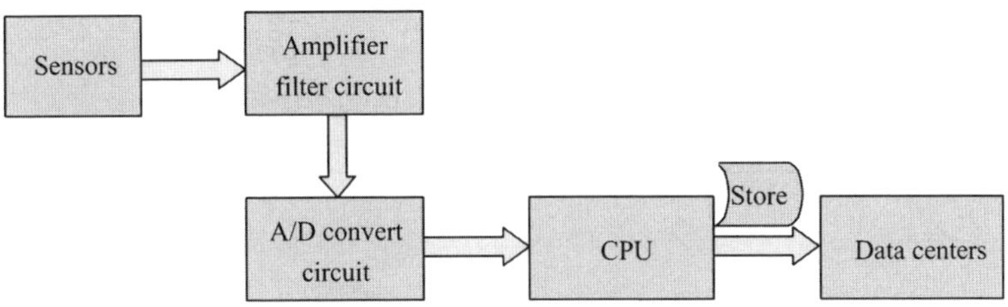

Figure 4.19 Structure schematic of the monitoring system

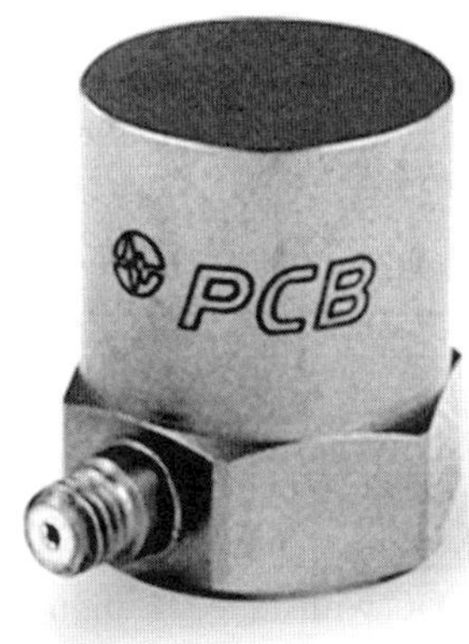

Figure 4.20 Acceleration sensor

anti-interference ability, PCB is very suitable for acceleration data collection in the system. The main parameters of the PCB acceleration sensors are listed in Table 4.3.

For this rotor monitoring system, to collect the displacement of the rotor, a displacement sensor is needed. To minimize the influence to the system, we need a non-contact sensor, in this case, an eddy current displacement sensor is very suitable. An eddy current displacement sensor is shown in Figure 4.21, and the main parameters of the PCB acceleration sensors are listed in Table 4.4.

Table 4.3 Main parameters of acceleration sensor

Performance	SI
Sensitivity	102 mV m^{-1} s^2
Sensitivity tolerance	±5%
Measurement range	±9800 m s^{-2} pk
Frequency range (±5%)	1–10 kHz
Resonant frequency	±70 kHz
Broadband resolution (1–10 kHz)	0.01 g rms
Non-linearity	≤1%
Transverse sensitivity	≤5%
Overload limit	±10 kg pk
Excitation voltage	18–30 VDC

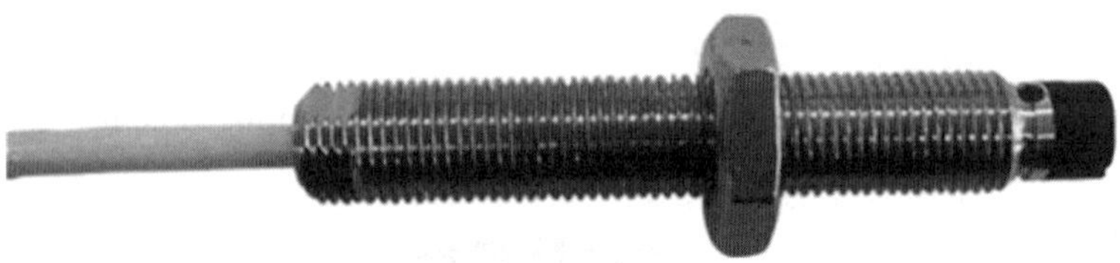

Figure 4.21 Eddy current displacement sensor

Table 4.4 Main parameters of displacement sensor

Performance	SI
Measurement range	0–4.45 mm
Input voltage	Regulated 12–24 V DC
Analog output voltage	0–22 V DC with 24 V DC input 0–10 V DC with 12 V DC input
Current (full load)	4.2 mA maximum
Impedance	50 Ω
Frequency response	0–10 kHz (±3 db)
Load current	100 mA maximum AC or DC
Load voltage	30 V rms, 42.4 V peak, or 60 V DC
On resistance	30 Ω minimum/50 Ω maximum
Frequency response	3.3 kHz
Resolution	<0.008% of measuring range using a 5CM sensor on a 4130 steel target at midscale, mid gain, and 12 V DC input

2. *DAQ device*

The recordings of all the data coming from accelerometers and displacement sensors are realized by a National Instruments NI-4472 and NI PXI-1042Q DAQ device, which are shown in Figures 4.22 and 4.23.

The National Instruments PXI-4472 is an eight-channel dynamic signal acquisition device for making high-accuracy audio-frequency measurements. It has

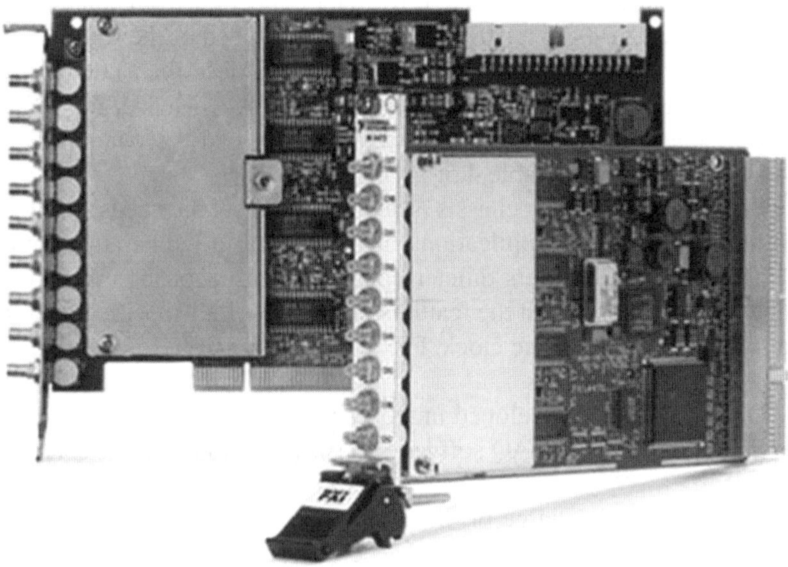

Figure 4.22 NI PXI-4472 dynamic signal acquisition device

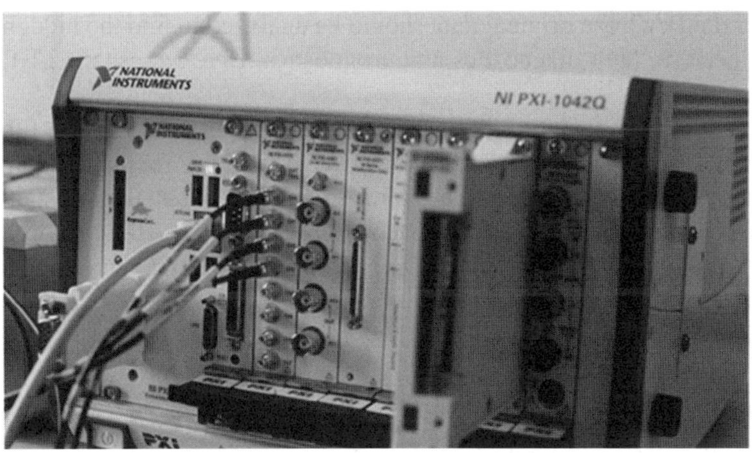

Figure 4.23 NI PXI-1042Q quiet eight-slot chassis

Table 4.5 Main parameters of NI PXI-4472

Bus	Analog inputs	Resolution	Sampling rate	Input range	Triggering	AC cutoff frequency
PCI, PXI	8	24 bits	102.4 kS s^{-1}	±10 V	Analog and digital	3.4 Hz

eight analog inputs, which is enough for data collection from four sensors. The sampling rate of PXI-4472 is 102.4 kS s^{-1}, the top speed of the rotor is no greater than 10 000 rpm, so the frequency of the signal is less than 200 Hz (from the Nyquist–Shannon sampling theorem discussed above). Hence, the PXI-4472 is absolutely capable of collecting enough data for the analysis. Main parameters of NI PXI-4472 are listed in Table 4.5.

The PXI-1042Q eight slot chassis is designed to meet the needs of a wide range of test and measurement applications, it operates in a temperature range up to 55 °C. The PXI-1042Q offers quieter operation, with acoustic emissions as low as 43 dBA. It incorporates all the features of the latest PXI specification, including the built-in 10 MHz reference clock, PXI trigger bus, star trigger, and local bus.

3. *Software*

The DAQ software is developed in the LabVIEW programing environment. As shown in Figure 4.24, the DAQ software consists of two parts: the server part and the client part.

The server part is in charge of the data collecting, the display panel can show four channels of data, two channels of acceleration data and two channels of displacement data. The four channels of data are transported to the client part as soon as collected, when the record button is pressed, the data will be stored. The experimental set-up of the whole system is shown in Figure 4.25.

4. *Signal processing*

After the DAQ, the original data should be analyzed to find the hidden information to perform fault diagnostics and prognostics. Here we use the FFT to do the analysis.

We can see from Figure 4.26, there are prominent peaks at the fundamental frequency of each group of data, and no peaks at other frequency domains, this indicates that the main fault of the rotor is imbalance. When the imbalance magnitude is increased, the amplitudes of each group of data are getting larger and larger, this result shows that the signal energy is proportional to the increasing imbalance magnitude.

4.4 Failure Prognosis

The composition and structure of machinery equipment are getting more and more complicated with higher and higher performance standards, which increases the

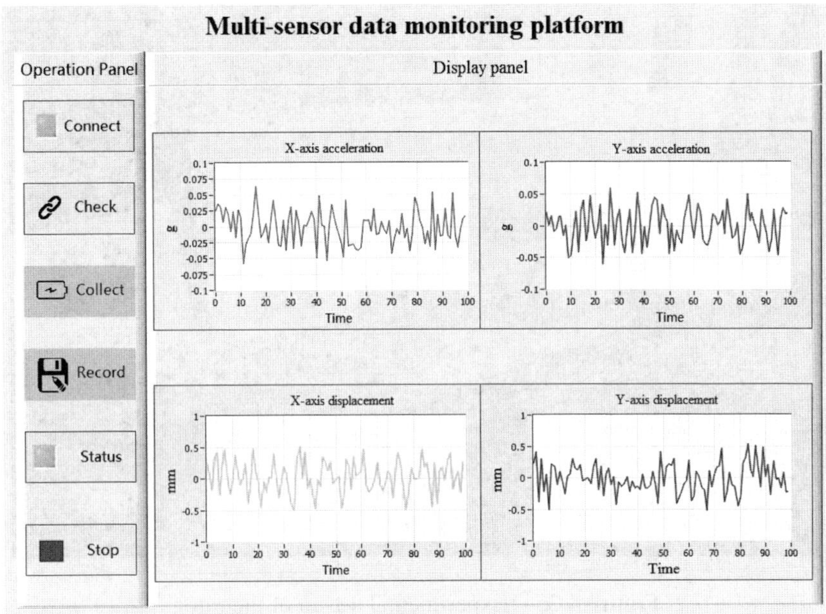

(a)

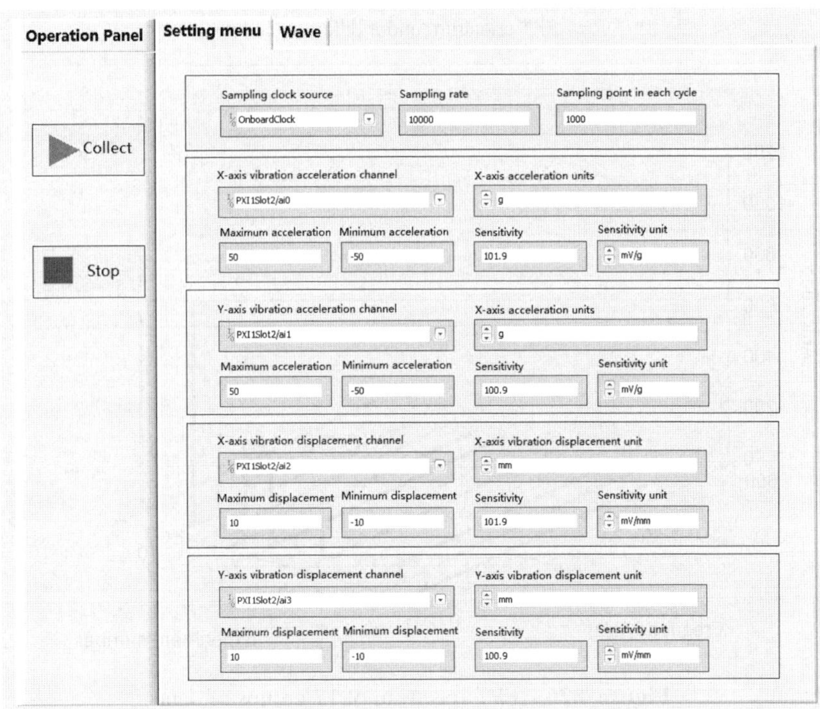

(b)

Figure 4.24 DAQ software

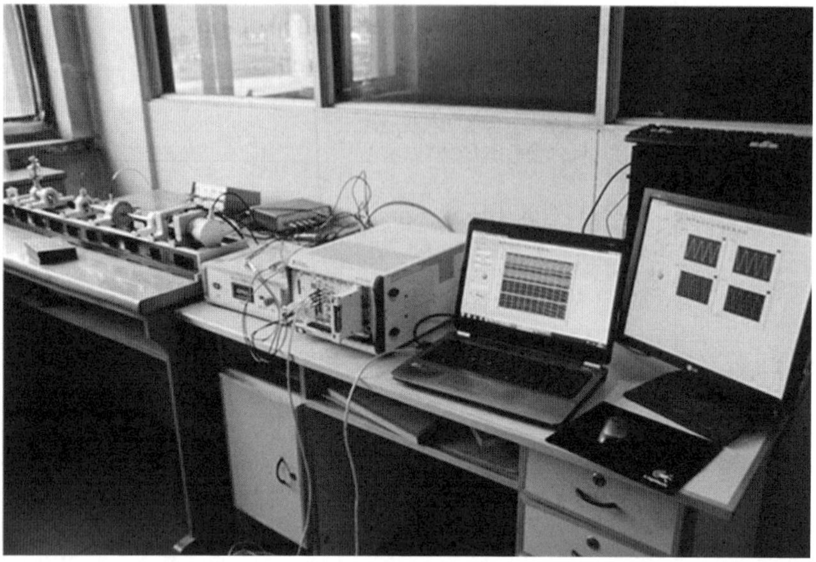

Figure 4.25 Experimental set-up of the rotor

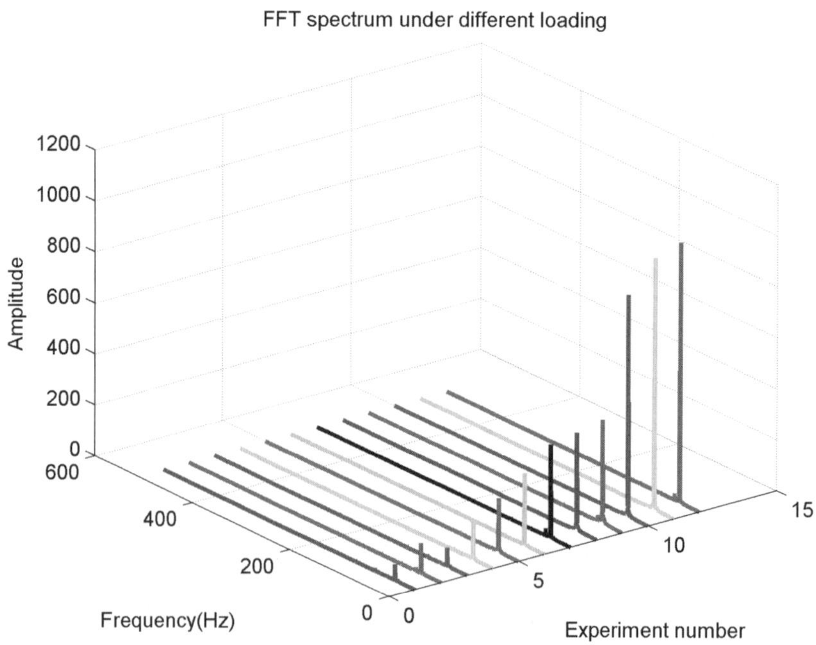

Figure 4.26 FFT spectrum of 12 groups of data

probability of potential failure occurrences. Once failures and faults occur in key components of equipment, the normal production of factories may be disturbed immediately, resulting in tremendous economic losses and even catastrophic consequences. Obviously, corrective and periodical maintenance, the early forms of maintenance, can no longer guarantee that large-scale complex equipment works normally, effectively, and safely. It is of great theoretical significance in science and practical value in engineering that those failures can be predicted and prevented prior to their occurrence through employing and studying advanced intelligent maintenance approaches and technologies.

There is a lack of one-to-one correspondence between failures and features of equipment, that is a type of failure may correspond to multiple types of features, and a type of feature may result from a variety of failures. For each type of equipment, its features change uniquely, which makes it a precondition of effective fault prognosis to discover precisely which features reflect the equipment condition. Therefore, feature selection is directly related to the precision of early stage fault diagnosis and the accuracy of fault prognosis.

Clustering analysis, which is an important data analysis technique, assists in obtaining better understanding of the global distribution pattern of signal features and the internal relationship among the features. Features that reflect equipment condition can be selected effectively by analyzing the characteristics of each cluster and then focusing on certain clusters with in-depth analysis. Instead of being studied comprehensively at different levels and from different perspectives, existing clustering algorithms are developed from the perspective of individual practicability. As to the uncertainty existing in the frequency domain features of non-stationary signals, a fuzzy transitive closure method could be utilized from the perspective of artificial intelligence.

4.4.1 Classification and Clustering

Classification is the actual or ideal arrangement together of those which are like, and the separation of those which are unlike. Classification is a type of supervised learning (background knowledge is known) and clustering is a type of unsupervised learning (no such knowledge is known). In classification, the input comes from a mixture of classes (supervised learning). Classification has labels for some points and wants a "rule" that will accurately assign labels to new points. Clustering is a well-known and widely used process for grouping items into different classes where the features of the target classes are not known in advance. Points are grouped into clusters based on how "near" they are to one another, which identifies structure in the data (unsupervised learning). In this manner clustering – in contrast to classification – is an unsupervised learning, where the identification of target classes is based on different features of the investigated objects. The structure of classification and clustering is shown in Figure 4.27.

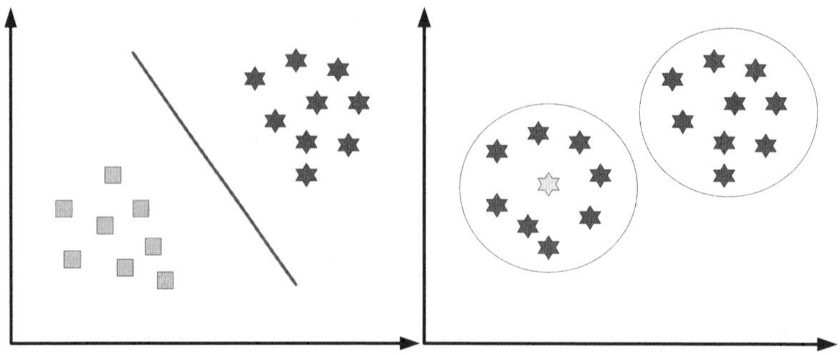

Figure 4.27 The structure of classification (a) and clustering (b)

4.4.2 Mathematical Model of the Classification Method

If we consider a database $D=\{t_1, t_2, \ldots, t_n\}$ and a group of classes $C=\{C_1, C_2, \ldots, C_m\}$, the classification problem is to define a mapping f:$D \rightarrow C$, where each t_i is assigned to one class. C_j contains all tuples mapped to the class, that is $C_j=\{t_i|f(t_i)=C_j, 1 \leq i \leq n$, and $t_i \in D\}$. From the definition, we could put the classification as a mapping from a database to a set of categories, and these classes are defined in advance without overlapping.

4.4.3 Mathematical Model of the Fuzzy C-Means Method

4.4.3.1 K-Means Clustering

The k-mean algorithm is one of the most important clustering algorithms. The function k-means partitions data into k mutually exclusive clusters, and returns the index of the cluster to which it has assigned each observation (see Figure 4.28). Unlike hierarchical clustering, k-means clustering operates on actual observations (rather than the larger set of dissimilarity measures), and creates a single level of clusters. The distinctions mean that k-means clustering is often more suitable than hierarchical clustering for large amounts of data.

K-means treats each observation in your data as an object having a location in space. It finds a partition in which objects within each cluster are as close to each other as possible, and as far from objects in other clusters as possible. You can choose from five different distance measures, depending on the kind of data you are clustering.

Each cluster in the partition is defined by its member objects and by its centroid, or center. The centroid for each cluster is the point to which the sum of distances from all objects in that cluster is minimized. K-means computes cluster centroids differently for each distance measure, to minimize the sum with respect to the measure that you specify.

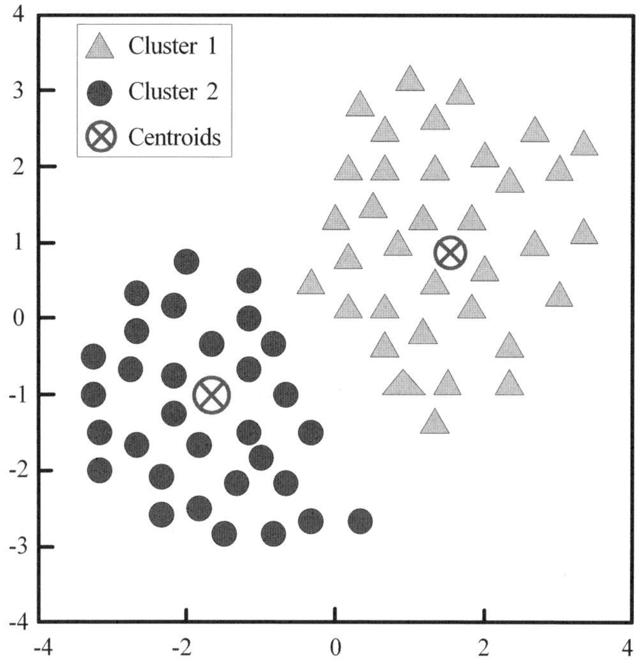

Figure 4.28 K-means clustering

K-means uses an iterative algorithm that minimizes the sum of distances from each object to its cluster centroid, over all clusters. This algorithm moves objects between clusters until the sum cannot be decreased further. The result is a set of clusters that are as compact and well-separated as possible. You can control the details of the minimization using several optional input parameters to k-means, including ones for the initial values of the cluster centroids, and for the maximum number of iterations.

Given a set of observations (x_1, $x_2, \ldots,$ x_n), where each observation is a d-dimensional real vector, k-means clustering aims to partition the n observations into k sets ($k \leq n$) $S = \{S_1, S_2, \ldots, S_k\}$ so as to minimize the within-cluster sum of squares:

$$d = \sum_{i=1}^{k} \sum_{x_j \in S_i} \|x_j - \mu_i\|^2 \tag{4.1}$$

where μ_i is the mean of points in S_i.

4.4.3.2 Fuzzy C-Means Clustering Method

Fuzzy c-means (FCM) (also known as fuzzy k-means) is a data clustering technique in which a dataset is grouped into k clusters with every data point in the dataset belonging to every cluster to a certain degree. For example, a certain data point that lies close to the center of a cluster will have a high degree of belonging or membership to that cluster and another data point that lies far away from the center of a cluster will have a low degree of belonging or membership to that cluster. It starts with an initial guess for the cluster centers, which are intended to mark the mean location of each cluster. The initial guess for these cluster centers is most likely incorrect. Next, FCM assigns every data point a membership grade for each cluster. By iteratively updating the cluster centers and the membership grades for each data point, FCM iteratively moves the cluster centers to the right location within a data set. This iteration is based on minimizing an objective function that represents the distance from any given data point to a cluster center weighted by that data point's membership grade. These clusters have "fuzzy" boundaries, in the sense that each data value belongs to each cluster to some degree or other. An important characteristic of the FCM algorithm is that it uses the squared Euclidian norm to measure the similarity between data points and cluster centroids.

If we consider a database $D = \{t_1, t_2, \dots, t_n\}$ of tuples and an integer value k, the clustering problem is to define a mapping f: $D\{1,.., k\}$, where each t_i is assigned to one cluster K_j, $1 \leq j \leq k$. A Cluster K_j contains precisely those tuples mapped to it. Unlike the classification problem, clusters are not known a priori (symmetry). The relationship between a data point and cluster representative is fuzzy. FCM clustering algorithms for interval-valued data are based on adaptive quadratic distances. The FCM clustering algorithms measure the fit between the clusters and their prototypes through an objective function. The algorithm is based on minimization of the following objective function:

$$J_m = \sum_{i=1}^{c} \sum_{j=1}^{n} \mu_{ij}^m (d_{ij})^2, \qquad m \in [1, +\infty] \tag{4.2}$$

where m represents the degree of fuzziness ($m > 1$), c indicates the number of clusters, n is the number of all components, and μ_{ij} indicates the fuzzy membership of the jth component in the ith cluster. d_{ij} is the Euclidian norm, which can be calculated as

$$d_{ij}^2 = \|x_j - p_i\|_A = (x_j - p_i)^{\mathrm{T}} A (x_j - p_i) \tag{4.3}$$

where x_j are the data points, p_i the clustering centroid of the ith cluster, and A is a positive definite symmetric matrix with degree $s \times s$.

Fuzzy partitioning is carried out through an iterative optimization of the objective function shown above, with the update of membership u_{ij} and the cluster centers c_j given by:

$$u_{ij} = \frac{1}{\sum_{k=1}^{C} \left(\frac{\|x_i - c_j\|}{\|x_i - c_k\|} \right)^{\frac{2}{m-1}}} \tag{4.4}$$

where $||x_i - c_j||$ is the distance from point i to the current cluster center j and $||x_i - c_k||$ is the distance from point i to the other cluster centers k.

$$c_j = \frac{\sum_{i=1}^{N} u_{ij}{}^m \cdot x_i}{\sum_{i=1}^{N} u_{ij}{}^m} \tag{4.5}$$

The iteration will stop when $\max_{ij}\{|u_{ij}{}^{(k+1)} - u_{ij}{}^{(k)}|\} < \varepsilon$, where ε is a termination criterion between 0 and 1 and k are the iteration steps. This procedure converges to a local minimum or a saddle point J_m.

4.4.4 Theory of Ant Colony Clustering Algorithm

In insect colonies, each insect seems to have its own agenda and yet the group as a whole appears to be highly organized. Apparently, the seamless integration of all individual activities does not require any supervision. In fact, scientists who study the behavior of social insects have found that cooperation at the colony level is highly self-organized: one of the most important and fascinating behaviors is their corpse accumulating, the data clustering based on the principle of the formation of an ant heap. It is known that an ant colony algorithm can get a satisfying clustering result. First, the basic ant colony clustering algorithm (ACCA) is introduced [20–22].

Clustering is a division of data into groups of similar objects, that is, minimizing intra-cluster similarity and maximizing inter-cluster similarity. The ant-based clustering algorithm works as follows: first, data objects are randomly projected onto a plane with a Cartesian grid; second, each ant chooses an object at random, and picks it up or moves or drops the object according to the picking-up or dropping probability with respect to the similarity of the current object within a local region. Finally, clusters are collected from the plane.

We assume that an ant is located at site r and finds an object o_i at the site. The local density $f(o_i)$ with respect to object o_i at r is given by

$$f(o_i) = \max\left\{0, \frac{1}{s^2} \sum_{o_j \in \mathrm{Neigh}_{s\times s}(r)} \left[1 - \frac{d\left(o_i, o_j\right)}{\alpha}\right]\right\} \tag{4.6}$$

where $f(o_i)$ is a measure of the average similarity density of object o_i with the other objects o_j present in the neighborhood of o_i. $\mathrm{Neigh}_{s\times s}$ (r) denotes a square of $s \times s$ sites surrounding site r. $\alpha(\in (0, 1])$ is a factor that defines the scale for dissimilarity. $d(o_i, o_j)$ is the distance between two objects o_i and o_j.

The cosine distance is defined by

$$d(o_i, o_j) = 1 - \text{sim}(o_i, o_j) \tag{4.7}$$

where

$$\text{sim}(o_i, o_j) = \frac{\sum_{k=1}^{m}(o_{ik} \cdot o_{jk})}{\sqrt{\sum_{k=1}^{m}(o_{ik})^2 \cdot \sum_{k=1}^{m}(o_{jk})^2}} \tag{4.8}$$

where o_{ik} represents the kth feature of an object o_i and m is the number of attributes.

The picking-up probability P_p for a randomly moving unloaded ant to pick up an object is given by

$$P_\mathrm{p} = 1 - \text{Sigmoid}(f(o_i)) \tag{4.9}$$

The dropping probability P_d for a randomly moving loaded ant to deposit an object is given by

$$P_\mathrm{d} = \text{Sigmoid}(f(o_i)) \tag{4.10}$$

The sigmoid function has a natural exponential form

$$\text{Sigmoid}(x) = \frac{1 - \mathrm{e}^{-cx}}{1 + \mathrm{e}^{-cx}} \tag{4.11}$$

where c is a slope constant and can speed up the algorithm convergence as it is increased.

4.4.5 Improved Ant Colony Clustering Algorithm

As social insects, ants exhibit great organization and establishment abilities by the colony behavior. It is known that the ant colony algorithm can obtain a satisfying clustering result, but the convergence speed is slow [23–26], which is not conducive to real-time analysis of data. Therefore, it is necessary to improve the ACCA.

4.4.5.1 Dynamic Adjustment Comparison Probability

In current studies, each ant picks up or drops down the sample according to comparing picking-up or dropping probability with a random probability. The randomness of the comparison probability is often inconsistent with environment change, affecting the correctness of ants picking-up or dropping samples. Therefore, in this part, an initial comparison probability is set to solve this problem, which could be further adjusted dynamically to environment changes. When the initial comparison probability is smaller and the speed of picking-up or dropping is higher, datasets can be roughly divided into several categories. With increase in the iterations, the comparison probability increases gradually, ants can subdivide samples more accurately, thus forming a more accurate clustering result.

Dynamic adjustment comparison probability can be described as follows:

1. *Initialization parameters*: initial comparison probability P_r, adjustment interval of comparison probability N_i, maximal comparison probability P_{max} ($P_{max} \leq 1$), maximum iteration number I_{max}, where I_{num} represents the iteration number.
2. if mod (I_{num}, I_{max}/N_i) = 0; (In the range of iterations to calculate the adjustment interval of the comparison probability)
3. $P_r = P_r + P_{max}/N_i$; (Calculate the comparison probability of the adjustment interval)
4. if $P_r \geq P_{max}$; (Whether the comparison probability of the adjustment interval is bigger than the maximal comparison probability)
5. $P_r = P_{max}$; (When the comparison probability of the adjustment interval is bigger than the maximal comparison probability, the comparison probability is the maximal comparison probability)
6. end if
7. end if
8. $P_r = (P_{max} - P_r)$*rand + P_r; (Produce a relatively greater than comparison probability of adjustment interval).

Finally, the improved ant colony clustering algorithm (IACCA) is depicted as a flowchart, shown in Figure 4.29.

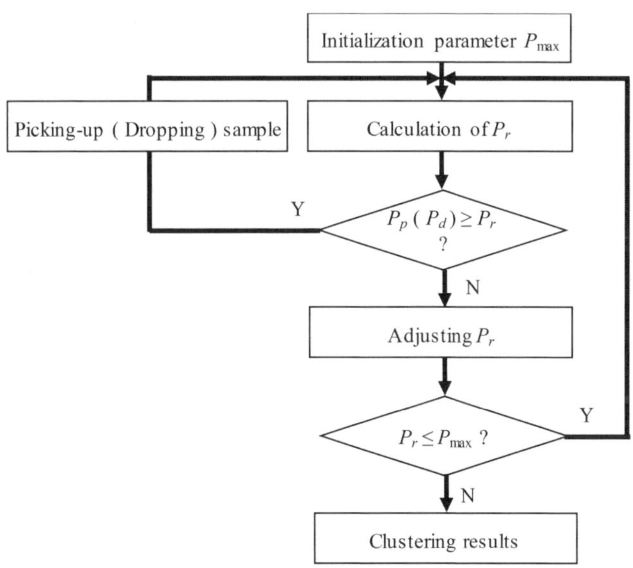

Figure 4.29 Flowchart of improved ant colony clustering algorithm

Through adjusting the comparison probability dynamically, the convergence of IACCA is strengthened, and the efficiency of the algorithm is improved to meet the requirements of real-time data analysis.

4.4.5.2 Outlier Detection

An outlier is an observation that appears to be inconsistent with the remainder of the dataset [27]. The purpose of outlier detection is to find the rare data whose behavior is very exceptional compared to other data. During a clustering procedure, there might be some outliers with dissimilarity to all other data elements. Since the ant carrying an outlier may never find a proper location to drop, and the ant keeps moving then this results in the consumption of computation time. If an ant is loaded still until an iterative process ends, the ant drops forcibly the sample in the position where it was picked-up, marks itself as unloaded and prepares for the next iteration, then the sample is marked as an outlier at the time of the condition. In addition, in Equation 4.6, the greater the value of c, the more outliers are dropped. Hence, c is increased gradually to help ants to drop the outliers at the later stage of the algorithm.

4.4.5.3 Numerical Simulation

In order to verify the effect of the IACCA, the ant-based clustering algorithms modifications (ACAM) [15], ACCA, and IACCA are applied to the Iris dataset [28], respectively. The Iris dataset is one of the well-known databases to be found in the pattern recognition literature. It consists of 150 data with four attributes and contains 3 classes of 50 instances each, where each class refers to a type of Iris plant. One class is linearly separable from the other two, and the others are not linearly separable from each other.

In order to classify samples into one category, the IACCA presented in Sections 4.4.5.1 and 4.4.5.2 are applied. Ten ants would be sufficient for this example. The number of ants should be selected moderately. The performance of the algorithm is no better with a larger value than with a smaller one. In order to obtain an optimal value of α, we ran a simulation of α from 0.1 to 0.4 with a step size of 0.01 and selected the best one 0.24 for the improved ACCA. The size of the grid is set to 30*30 based on the size of cluster data according to empirical analysis. The neighbor may be set 3*3, or 5*5, or 7*7. The neighbor area of the latter two is larger, resulting in the consumption of computation time. The neighbor area of the first is optimal. The maximal comparison probability is limited within the interval (0, 1]. According to Section 4.4.5.1, the maximal comparison probability $P_{\max} = 0.9$. Figure 4.30a shows the initial random distribution of the samples in the grid. The clustering result is shown in Figure 4.30b.

However, the results of the clustering algorithm ought to be evaluated using an informative quality measure that reflects the "goodness" of the resulting clusters. An external evaluation criterion called the F-measure [29] is used as the quality

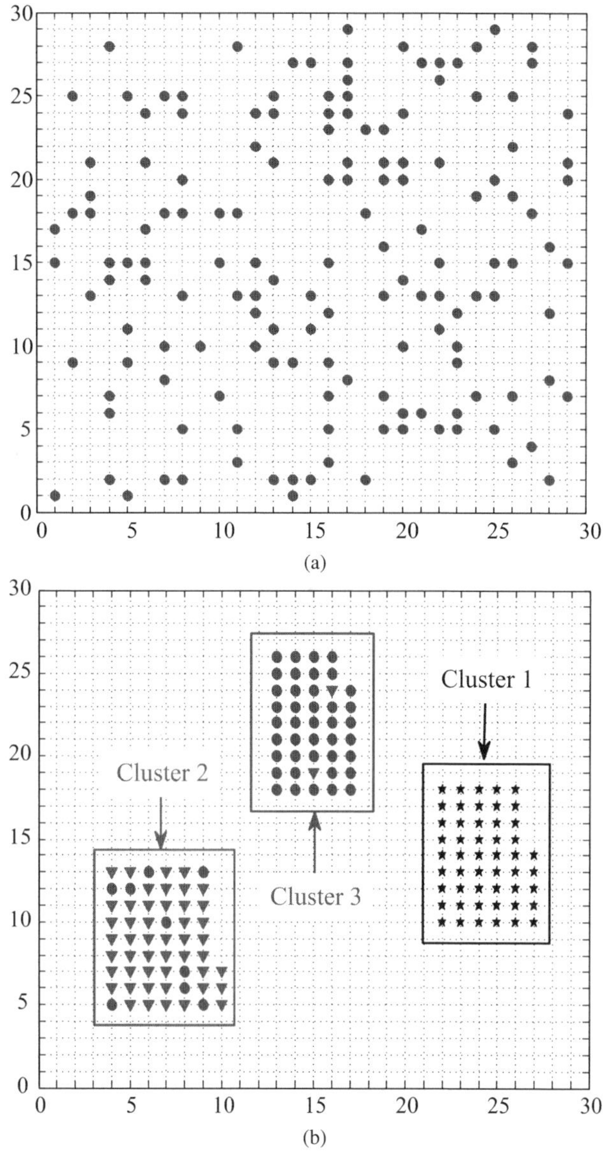

Figure 4.30 Clustering: (a) the initial random distribution of the samples in the grid, (b) the clustering results

measure here. The F-measure combines the ideas of precision and recall from the information retrieval literature. The value of the F-measure is limited within the interval [0, 1], and the higher the value, the better the clustering result. The clustering results of Iris datasets are listed in Table 4.6.

Table 4.6 indicates that, compared with ACCA, iterations of the IACCA are reduced to 2000 times and the better clustering result is obtained by the IACCA. It is obvious

Table 4.6 Result comparison of fuzzy c-means (FCM), ACAM [15], ACCA, and IACCA on Iris dataset

	FCM	ACAM [15]	ACCA	IACCA
Ant number	/	10	10	10
Iterations	/	1 000 000	10 000	2 000
F-measure	0.894	0.842	0.916	0.927

Ant number, iterations, and the value of F-measure of ACAM are given in Ref. [23].

that IACCA is better than ACAM [15] and ACCA in iterations and the value of the F-measure. Moreover, IACCA shows its superiority to FCM, which algorithm is a soft extension of hard k-means and also a very popular clustering algorithm through minimizing the distance-based objective function, because it has a higher value of F-measure on Iris datasets.

4.4.6 Intelligent Fault Diagnosis Method

The key procedure of fault diagnosis is extracting major features that can be used for diagnosing the current operation conditions of equipment. Feature extraction [30] and feature selection [31] are used to mine feature components containing crucial information and discard those providing little information, which contributes to reducing the dimension of features and extracting the optimal features for the classification process. Feature extraction from the original data is an important step in the fault classification process because it can remove the redundancy and avoid the curse of dimensionality. After feature extraction, there is still irrelevant or redundant information in these extracted features. Feature selection can solve the problem of irrelevant information in feature space, which not only makes information able to be dealt with intuitively by simplifying and compression, but also accesses the system attributes by excavating the implicit relationships hidden in signals. Moreover, reducing the number of features increases comprehensibility and contributes further to decision-making. Finally, the Euclidean nearness degree is used to recognize relationships between the equipment's current operation conditions and the major features extracted from online data. The specific procedures of the intelligent fault diagnosis method are shown in Figure 4.31.

The procedure of the proposed fault diagnosis method can be described as follows:

Step 1: We extract the features using WPT and then calculate the energy of all sub-bands to reduce the dimensionality. Wavelet packet coefficients obtained by WPD have effective feature information. The most useful features must be extracted from those coefficients to reduce the dimension of feature vectors. Usually, direct evaluation from all wavelet packet coefficients results

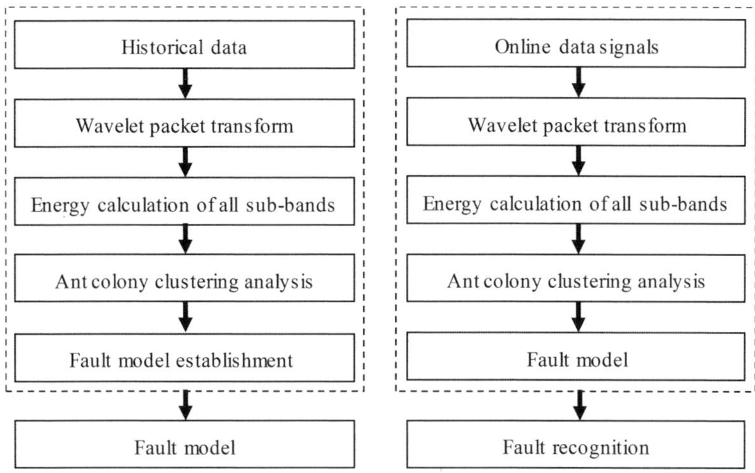

Figure 4.31 The procedure of intelligent fault diagnosis method. (a) model training, (b) fault diagnosis

in an inaccurate decision. For non-stationary signals, the frequency band energy spectrum provides a more robust signal feature than using coefficients directly. Therefore, the frequency band energy spectrum is defined as an individual feature component and is used as a robust exploration of the specific signal features that provide useful information for fault diagnosis [32, 33].

Step 2: Feature selection is performed using ant colony clustering analysis to remove the irrelevant features which are redundant and even degrade the performance of the classifier. The proposed IACCA, which can cluster similar relationships among information to mine useful information hidden in signals, is introduced to mine major features from the pattern of the frequency band perspective. The IACCA has been discussed in Section 4.4.5. Realization of a fault diagnosis model depends on these features extracted by IACCA.

Step 3: The goal of fault diagnosis is to establish the most suitable model to recognize different defects of the equipment. After feature extraction and feature selection, the major features are extracted from the training data. These features are the major source of information regarding the health of the equipment. Two types of fault patterns can be reflected by five features extracted, as shown in Figure 4.32a. According to the two given faults of the equipment from historical data, the fault diagnosis model is trained based on training data. Finally, the fault diagnosis model is established to combine the extracted major features with given fault prototypes, as shown in Figure 4.32a, where each solid line represents one type of fault, and each node represents one feature.

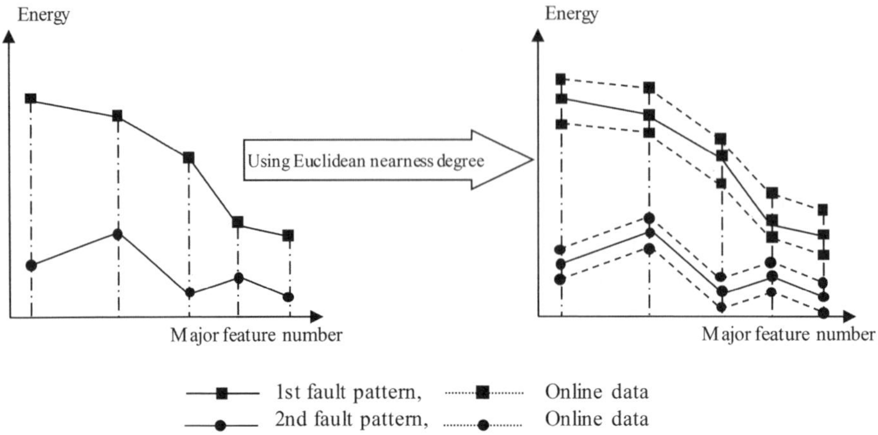

Figure 4.32 Schematic diagram of fault diagnosis based on the established model. (a) Fault model established, (b) fault recognition

Step 4: The classification process for fault diagnosis is carried out using the Euclidean nearness degree based on the fault model established. The Euclidean nearness degree based on the Euclidean distance can be defined by:

$$En(Fc_i, Ts_j) = 1 - \sqrt{\frac{1}{n}\sum_{k=1}^{n}(Fc_{ik} - Ts_{jk})^2} \tag{4.12}$$

where Fc_{ik} represents the vector of each fault category (i is the fault category number, k is the number of attributes), Ts_{jk} represents the vector of the online data (j is the online data number).

After the diagnosis model is constructed, the model can be used for diagnosis online. As illustrated in Figure 4.31b, first, online data are decomposed by WPT and the energy value of each feature is calculated. Then, the features obtained are clustered by the improved ant colony algorithm, and each cluster is analyzed in the frequency domain to extract major features. Fault patterns of four online data can be reflected by five features extracted, as shown in Figure 4.32b, where each dashed line represents one online data, and each node represents one feature. According to Equation 4.7, the values of the Euclidean nearness degree are calculated by online data and the fault model established, and the maximum value of each online data is selected representing one category fault. Finally, four online data are divided into two types of faults, and the fault recognition results are shown in Figure 4.32b, where each solid line represents one type of fault.

4.5 Physics-Based Prognosis Models

Technical approaches to building models in prognostics can be categorized into data-driven approaches, model-based approaches, and hybrid approaches. In the following sections we will discuss these approaches separately.

Physical model-based approaches usually employ mathematical models that are directly tied to physical processes that have direct or indirect effects on the health of related components. Physical models are usually developed by domain experts, and the parameters in the model are validated by large sets of data in the product design stage. Physical model-based approaches used for prognostics require specific mechanistic knowledge and theories relevant to the monitored systems [34]. A general flowchart of a model-based approach CBM (condition-based maintenance) system is shown in Figure 4.33.

These methods use residuals as features, where the residuals are the outcomes of consistency checks between the sensed measurements of a real system and the outputs of a mathematical model. The premise is that the residuals are large in the presence of malfunctions and small in the presence of normal disturbances, noise, and modeling errors. Statistical techniques are used to define the thresholds to detect the presence of faults. The three main ways of generating the residuals are based on parameter estimation, observers (e.g., Kalman filters, reduced-order unknown input observers, interacting multiple models (IMMs)), and parity relations.

The main advantage of a model-based approach is its ability to incorporate a physical understanding of the system for monitoring. Another advantage is that, in many situations, the changes in the feature vector are closely related to model parameters. Therefore, it can also establish a functional mapping between the drifting parameters and the selected prognostic features. Moreover, as the understanding of the system degradation improves, the model can be adapted to increase its accuracy and to address subtle performance problems [35].

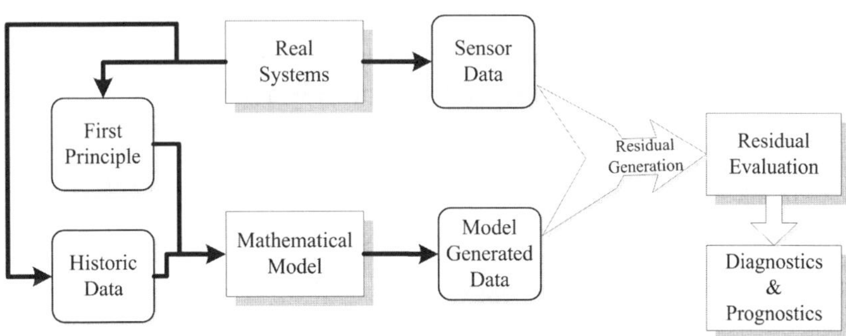

Figure 4.33 General flowchart of a model-based approach CBM system

Generally, with respect to the applied objects, model-based methods can be fulfilled at component and system levels. For the component level, the model-based methods are usually utilized for damage propagation. Dynamic equations define relations between the damage of a component and operational conditions, such as environmental stress and load profiles. There are several famous crack propagation laws, such as Paris' law, Walker' law, Forman' law, and so on, which will be discussed in the next chapter. From the view of a system level, the researchers trade all the components as a whole system. The system can be modeled by a simplified mathematical model considering the main parameters which have strong influence on the system performance. Here we refer to the literature to show the procedure of using the physics-based model in a system level.

4.5.1 Model-Based Methods for Systems

Model-based approaches to prognosis require specific mechanistic knowledge and theory relevant to the monitored machine [36]. From the perspective of dynamical systems theory, an evolving machine can be viewed as a hierarchical dynamical system consisting of a "fast time" directly observable subsystem coupled to a "slow time" damage subsystem. We consider a degradation model of a dynamic system with the following form:

$$\begin{aligned} \dot{X} &= f(X, \lambda(\theta), u) \\ \dot{\theta} &= \varepsilon g(X, \theta) \\ y &= CX + Du + v \end{aligned} \tag{4.13}$$

where $X \in R^n$ is the set of state variables associated with the fast dynamic behavior of the system; $\theta \in R^m$ is the set of slow dynamic variables related to system damage (degradation); $u \in R^l$ is the input vector; the parameter vector $\lambda \in R^q$ is a function of θ; the rate constant $0 < \varepsilon \ll 1$ defines the time-scale separation between the fast dynamics and the slow drift; $y \in R^p$ is the output vector and v is the measurement noise. Since ε is very small, Equation 4.13 can be considered as a system with slowly drifting parameters. For ease of exposition, in this research we consider the system of Equation 4.13 with scalar quantities defined as $g \equiv \mathrm{g}$, $\lambda = \lambda$, $\varepsilon = \epsilon$ and $\theta \equiv \theta$. This is a valid assumption if the scalar damage is independent of other damage variables.

From a stochastic fatigue point of view, the damage variable θ is often related to crack growth and its value is equal to crack size. A widely used crack growth model is the Paris–Erdogan law:

$$\frac{\mathrm{d}\theta}{\mathrm{d}n} = C(\Delta K)^{\gamma} \tag{4.14}$$

where $\Delta K = Y(\theta)(\Delta K)\sqrt{\pi\theta}$ is the stress intensity factor, $Y(\theta)$ accounts for the geometry of the crack of the specimen, C and γ are material constants. Typically, C is a small number ($0 < C \ll 1$) and γ is in the range of 2 to 4. We can easily see that Equation 4.14 can be written in the following general form:

$$\frac{d\theta}{dn} = \varepsilon\phi(\theta)\varphi(p) \tag{4.15}$$

where $\varepsilon = C$, $\phi(\theta) = (Y(\theta)\sqrt{\pi\theta})^{\gamma}$, $p = \Delta s$, and $\varphi(p) = p^{\gamma}$. The initial damage in the above equation is $\theta(0) = \theta_0$.

The damage development law in Equation 4.15 is a special case of that modeled in Equation 4.13 if the parameter p can be represented as a function of X, that is $p = h(X)$. $g(X, \theta) = \phi(\theta)\varphi(h(X))$ in Equation 4.13.

The value of the damage variable θ can be arbitrary. To facilitate analysis, it is convenient to use a damage measure ξ which takes values in the unit interval [0 1]. Defining the damage measure as $\xi = \theta/(\theta^* - \theta_0)$, where θ^* is the critical damage which is considered system failure. Equation 4.15 is rewritten as

$$d\xi/dn = \eta\phi[(\theta^* - \theta_0)\xi]\varphi(p) \tag{4.16}$$

where $\eta = \varepsilon/(\theta^* - \theta_0)$, $\phi[(\theta^* - \theta_0)\xi]\varphi(p)$ is a non-negative function and n is the number of cycles. The load parameter p varies with cycles. Then, for the ith cycle, we have a modified prognostic model in terms of damage measure

$$\begin{aligned} \dot{X} &= f(X, \lambda(\xi), u) \\ \xi_i &= \eta\phi(\xi_{i-1})\varphi(p_i) + \xi_{i-1} \\ y &= CX + Du + v \end{aligned} \tag{4.17}$$

The function $\lambda(\xi)$, which maps the degradation measure to a system parameter, is often assumed to be a polynomial: $\lambda(\xi) = \sum_{i=0}^{K} \alpha_i \xi^i$.

Monte-Carlo simulations were used to accomplish the evolution of system dynamics. We obtain the updated degradation measure as

$$\xi_i - \xi_{i-1} = n_i\bar{q} \Rightarrow \xi_i = \eta\phi(\xi_{i-1})\sum_{j=1}^{n_i} \varphi(p_i^j) + \xi_{i-1}$$

Based on the degradation measure, prognostics modeling was performed. Then, since the hidden variable ξ is unobserved, the input/output data $\{y, u\}$ were used to estimate it. After tracking the degradation measure, the remaining life was predicted. Details can be found in Ref. [36]. Other literature [37–39] also adopted non- linear damage prediction methods to forecast the remaining life in structure dynamic systems. This method requires physics knowledge about the system and dynamic modeling methods which limited the application in practice.

4.6 Data-Driven Prognosis Models

Data-driven techniques utilize monitored operational data related to the system health. Data-driven approaches are appropriate when understanding of the first principles of system operation is not comprehensive or when the system is sufficiently complex that developing an accurate model is prohibitively expensive. They are built on history records and produce prediction outputs directly in terms of health monitoring data.

The conventional data-driven methods include simple projection models, such as exponential smoothing and an autoregressive model. One major advantage of these techniques is the simplicity of their calculations, which can be carried out on a programmable calculator. However, most of these trend forecasting techniques assume that there is some underlying stability in the monitored system. They also rely on past patterns of degradation to project future degradation.

This reliance could lead to inaccurate forecasts in times of change. Most of these models follow the changing pattern with a time lag of at least one observation. Cempel [40] introduced the tribo-vibro acoustical (TVA) model, which can estimate the time to failure of a machine as well as forecasting the vibration amplitude or condition. The model was compared with a constant trend parabolic model, an exponential trend model, and an adaptive trending model in predicting a rolling bearing's peak vibration acceleration. It was reported that none of the forecasting techniques was able to predict the sudden change in the life curve [41].

The fuzzy logic systems (FLSs) [42], the support vector machine (SVM) [43], the gray model (GM) [44], particle filtering [45], Bayesian network [46], and so on, are artificial intelligence techniques that have been increasingly applied to machine prognostics and shown improved performance over conventional approaches. The most popular AI technique currently is artificial neural networks (ANNs), the typical structure of which can be seen in Figure 4.34. An ANN is a computational model that mimics the human brain structure and consists of three types of layers: input layer,

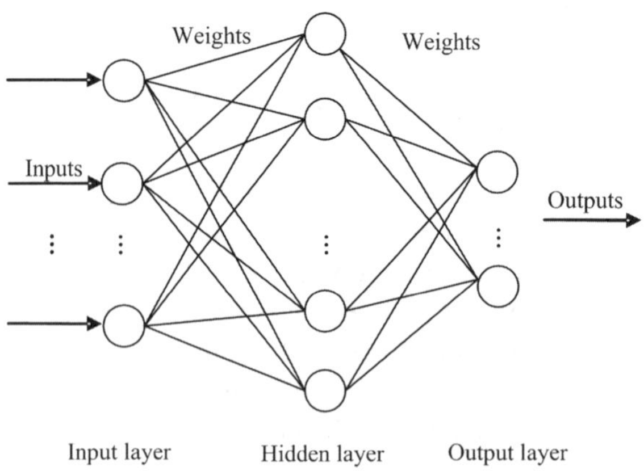

Figure 4.34 Typical structure of a multilayer neural network

hidden layer, and output layer. Each layer has a number of simple, neuron-like processing elements called "nodes" or "neurons" that interact with each other by using numerically weighted connections. The ANN learns the unknown function by adjusting its weights with observations of input and output. This process is usually called training of an ANN.

Numerous studies across various disciplines have demonstrated the merits of ANNs, including the abilities to (i) perform faster than system identification techniques in multivariate prognosis; (ii) perform at least as well as the best traditional statistical methods, without requiring untenable distributional assumptions; and (iii) capture complex phenomenon without a priori knowledge. A widely known limitation of ANNs is the lack of transparency, or rather the lack of documentation on how decisions are reached in a trained network. Even though these limitations lead to non-standardly trained neural networks, the ANN models have been widely used in fault prognostics for their excellent capability in modeling complex phenomena.

There are two types of applications of ANN for prognostics. One is to be used as a non-linear function approximator to predict system failure features and trends by estimating and classifying applications. The other is to be used with feedback connections to model dynamic processes of system degradation and give an expectation of the remaining useful life (RUL). Tian *et al.* [47] developed an ANN approach utilizing both failure and suspension condition monitoring histories. The ANN model uses age and condition monitoring data as the inputs and the life percentage as the output. For each suspension history, the optimal predicted life is determined which can minimize the validation mean square error in the training process using the suspension history and the failure histories. Then the ANN is trained using the failure histories and all the suspension histories with the obtained optimal predicted life values, and the trained ANN can be used for RUL prediction of other equipment. Mahamad *et al.* [4] adopted time and fitted measurements of Weibull hazard rates of RMS and kurtosis from the present and previous points as input of the ANN model. The normalized life percentage was used as output. The feed forward neural network (FFNN) with Levenberg Marquardt of the training algorithm was utilized as the training algorithm. The proposed ANN model shows good performance in the bearing RUL prediction. Tse and Atherton [48] used recurrent neural networks to trend CM indices and forecast the successive index value at the next time step. Gebraeel *et al.* [49] developed neural-network-based models for predicting bearing failures and concluded that the weighted average of the exponential parameters gives the best estimate of bearing failure times. Zhang and Ganesan [50] used a self-organizing neural network for multivariable trending of fault development to estimate the RUL of a bearing system.

A FLS is unique in that it is able to simultaneously handle numerical data and linguistic knowledge. It is a non-linear mapping of an input data (feature) vector into a scalar output. FLS can be considered as a universal approximator. This means that with sufficient training on appropriate input/output data a FLS can represent arbitrarily closely any continuous vector map. However, the "training" of the FLS from the

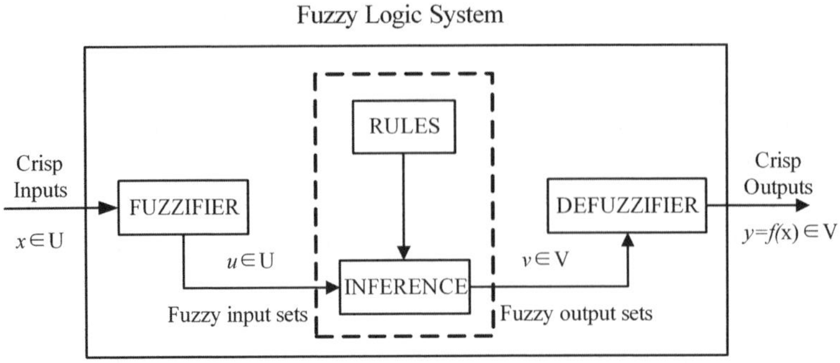

Figure 4.35 Fuzzy logic system

system data is typically not straightforward, there is still a high degree of "art" associated with selecting and preprocessing data for this purpose. This "model-free" type of identification contrasts significantly with many of the standard identification methods which usually require not only that the system be linear but also, in many cases, that the order and structure of the system be known in advance [51].

Figure 4.35 depicts a FLS that is widely used in fuzzy logic controllers and signal processing applications. A FLS maps crisp inputs into crisp outputs. It contains four components: rules, fuzzifier, inference engine, and defuzzifier. Once the rules have been established, a FLS can be viewed as a mapping from inputs to outputs, and this mapping can be expressed quantitatively as $y = f(x)$. One of the major goals of FLS is to obtain explicit formulas for the non-linear mapping between x and y.

Rules may be provided by experts or can be extracted from numerical data. In either case, engineering rules are expressed as a collection of IF–THEN statements. The fuzzifier maps crisp numbers into fuzzy sets. It is needed in order to activate rules which are in terms of linguistic variables, which have fuzzy sets associated with them. The inference engine of the FLS maps fuzzy sets into fuzzy sets. It handles the way in which rules are combined. Just as we humans use many different types of inferential procedures to help us understand things or to make decisions, there are many different fuzzy logic inferential procedures. Only a very small number of them are actually being used in engineering applications of FLS. In many applications, crisp numbers must be obtained at the output of a FLS. The defuzzifier maps output sets into crisp numbers. In a signal processing application, such a number could correspond to the prediction of next year's sunspot activity, a financial forecast, or the location of a target [52].

Other AI techniques used in RUL prediction include FLSs. But this (data-driven) technique needs a large amount of data to make the system as close to real application as possible. Data-driven models may often be the more available solution in many practical cases in which it is easier to gather data than to build accurate system physics models.

4.7 Hybrid Prognosis Models

As described previously, the model-based methods are applicable in situations where accurate mathematical models can be constructed from first principles. They incorporate a physical understanding of the system to be monitored. As the understanding of the system degradation improves, the model can be adapted to increase its accuracy and to address subtle performance problems. Data-driven methods can capture the complex relationships and learn trends available in the data without knowing the failure mechanism. Therefore, it is necessary to develop integrated prognostic methods to take advantage of the merits of both the model-based and data-driven methods.

Hybrid approaches attempt to leverage the strength from both data-driven approaches and model-based approaches [53, 54]. In reality, it is rare that the fielded approaches are completely either purely data-driven or purely model-based. More often than not, model-based approaches include some aspects of data-driven approaches and data-driven approaches glean available information from models. An example for the former would be where model parameters are tuned using field data. An example for the latter is when the set-point, bias, or normalization factor for a data-driven approach is given by models. Hybrid approaches can be categorized broadly into two categories: pre-estimate fusion and post-estimate fusion.

1. *Pre-estimate fusion of models and data*
   The motivation for pre-estimate aggregation may be that no ground truth data are available. This may occur in situations where diagnostics does a good job in detecting faults that are resolved (through maintenance) before system failure occurs. Therefore, there are hardly any run-to-failure data. However, there is an incentive to know better when a system would fail in order to better leverage the RUL, while at the same time avoiding unscheduled maintenance (unscheduled maintenance is typically more costly than scheduled maintenance and results in system downtime). Another way to accomplish the pre-estimate aggregation is by a combined off-line process and on-line process: in the off-line mode, one can use a physics-based simulation model to understand the relationships of sensor response to fault state; in the on-line mode, one can use data to identify current damage state, then track the data to characterize damage propagation, and finally apply an individualized data-driven propagation model for remaining life prediction.
2. *Post-estimate fusion of model-based approaches with data-driven approaches*
   Motivation for post-estimate fusion is often consideration of uncertainty management. That is, the post-estimate fusion helps to narrow the uncertainty intervals of data-driven or model-based approaches. At the same time, the accuracy improves. The underlying notion is that multiple information sources can help to improve the performance of an estimator. This principle has been successfully applied within the context of classifier fusion where the output of multiple classifiers is used to arrive at a better result than any classifier alone. Within the context

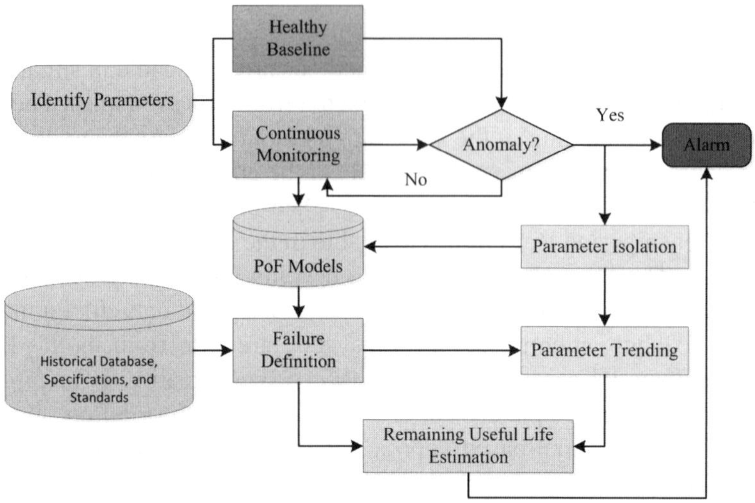

Figure 4.36 RUL prediction by fusion PHM method

of prognostics, fusion can be accomplished by employing quality assessments that are assigned to the individual estimators based on a variety of inputs, for example, heuristics, a priori known performance, prediction horizon, or robustness of the prediction.

Cheng and Pecht [55] presented a fusion method which fuses data-driven methods and the physics-based failure methods to predict the RUL of electronic products. The flowchart of the proposed method can be cited here as Figure 4.36.

Nine steps are included to implement the fusion prognostics method.

Step 1: Parameter identification
Step 2: Parameter monitoring
Step 3: Feature extraction and healthy baseline creation
Step 4: Anomaly detection
Step 5: Parameter isolation
Step 6: PoF models
Step 7: Failure definition
Step 8: Parameter trending
Step 9: RUL prediction.

In this implementation method, the PoF method is used to identify the critical parameters, identify and prioritize the potential failure mechanisms, identify the failure models, and define the failure criteria in terms of the isolated parameters or a function of the isolated parameters. The data-driven method is used to extract the features from the monitored parameters, create a healthy baseline, and compare the monitored parameters with the baseline to conduct anomaly detection and trend the isolated parameters. In this method, one of the most important steps is the identification of the potential failure mechanisms of the monitored product under the field environmental and operational conditions. However, it is difficult to know the exact failure mechanisms during the monitoring of the product. The practical method is using the PoF-based method to identify the potential failure mechanisms. The potential failure mechanisms then help to isolate the parameters to monitor, trend, and define the failure. If the failure models for the potential failure mechanisms are identified, the definition of the failure can be defined based on the models. If the failure models are not identified, the failure can be defined from the historical database. In this case, the failed data in the database should be classified based on the identified failure mechanisms. It is assumed that the failure analysis was conducted for all the failed products in the historical database to identify the exact failure mechanisms. Thus, the failure definition for the failure mechanisms can be obtained by statistical methods (such as the distribution of the failure). If the environmental conditions are different but the failure mechanisms are the same, an accelerated factor should be identified to transfer the failure definition from the historical conditions to the field conditions.

Following the procedure, RUL prediction of flexible-termination MLCCs with precious metal electrodes made of silver–palladium was performed. The results show the fusion prognostics method can provide reasonable RUL prediction.

Another example of hybrid prognostics models was provided by Goebel *et al.* [56]. One method uses first principles to model fault propagation through consideration of the physics of the system. The other method is an empirical model using data from experiments at known conditions and component damage level to estimate condition-based fault propagation rate. These two approaches are fused to produce a result that is more accurate and more robust than either method alone. The fusion method employs a Dempster–Shafer regression that – in addition to the damage estimates – takes advantage of subjective quality assessments that quantify the uncertainty of the estimates at any time. The experiment was set up on a rig where a bearing was run under typical mission flight profiles. Spall was initiated and bearing spall growth was carefully monitored.

References

1. Kazzaz, A. and Singh, G.K. (2003) Experimental investigations on induction machine condition monitoring and fault diagnosis using digital signal processing techniques. *Electric Power Systems Research*, **65** (3), 197–221.
2. Zhao, R., Yan, R. and Gao, R.X. (2013) Dual-scale cascaded adaptive stochastic resonance for rotary machine health monitoring. *Journal of Manufacturing Systems*, **32** (4), 529–535.
3. Tran, V.T., Thom Pham, H., Yang, B.S. *et al.* (2012) Machine performance degradation assessment and remaining useful life prediction using proportional hazard model and support vector machine. *Mechanical Systems and Signal Processing*, **32**, 320–330.
4. Mahamad, A.K., Saon, S. and Hiyama, T. (2010) Predicting remaining useful life of rotating machinery based artificial neural network. *Computers & Mathematics with Applications*, **60** (4), 1078–1087.

5. Qiu, H., Lee, J., Lin, J. *et al.* (2003) Robust performance degradation assessment methods for enhanced rolling element bearing prognostics. *Advanced Engineering Informatics*, **17** (3), 127–140.
6. Djurdjanovic, D., Lee, J. and Ni, J. (2003) Watchdog Agent – an infotronics-based prognostics approach for product performance degradation assessment and prediction. *Advanced Engineering Informatics*, **17** (3), 109–125.
7. Lee, J., Wu, F., Zhao, W. *et al.* (2013) Prognostics and health management design for rotary machinery systesm -- reviews, methodology and applications. *Mechanical Systems and Signal Processing*, **42**, 314–334.
8. Lee, J., Ni, J., Djurdjanovic, D. *et al.* (2006) Intelligent prognostics tools and e-maintenance. *Computers in Industry*, **57** (6), 476–489.
9. Loutas, T.H., Sotiriades, G., Kalaitzoglou, I. and Kostopoulos, V. (2009) Condition monitoring of a single-stage gearbox with artificially induced gear cracks utilizing on-line vibration and acoustic emission measurements. *Applied Acoustics*, **70** (9), 1148–1159.
10. Ottewill, J.R. and Orkisz, M. (2013) Condition monitoring of gearboxes using synchronously averaged electric motor signals. *Mechanical Systems and Signal Processing*, **38**, 482–498.
11. Hameed, Z., Hong, Y.S., Cho, Y.M. *et al.* (2009) Condition monitoring and fault detection of wind turbines and related algorithms: a review. *Renewable and Sustainable Energy Reviews*, **13** (1), 1–39.
12. García Márquez, F.P., Tobias, A.M., Pinar Pérez, J.M. *et al.* (2012) Condition monitoring of wind turbines: techniques and methods. *Renewable Energy*, **46**, 169–178.
13. Yu, Y., Zhao, X., Shi, Y. *et al.* (2013) Design of a real-time overload monitoring system for bridges and roads based on structural response. *Measurement*, **46**, 345–352.
14. Ko, J.M. and Ni, Y.Q. (2005) Technology developments in structural health monitoring of large-scale bridges. *Engineering Structures*, **27** (12), 1715–1725.
15. Ertunc, H.M., Loparo, K.A. and Ocak, H. (2001) Tool wear condition monitoring in drilling operations using hidden Markov models (HMMs). *International Journal of Machine Tools and Manufacture*, **41** (9), 1363–1384.
16. Zhu, K., Wong, Y.S. and Hong, G.S. (2009) Wavelet analysis of sensor signals for tool condition monitoring: a review and some new results. *International Journal of Machine Tools and Manufacture*, **49** (7), 537–553.
17. Zhang, C. and Wang, N. (2012) Aero-engine condition monitoring based on support vector machine. *Physics Procedia*, **24**, 1546–1552.
18. Liu, J., Seraoui, R., Vitelli, V. *et al.* (2013) Nuclear power plant components condition monitoring by probabilistic support vector machine. *Annals of Nuclear Energy*, **56**, 23–33.
19. Hashemian, H.M. (2011) On-line monitoring applications in nuclear power plants. *Progress in Nuclear Energy*, **53** (2), 167–181.
20. Deneubourg, J.L., Goss, S., Franks, N. *et al.* (1991) The dynamics of collective sorting: robot-like ants and ant-like robots, in *Proceedings of the First International Conference on Simulation of Adaptive behavior: From Animal to Animats*, MIT Press, Cambridge, MA, pp. 356–363.
21. Lumer, E.D. and Faieta, B. (1994) Diversity and adaptation in populations of clustering ants, in *Proceedings of the Third International Conference on Simulation of Adaptive Behavior: From Animals to Animats*, MIT Press, Cambridge, MA, pp. 501–508.
22. Yang, Y. and Kamel, M. (2003) Clustering ensemble using swarm intelligence. Proceedings of the IEEE Swarm Intelligence Symposium (SIS), Indiana, pp. 65–71.
23. Boryczka, U. (2009) Finding groups in data: cluster analysis with ants. *Applied Soft Computing*, **9** (1), 61–70.
24. Chen, L., Xu, X.H., Chen, Y.X., and He, P. (2004) A novel ant clustering algorithm based on cellular automata. Proceedings of the IEEE/WIC/ACM International Conference on Intelligent Agent Technology (IAT), Washington, DC, pp. 148–154.
25. Qu, J.H. and Liu, X.Y. (2007) A quick ant clustering algorithm. *Proceedings of the Fourth International Conference on Fuzzy Systems and Knowledge Discovery (FSKD 2007)*, IEEE Computer Society, Washington, DC, vol. 1, pp. 722–725.

26. Xu, X.H., Chen, L., and Chen, Y.X. (2004) A^4C: an adaptive artificial ants clustering algorithm. Proceedings of the IEEE Symposium on Computational Intelligence in Bioinformatics and Computational Biology (CIBCB), California, pp. 268–275.
27. Barnett, V. and Lewis, T. (1994) *Outliers in Statistical Data*, 3rd edn, John Wiley & Sons, Inc., New York.
28. UCI (0000) UCI Repository for Machine Learning Databases retrieved from the World Wide Web, http://www.ics.uci.edu/~mlearn/MLRepository.html (accessed 09 June 2014).
29. Larsen, B. and Aone, C. (1999) Fast and effective text mining using linear-time document clustering. Proceedings of the Fifth ACM SIGKDD International Conference on Knowledge Discovery and Data Mining, San Diego, CA, pp. 16–22.
30. Zhang, P., Bui, T.D. and Suen, C.Y. (2004) Feature dimensionality reduction for the verification of handwritten numerals. *Pattern Analysis & Applications*, **7** (3), 296–307.
31. Zeng, H. and Cheung, Y.M. (2009) A new feature selection method for Gaussian mixture clustering. *Pattern Recognition*, **42**, 243–250.
32. Hu, Q., He, Z.J., Zhang, Z.S. and Zi, Y.Y. (2007) Fault diagnosis of rotating machinery based on improved wavelet package transform and SVMs ensemble. *Mechanical Systems and Signal Processing*, **21** (2), 688–705.
33. Uyar, M., Yildirim, S. and Gencoglu, M.T. (2008) An effective wavelet-based feature extraction method for classification of power quality disturbance signals. *Electric Power Systems Research*, **78** (10), 1747–1755.
34. Peng, Y., Dong, M. and Zuo, M.J. (2010) Current status of machine prognostics in condition-based maintenance: a review. *The International Journal of Advanced Manufacturing Technology*, **50** (1–4), 297–313.
35. Luo, J., Pattipati, K.R., Qiao, L. *et al.* (2008) Model-based prognostic techniques applied to a suspension system. *IEEE Transactions on Systems, Man, and Cybernetics Part A: Systems and Humans*, **38** (5), 1156–1168.
36. Luo, J., Bixby, A., Pattipati, K. *et al.* (2003) An interacting multiple model approach to model-based prognostics. IEEE International Conference on Systems, Man and Cybernetics, 2003, IEEE, Vol. 1, pp. 189–194.
37. Adams, D.E. and Nataraju, M. (2002) A nonlinear dynamical systems framework for structural diagnosis and prognosis. *International Journal of Engineering Science*, **40** (17), 1919–1941.
38. Cusumano, J.P. and Chatterjee, A. (2002) A dynamical systems approach to damage evolution tracking, part 1: description and experimental application. *Journal of Vibration and Acoustics*, **124** (2), 250–257.
39. Daigle, M. and Goebel, K. (2011) Multiple damage progression paths in model-based prognostics. 2011 IEEE Aerospace Conference, March 2011, IEEE, pp. 1–10.
40. Cempel, C. (1987) Simple condition forecasting techniques in vibroacoustical diagnostics. *Mechanical Systems and Signal Processing*, **1** (1), 75–82.
41. Heng, A., Zhang, S., Tan, A.C. *et al.* (2009) Rotating machinery prognostics: state of the art, challenges and opportunities. *Mechanical Systems and Signal Processing*, **23** (3), 724–739.
42. Fanegan, J., Ralescu, A., and Ueda, F. (2007) A Fuzzy model for estimating the remaining lifetime a diesel engine. Fuzzy Information Processing Society, 2007. NAFIPS'07. Annual Meeting of the North American, June, 2007, IEEE, pp. 473–477.
43. Widodo, A. and Yang, B.S. (2011) Machine health prognostics using survival probability and support vector machine. *Expert Systems with Applications*, **38** (7), 8430–8437.
44. Ku, L.L. and Huang, T.C. (2006) Sequential monitoring of manufacturing processes: an application of grey forecasting models. *The International Journal of Advanced Manufacturing Technology*, **27** (5–6), 543–546.
45. Zio, E. and Peloni, G. (2011) Particle filtering prognostic estimation of the remaining useful life of nonlinear components. *Reliability Engineering & System Safety*, **96** (3), 403–409.

46. Gebraeel, N.Z., Lawley, M.A., Li, R. *et al.* (2005) Residual-life distributions from component degradation signals: a Bayesian approach. *IIE Transactions*, **37** (6), 543–557.
47. Tian, Z., Wong, L. and Safaei, N. (2010) A neural network approach for remaining useful life prediction utilizing both failure and suspension histories. *Mechanical Systems and Signal Processing*, **24** (5), 1542–1555.
48. Tse, P.W. and Atherton, D.P. (1999) Prediction of machine deterioration using vibration based fault trends and recurrent neural networks. *Journal of Vibration and Acoustics*, **121** (3), 355–362.
49. Gebraeel, N., Lawley, M., Liu, R. *et al.* (2004) Residual life predictions from vibration-based degradation signals: a neural network approach. *IEEE Transactions on Industrial Electronics*, **51** (3), 694–700.
50. Zhang, S. and Ganesan, R. (1997) Multivariable trend analysis using neural networks for intelligent diagnostics of rotating machinery. *Journal of Engineering for Gas Turbines and Power*, **119** (2), 378–384.
51. VanLandingham, H. and Chrysanthakopoulos, G. (1995) Data driven fuzzy logic systems for system modeling. IEEE International Conference on Systems, Man and Cybernetics, 1995. Intelligent Systems for the 21st Century, Vancouver, BC, vol. 1, pp. 841–884.
52. Mendel, J.M. (1995) Fuzzy logic systems for engineering: a tutorial. *Proceedings of the IEEE*, **83** (3), 345–377.
53. Pecht, M. and Jaai, R. (2010) A prognostics and health management roadmap for information and electronics-rich systems. *Microelectronics Reliability*, **50** (3), 317–323.
54. Liu, J., Wang, W., Ma, F. *et al.* (2012) A data-model-fusion prognostic framework for dynamic system state forecasting. *Engineering Applications of Artificial Intelligence*, **25** (4), 814–823.
55. Cheng, S. and Pecht, M. (2009) A fusion prognostics method for remaining useful life prediction of electronic products. IEEE International Conference on Automation Science and Engineering, 2009. CASE 2009, August 22-25, 2009, Bangalore, IEEE, pp. 102–107.
56. Goebel, K., Eklund, N., and Bonanni, P. (2006) Fusing competing prediction algorithms for prognostics. 2006 IEEE Aerospace Conference, Big Sky, MT, IEEE, p. 10.

5

Prediction of Remaining Useful Life

5.1 Formulation of Problem

Prognosis targets the prediction of remaining useful life (RUL) in order to minimize the breakdown time and maintenance costs. RUL, also called residual service life, refers to the time left before the target of interest loses its specified function given the current machine age and condition, and the past operation profile. It can be defined as the conditional random variable $\{T - t|T > t, Z(t)\}$, where T denotes the random variable for time to failure, t is the current age and $Z(t)$ is the past condition profile up to the current time. In some cases, RUL prediction means finding the distribution of RUL. In some other cases, it just means the expectation of RUL, noted as $E[T - t| T > t, Z(t)]$. It should be noted that a proper definition of failure is crucial to correct interpretation of RUL. Although there is a controversy in current industrial practice, a formal definition of failure can be found in many reliability textbooks. To carry out prognosis, in addition to knowledge (or data) on the fault propagation process, knowledge (or data) on the failure mechanism must be available. The fault propagation process is usually tracked by a trending or forecasting model for certain condition variables. There are two ways to describe the failure mechanism. The first one assumes that failure depends only on the condition variables, which reflect the actual fault level, and the predetermined boundary. The most commonly used failure definition in this case is simple: failure occurs when the fault reaches a predetermined level. The second one builds a model for the failure mechanism using available historical data [1].

As one vital step of prognosis, RUL prediction has become an attractive research field worldwide. Many prediction models have been developed to forecast the RUL and they can be categorized as prediction based on probability, dynamic prediction with time series and prediction by crack-growth criterion. These various methods show good prediction performance in different applications [2–4]. Generally, prediction models are selected or trained based on the researchers' experiences and

Machinery Prognostics and Prognosis Oriented Maintenance Management, First Edition. Jihong Yan.

measurements. In most of the previous research, the established models are static once they have been trained by historical data, which means the parameters of these models are never changed in the future. However, in fact as time passes, more and more data are collected which provides new information to the trained models. When new information is available, the prediction model does not learn from the new data, which leads to error in the prediction results. It is necessary to update these models in order to fully take advantage of the new information so that the models can capture the developing trend of the monitored system more accurately; this is called the dynamic prediction method. How to implement the update is still a new and interesting topic in the research on RUL prediction.

In the following sections, we will introduce these three main categories of RUL prediction methods and for some of them we will provide application examples.

5.2 Methodology of Probabilistic Prediction

In most research work, the parameters used in the models for remaining life prediction were treated as single values. However, during the remaining life prediction, many factors related to the prediction process are random variables which introduce uncertainties into the results. For instance, in the health prognosis methods for damage propagation, due to material variation, experimental errors, measurement inaccuracy as well as variations of operating condition, failure times are different for different units which should take the form of a statistical distribution rather than a single value. Also uncertainties can be generated by data collecting equipment such as sensors, A/D converters, data recording, and transmission devices. So the prognosis of equipment future condition or component failure time should be studied in a probabilistic framework. Different from the methods which only focus on the accuracy of the prediction results and only provide a single value of RUL, probability prediction methods can provide more information including both the accuracy and the confidence in the results to form a decision or corrective. These methods require less detailed information than model-based techniques because the information needed for prognosis resides in various probability density functions (PDFs), not in dynamic differential equations. Advantages are that the required PDFs can be found from observed statistical data and that the PDFs are sufficient to predict the quantities of interest in prognosis. The problem of using these probability methods is that sufficient data are required to completely characterize the true remaining life PDF of a given component empirically in all possible damage conditions.

Mathematically the probability estimation of RUL can be described as follows. Consider a non-negative random variable X_t which represents RUL at time t, then the PDF of X_t conditional on Y_t is denoted as $f(X_t|Y_t)$ where Y_t is the history of the operation profiles and condition monitoring information up to t. Therefore estimating the PDF $f(X_t|Y_t)$ or $E(X_t|Y_t)$ is very important. If Y_t is not available then the estimation of

$f(X_t|Y_t)$ is more likely to be the PDF in the reliability field since

$$f(X_t|Y_t) = f(X_t) = \frac{f(t+X_t)}{R(t)} \tag{5.1}$$

where $f(t+X_t)$ is the PDF of the life at $t+X_t$ and $R(t)$ is the survival function at time t.

If Y_t is available, then it is a non-trivial task to estimate $f(X_t|Y_t)$ which incorporates the condition monitoring data Y_t into the estimation of X_t [5]. For the first case, Weibull distribution is the most widely used probability density function. If considering Y_t, Bayesian analysis is more suitable to estimate the failure times of products and systems.

5.2.1 Theory of Weibull Distribution

Reliability analysis of a wide variety of engineering products and systems suggests that time-to-failure data tend to fit well a Weibull distribution. Especially, a Weibull distribution has more reliable values than other distributions in fatigue data evaluations from the point of view of variables in life and strength parameters. Therefore, Weibull distribution will be useful in the remaining life prediction of failing components. The popular forms of this distribution are two- and three-parameter Weibull distributions. A general form of the three-parameter Weibull distribution can be described as follows.

The hazard rate

$$h(t) = \frac{\beta}{\eta}\left(\frac{t-\gamma}{\eta}\right)^{\beta-1} \qquad t \geq \gamma;\ \beta, \eta > 0 \tag{5.2}$$

The probability density function (PDF)

$$f(t) = \frac{\beta}{\eta}\left(\frac{t-\gamma}{\eta}\right)^{\beta-1} \exp\left[-\left(\frac{t-\gamma}{\eta}\right)^{\beta}\right] \qquad t \geq \gamma;\ \beta, \eta > 0 \tag{5.3}$$

where η is the characteristic life, β is the shape factor, and γ is the location parameter. The influence of the shape factor β is shown in Figure 5.1.

It can be clearly seen that the shape factor β decides the shape of the PDF dramatically. When $\beta > 1$, the PDF curve shows the property of one-peak, and as β decreases, the peak value decreases; when $\beta = 3 \sim 4$, the PDF is very similar to that of normal distribution in that $\beta > 1$ represents wear-out failure mode with increasing failure rate. The PDF remains constant at $\beta = 1$ to indicate a failure mode with a constant and lower failure rate, which has the characteristics of an exponential distribution. As for the value of $\beta < 1$, the failure rate decreases with operating time to give an early failure mode. Therefore, the failure mode can be determined from the shape parameter or the relationships between the failure rate and operating time sequence.

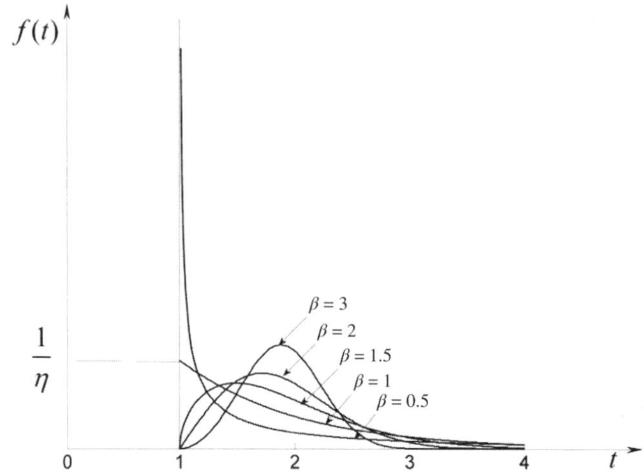

Figure 5.1 PDF of Weibull distribution for varying shape factors ($\eta = 1,\ \gamma = 1$)

The location parameter γ reflects the starting point of the PDF curve in the horizontal axis. In the reliability analysis, γ represents the limits of the fatigue and life of components, which means before the moment $t = \gamma$ the component does not fail. Hence, γ is also called the minimum guaranteed life. When $\gamma = 0$, the two-parameter distribution is obtained.

The advantages of a two-parameter Weibull distribution are as follows [5]:

1. It can be explained with a simple function and applied easily.
2. It is used frequently in the evaluation of fatigue life of composites.
3. Its usage is easy having present graphics and simple calculation methods.
4. It gives some physical rules concerning failure when the slope of the Weibull probability plots is taken into account.

The cumulative probability distribution can be calculated by integrating the density function over time t. This distribution provides the probability $F(t)$ that a future failure will occur at any time. Consequently, the probability of survival or reliability $R(t)$ can be calculated. If γ is set to zero, we obtain the two-parameter Weibull distribution. The reliability curve of the Weibull distribution for $\eta = 1,\ \gamma = 1$ is shown in Figure 5.2.

$$F(t) = 1 - \exp\left[-\left(\frac{t-\gamma}{\eta}\right)^{\beta}\right] \qquad t \geq \gamma;\ \beta, \eta > 0 \tag{5.4}$$

$$R(t) = 1 - F(t) = \exp\left[-\left(\frac{t-\gamma}{\eta}\right)^{\beta}\right] \qquad t \geq \gamma;\ \beta, \eta > 0 \tag{5.5}$$

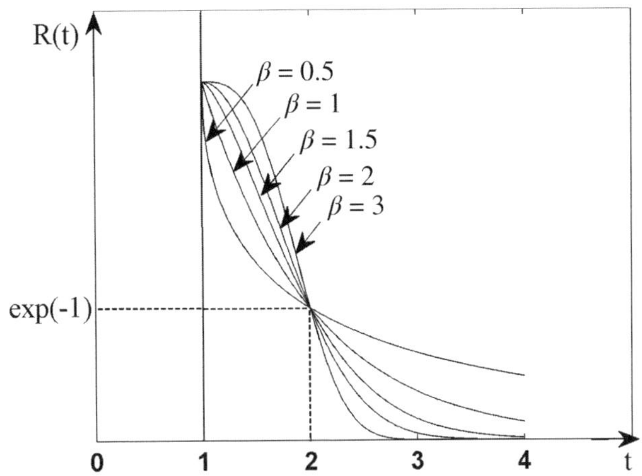

Figure 5.2 Reliability function of Weibull distribution($\eta = 1,\ \gamma = 1$)

There are several methods to estimate the parameters in a Weibull distribution by taking advantage of failure data. Three principal methods are least squares, maximum likelihood, and moments. These methods are called data fitting methods which treat the Weibull distribution parameters as constants. Another method to obtain the parameters is Bayesian analysis which regards the model parameters as random variables. Since Weibull distribution is more suitable to describe the rule of component failures, it has been widely used in fatigue life prediction.

5.2.2 Bayesian Theorem

The Bayesian method is an efficient analytical tool to consider uncertainties in the remaining life prediction. In principle, Bayesian analysis is grounded on a probabilistic generative model of a process. With the generative model, Bayes' theorem provides an approach to inferring one or more parameters in a process from the observed data, where the parameters are supposed to characterize the process of interest. In the Bayesian viewpoint, probability can be used to quantify degrees of belief of inference with given assumptions. Thus, Bayesian inference deals with uncertainty of unknown parameters or hypotheses of interest in probabilistic forms. Under a Bayesian framework, the unknown quantities are modeled as random variables, instead of constants or fixed values. When new information is obtained, prior knowledge about the unknown quantities of interest is revised accordingly. In this regard, Bayes' theorem provides a formal mechanism to revise or update prior beliefs in the light of new data to yield posterior probability statements about the unknown parameters or hypotheses. The general paradigm of a Bayesian inference analysis can be sketched as the hierarchical flow chart displayed in Figure 5.3 [6].

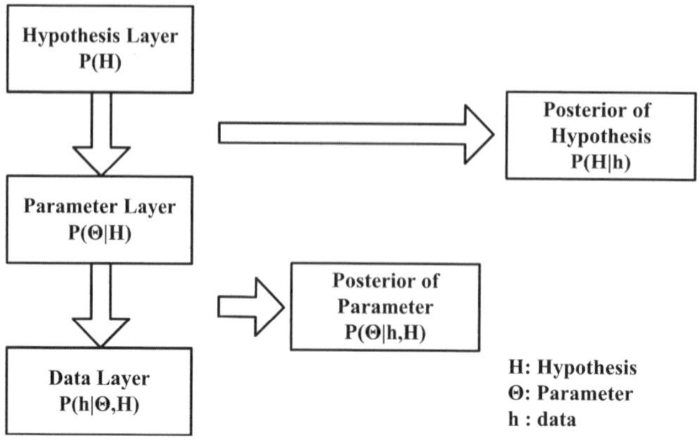

Figure 5.3 A three-layer hierarchical Bayesian analysis model [7]

On the top of the Bayesian network is the hypothesis or model layer, which defines a hypothesis or model with its associated parameter set. Presumably, the observed data is sampled from this generative model. Before observing the data, there is some subjective belief of the hypothesis or model along with its associated parameter set, which is termed as "prior". In order to understand the accurate meaning of probability expressions, it is necessary to learn some terminology used in the Bayesian theorem [7].

The probability that a proposition x has a particular value is denoted by $P(x|I)$, where "$|I$" indicates that the probability is conditional on some background information I. That is, the probability of anything to the left of "|" is conditional on anything to the right of "|". In addition, care is taken to declare the appropriate information on which the probability is based. This underscores an important property of a consistent reasoning process, that in order to make an inference concerning a particular proposition, the available and appropriate information must be declared and taken into account.

An important property of probabilities $P(x|I)$ is that they are bounded below by 0 and above by 1, such that $0 \leq P(x|I) \leq 1$, where $x \in \theta$ for a complete set of propositions or hypotheses. This property asserts the positivity property of probabilities. For example, suppose $x \cup \overline{x}$ where $\overline{x}$ represents the proposition of x not true, then the probabilities must be normalized to unity over Θ to satisfy the above-mentioned property,

$$P(x|I) + P(\overline{x}|I) = 1 \tag{5.6}$$

In general, for a complete set of N independent probabilities, we expect them to be normalized such that $\sum_{i=1}^{N} P(x_i|I) = 1$.

1. *Product rule*

   The product rule for probabilities defines the joint probability of two or more propositions. Given the two propositions, x and y, the probability that x and y are both true is the probability that one, say x, is true multiplied by the probability that y is true, given the truth of x,

$$P(x, y|I) = P(x|I)P(y|x, I) \tag{5.7}$$

Since x and y are interchangeable, we also have,

$$P(x, y|I) = P(y|I)P(x|y, I) \tag{5.8}$$

where $P(x, y|I)$ reads the probability of "x and y" conditional on I. The product rule enables a joint probability to be decomposed into its constituents, and demonstrates that such conditions are in fact symmetrical. In the case of probabilistic independence, where $P(x|y, I) = P(x|I)$ and $P(y|x, I) = P(y|I)$, the equations become

$$P(x, y|I) = P(y|I)P(x|I) \tag{5.9}$$

2. *Addition rule or "marginalization"*
   Now suppose we have a set of propositions $\{x_i;\ i = 1, 2, \ldots, M\}$ and $\{y_i;\ i = 1, 2, \ldots, N\}$, respectively, and where $M \neq N$. The generalization of the additivity properties can be expressed as

$$P(\{y_i\}|I) = \sum_{i=1}^{M} P(\{y_i\},\ \{x_i\}|I) \tag{5.10a}$$

$$= \sum_{i=1}^{M} P(\{x_i\}|I)P(\{y_i\}|\ \{x_i\},\ I) \tag{5.10b}$$

where we have used the product rule to decompose the joint probability. Also by symmetry, we have

$$P(\{x_i\}|I) = \sum_{j=1}^{N} P(\{x_i\},\ \{y_i\}|I) \tag{5.11a}$$

$$= \sum_{j=1}^{N} P(\{y_i\}|I)P(\{x_i\}|\ \{y_i\},\ I) \tag{5.11b}$$

In the above cases, we have defined marginalization of joint probabilities for a discrete set of variables. Both Equations 5.10b and 5.11b are also known as the total probability theorem. The same holds for continuous variables, such that $x \in X$, $y \in Y$ and $X, Y \subseteq R$,

$$P(x|I) = \int_{Y} P(x,\ y|I)\mathrm{d}y \tag{5.12}$$

$$P(y|I) = \int_{X} P(x,\ y|I)\mathrm{d}x \tag{5.13}$$

3. *Bayes theorem*

Mathematically, assuming a hypothesis or model H is given and we denote the observed data by $\mathbf{h}$, the Bayesian formula to infer the parameter set $\boldsymbol{\theta}$ is given by

$$P(\boldsymbol{\theta}|\mathbf{h}, H) = \frac{P(\mathbf{h}|\boldsymbol{\theta}, H)P(\boldsymbol{\theta}|H)}{P(\mathbf{h}|H)} \tag{5.14}$$

where the denominator $P(\mathbf{h}|H) = \int_{\boldsymbol{\theta}} P(\mathbf{h}|\boldsymbol{\theta}, H)P(\boldsymbol{\theta}|H)\mathrm{d}\boldsymbol{\theta}$.

The left-hand side of Equation 5.14 asserts the plausibility of $\boldsymbol{\theta}$ given the data $\mathbf{h}$. This is termed the posterior probability of $\boldsymbol{\theta}$ conditional on $\mathbf{h}$ and H. In other words, $P(\boldsymbol{\theta}|\mathbf{h}, H)$ quantifies a scientist's state of knowledge "after" performing the experiment and obtaining the data. On the right-hand side, the prior information is defined by $P(\boldsymbol{\theta}, H)$, which asserts the plausibility of $\boldsymbol{\theta}$ "before" the experiment has been conducted. The likelihood probability, $P(\mathbf{h}|\boldsymbol{\theta}, H)$ quantifies the plausibility of the data $\mathbf{h}$, conditional on $\boldsymbol{\theta}$ and H. An important observation to make regarding Equation 5.14 is the role the prior term plays in reversing the statement asserting "the plausibility of the data $\mathbf{h}$, given $\boldsymbol{\theta}$ and H" to asserting "the plausibility of $\boldsymbol{\theta}$ conditional on $\mathbf{h}$ and H". Logically, these statements are not equal, and it is the assertions of the prior which plays a critical role. In many applications of Bayesian analysis, such as parameter estimation, it is sufficient to state

$$P(\boldsymbol{\theta}|\mathbf{h}, H) \propto P(\boldsymbol{\theta}|H)P(\mathbf{h}|\boldsymbol{\theta}, H) \tag{5.15}$$

and ignore the denominator, since it plays the role of a normalization constant. The resulting equation can be used to determine the most probable parameter value, say $\widehat{\boldsymbol{\theta}}$, such that $\frac{\mathrm{d}P(\boldsymbol{\theta}|\mathbf{h}, H)}{\mathrm{d}\boldsymbol{\theta}} = 0$ for $\boldsymbol{\theta} = \widehat{\boldsymbol{\theta}}$.

Bayes discovered the way to combine prior information for a hypothesis with the probability of the observed data if the hypothesis were true to give the probability of the hypothesis itself.

5.3 Dynamic Life Prediction Using Time Series

5.3.1 General Introduction

As mentioned previously, most of the existing prediction models are static, which means these models do not update with time. This will generate large errors in long-term RUL prediction. A better option is to re-train the models with new data, which is called dynamic life prediction. First we will introduce the procedure of regular RUL prediction using a time series before the dynamic RUL prediction is discussed.

A time series is a sequence of data points measured typically at successive points in time spaced at uniform time intervals. In remaining life prediction, a time series

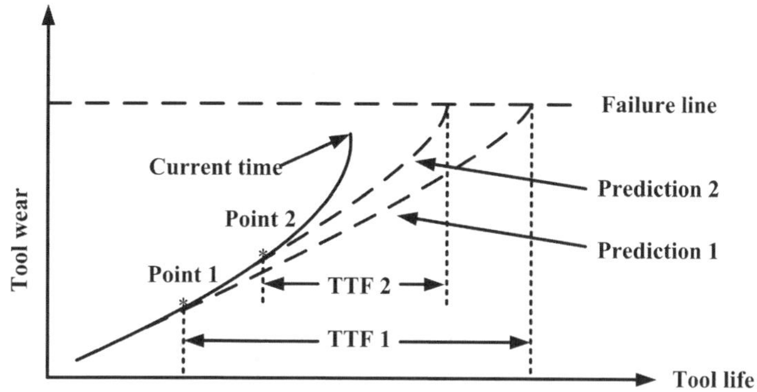

Figure 5.4 Prediction time to failure at each moment

is the most convenient and suitable type of data to adopt, such as vibration, pressure, and temperature signals. Degradation indices extracted from these signals are still in the form of a time series. Based on these indices, prediction models can be built. It is noted that the model training process adopts the historical samples offline. The time series based RUL prediction is always performed by the continuous single-step ahead method. The diagram is shown in Figure 5.4.

At the moment of point 1, the corresponding prediction trajectory is shown as a dashed curve prediction 1, and TTF1 is the time to failure of the moment. The prediction tendency and time to failure of point 2 are also shown in Figure 5.4. At each moment, the predicted tendency and time to failure are calculated by the continuous single-step ahead method as shown in Figure 5.5.

According to Figure 5.5, in order to predict the RUL at moment t_1, $N-1$ points before t_1 of the time series $d_{t_1-N+1}\ d_{t_1-N+2}\ \cdots\ d_{t_1-1}$ are used as inputs of the prediction model and the output $\hat{d}_{t_1}$ is the predicted indicator value. In step 2, the inputs are updated by removing the first value d_{t_1-N+1} and adding the new value $\hat{d}_{t_1}$ as the last data. The output in this step is $\hat{d}_{t_1+1}$. Then, following the same updating method, we get a series of predicted data until the last predicted value overcomes a preset failure line. This process corresponds to the dashed lines in Figure 5.4 and the RUL can be calculated for moment t_1. By comparing the predicted RULs with historical records, the best parameter set is chosen for the prediction model. This whole process can be performed offline. Finally, this trained model can be used for online RUL prediction when the online time series is available.

However, this traditional prediction procedure does not take advantage of the online information. As time goes on, more and more online data are collected which can be used to improve the model accuracy. If online model parameter identification is implemented using a real-life performance index, then the prediction is called dynamic life prediction.

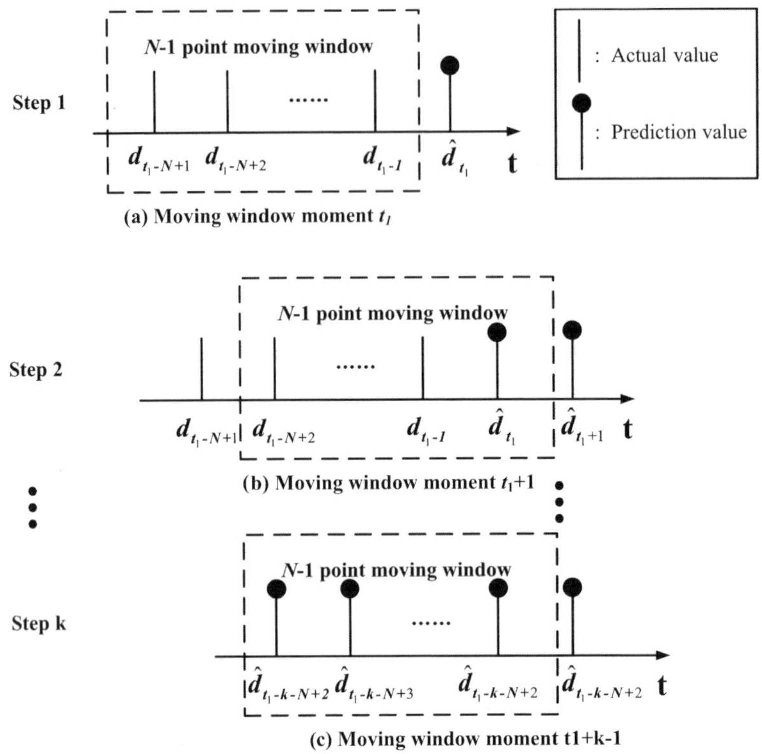

Figure 5.5 Prediction procedure for moment t_1

5.3.2 Prediction Models

In this section several commonly used RUL prediction models, such as the auto-regressive and moving average (ARMA) model, the grey model (GM), the artificial neural network (ANN), the hidden Markov model (HMM), the logistic regression (LR), and the support vector machine (SVM), will be introduced for time-series prediction.

5.3.2.1 ARMA Model

The ARMA (p, q) or Box–Jenkins model is one of the most traditional techniques in statistical time-series analysis. The ARMA prediction model essentially consists of feed-forward and feed-back linear combiners. The feed-forward portion acts as a moving average (MA) or all-zero network whereas the feed-back portion functions as an auto-regressive (AR) or all-pole network. Thus the ARMA model contains both feed-forward and feed-back coefficients which need to be properly trained using an appropriate learning algorithm. The general framework is shown in Figure 5.6 [8].

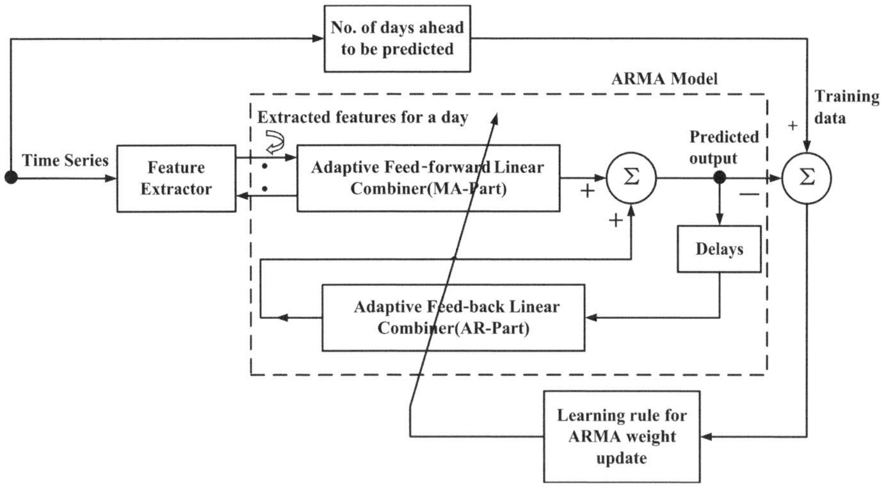

Figure 5.6 A generalized ARMA prediction model [8]

Generally the ARMA model is of the form:

$$x_t = \alpha_1 x_{t-1} + \cdots + \alpha_p x_{t-p} + \epsilon_t - \beta_1 \epsilon_{t-1} - \cdots \beta_q \epsilon_{t-q} \tag{5.16}$$

where x_t is the output of a stationary ARMA (p, q) process, p the order of the autoregressive part, q the order of the moving-average part, $\alpha_1, \cdots, \alpha_p$ are the autoregressive parameters, and $\beta_1, \cdots, \beta_q$ are the moving-average parameters; ϵ_t denotes the series of errors.

Equation 5.16 can be expressed as [9]:

$$x_t = \sum_{k=1}^{p} \alpha_k x_{t-k} - \sum_{k=0}^{q} \beta_k \epsilon_{t-k} \tag{5.17}$$

Note that if all β_k are zero except β_0; then the ARMA model reduces to the AR model. If all α_q are zero, then the model reduces to the MA model. The coefficients β_k are referred to as the MA coefficients. It has been established that determination of the AR coefficients is a linear problem whereas determination of the MA coefficients is a non-linear problem, since the model error $X^{(0)}$, and hence the MA coefficients β_k, cannot be computed until the model has been fitted and the AR coefficients have been determined. Thus, the AR technique has a computational advantage over the ARMA technique.

It is convenient to express Equation 5.16 in terms of a finite number of ARand/or MA components. An AR model seeks to represent a time series x by a linear regression of x on itself plus an error series assumed to be noise with a Gaussian distribution.

The way of approaching the modeling of such an ARMA (p, q) process is to first determine the model orders p and q. This part is done offline. The specific procedure is as follows [10]:

1. Performance calculation using Equation 5.16 a series of performance indices is obtained.
2. Choose suitable p, q:

```
Do {
     ARMA model order (p, q) selection
     ARMA model validation
   } while ARMA model is rejected;
```

After p and q are determined, the online ARMA model parameters identification is implemented using a real-life performance index; prediction can then be done based on the built dynamic ARMA model.

5.3.2.2 Grey Model

Grey system theory was originally proposed by Deng. It is able to deal effectively with incomplete data for system analysis, modeling, prediction, decision-making, and controlling. Grey system theories have been successfully applied in many fields such as management, economics, engineering, and finance. Within a grey system, the information is not completely clear or unknown as in a white or black system. Grey systems set each stochastic variable as a grey quantity that changes within a given range. They deal directly with the original data and search the intrinsic regularity of data [11]. The gray forecasting model can be effectively applied to various cases with the minimum data. For instance, GM(1, 1) is a time-series forecasting model which is the most widely used in the literature, pronounced as "Grey Model First Order One Variable". The differential equations of the GM(1,1) model have time-varying coefficients. In other words, the model is renewed as new data become available to the prediction model. The GM(1,1) model can only be used in positive data sequences and it has five basic operations [12]:

1. obtain the original data series: $X^{(0)}$
2. do accumulated generating operation (AGO) to obtain data series: $X^{(1)}$
3. estimate parameters
4. predict future point $X^{(1)}$
5. and apply inverse accumulated generating operation (IAGO) to predict values for original data series $X^{(0)}$.

The gray forecasting model uses accumulated operations to construct differential equations. For an initial time sequence $X^{(0)} = \{X^{(0)}(1), X^{(0)}(2), \ldots, X^{(0)}(i), \ldots, X^{(0)}(n)\}$, where $X^{(0)}$ (i) is the time-series data at time i. AGO is used to transform an original set of data into a new set that highlights trends but has less noise and randomness. The equation used in generating the AGO series is:

$$X^{(1)}(k) = \sum\nolimits_{i=1}^{k} X^{(0)}(i) \tag{5.18}$$

Where $X^{(1)} = \{X^{(1)}(1), X^{(1)}(2), \ldots, X^{(1)}(i), \ldots, X^{(1)}(n)\}$. After $X^{(1)}$ is obtained, the grey differential equation with one variable is built as:

$$\frac{\mathrm{d}X^{(1)}}{\mathrm{d}t} + aX^{(1)} = b \tag{5.19}$$

where coefficients a and b express the relationship between $\mathrm{d}X/\mathrm{d}t$ (how fast the current state changes) and X (the current state). a and b can be determined by the least-squares method. Then, the predicted data points for the AGO series are calculated. Let $X^{(1)}$ represent the predicted AGO series. IAGO is used to transform the forecasted AGO data series back into the original data series with the equation $\underline{X}^{(0)}(i+1) = \underline{X}^{(0)}(i+1) - \underline{X}^{(0)}(i)$, where $X^{(0)}$ is the predicted original data series.

Generally speaking, grey system theory is a very important method in the field of prediction and decision-making. However, the prediction accuracy of the GM(1, 1) model is always limited by the boundary value, the background value, and the initial value [13]. In Ref. [14] a genetic algorithm was used to optimize the background value and translational parameter of the GM(1, 1) model and the residual model. But this way still has its limitation because not all models can build their residual models. In the process of modeling, we use a sine function to deal with sequence, introduce boundary value parameters approximately and optimize parameters by using an improved genetic algorithm. Finally, we correct the predicted sequence by building a metabolism model through which we can effectively increase prediction precision.

5.3.2.3 Fuzzy Regression Model

Statistical models use the concept of measurement error to deal with the difference between estimations and observations, but these data are precise values and do not include measurement errors. It is also the same for the basic concept of the fuzzy regression model as suggested by Tanaka and Ishibuchi. The basic concept of the fuzzy theory of fuzzy regression is that the residuals between estimations and observations are not produced by measurement errors, but rather by the parameter uncertainty in the model, and the possibility distribution is used to deal with real observations. The following is a generalized model of fuzzy linear regression [15]:

$$\widetilde{Y} = \widetilde{\beta}_0 + \widetilde{\beta}_1 x_1 + \cdots + \widetilde{\beta}_n x_n = \sum_{i=0}^{n} \widetilde{\beta}_i x_i = X'\widetilde{\beta} \tag{5.20}$$

where X is the vector of independent variables, prime ($'$) denotes the transposition operation, n is the number of variables, and $\widetilde{\beta}_i$ represents fuzzy sets representing the

ith parameter of the model. Instead of using a crisp, fuzzy parameter $\widetilde{\beta_i}$ in the form of the L-type fuzzy numbers of Dubois and Prade, $(\alpha_i, c_i)_L$ the possibility distribution is:

$$\mu_{\widetilde{\beta}_i}(\widetilde{\beta_i}) = L\left\{\frac{\alpha_i - \beta_i}{c}\right\} \tag{5.21}$$

where L is a function type. Fuzzy parameters in the form of triangular fuzzy numbers are used:

$$\mu_{\widetilde{\beta}_i}(\widetilde{\beta_i}) = L\begin{cases} 1 - \dfrac{|\alpha_i - \beta_i|}{c_i} & \alpha_i - c_i \le \beta_i \le \alpha_i + c_i, \\ 0 & \text{otherwise,} \end{cases} \tag{5.22}$$

where $\mu_{\widetilde{\beta}_i}(\beta_i)$ the membership function of the fuzzy set is represented by a parameter, α_i is the center of the fuzzy number and c_i is the width or spread around the center of the fuzzy number. Using the extension principle, the membership function of the fuzzy number $\widetilde{y}_t = x'_t\widetilde{\beta}$ can be defined using a pyramidal fuzzy parameter as follows:

$$\mu_{\widetilde{y}}(y_t)\begin{cases} 1 - \dfrac{|y_t - X_t\alpha|}{c'|X_t|} & \text{for}\, X_t \ne 0, \\ 1 & \text{for}\, X_t = 0, y_t = 0, \\ 0 & \text{for}\, X_t = 0, y_t \ne 0, \end{cases} \tag{5.23}$$

Where α and c denote vectors of model values and spreads for all model parameters, respectively; and t is the number of observations, $t = 1, 2, \ldots, k$. Finally, the method uses the criterion of minimizing the total vagueness, S, defined as the sum of individual spreads of the fuzzy parameters of the model:

$$\text{Minimize} \quad S = \sum_{t=1}^{k} c'|X_t| \tag{5.24}$$

At the same time, this approach takes into account the condition that the membership value of each observation y_t is greater than an imposed threshold, h-level, $h \in [0, 1]$. This criterion data simply express the fact that the fuzzy output of the model should be over all the data points $y_1, y_2, \ldots y_k$ to a certain h-level. The choice of the h-level value influences the widths c of the fuzzy parameters:

$$\mu_{\widetilde{y}}(y_t) \ge h \quad \text{for}\, t = 1, 2, \ldots, k. \tag{5.25}$$

The index t refers to the number of non-fuzzy data used in constructing the model. The problem of finding the fuzzy regression parameters was formulated by Tanaka and Ishibuchi [12] as a linear programing problem:

$$\text{Minimize} \quad S = \sum_{t=1}^{k} c'|X_t|,$$

$$\text{subject to} \quad \begin{cases} X_t'\alpha + (1-h)\,c'|X_t| \geq y_t, & t = 1,2,\ \ldots\ ,k. \\ X_t'\alpha - (1-h)c'|X_t| \leq y_t, & t = 1,2,\ \ldots\ ,k. \\ c \geq 0, \end{cases} \tag{5.26}$$

where $\alpha' = (\alpha_{1,}\alpha_{2,}\ \ldots\ ,\alpha_n)$ and $c' = (c_{1,}c_{2,}\ \ldots\ ,c_n)$ are vectors of unknown variables and S is the total vagueness as previously defined.

5.3.2.4 ANN Model

Artificial neural networks are flexible computing frameworks for modeling a broad range of non-linear problems. One significant advantage of the ANN models over other classes of non-linear models is that ANNs are universal approximators that can approximate a large class of functions with a high degree of accuracy. Their power comes from the parallel processing of the information from the data. No prior assumption of the model form is required in the model building process. Instead, the network model is largely determined by the characteristics of the data. A single hidden layer feed-forward network is the most widely used model form for time series modeling and forecasting. The model is characterized by a network of several layers of simple processing units connected by an acyclic link, as shown in Figure 5.7.

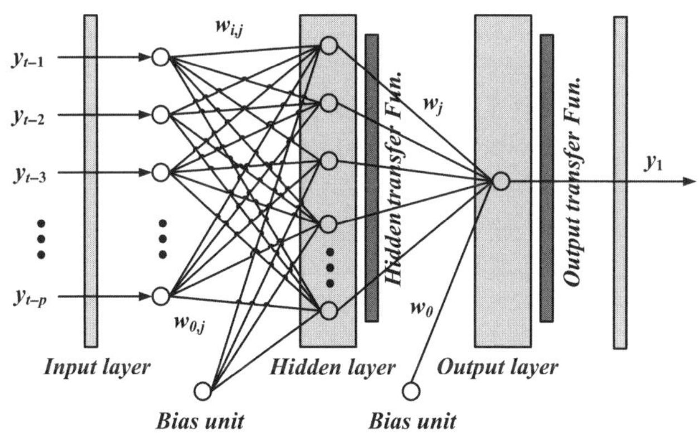

Figure 5.7 Structure of ANN

The relationship between the output (y_t) and the inputs ($y_{t-1}, y_{t-2}, \ldots, y_{t-p}$) has the following mathematical representation:

$$y_t = \omega_0 + \sum_{i=1}^{Q} \omega_j g\left(\omega_{oj} + \sum_{i=1}^{P} \omega_{ij} y_{t-1}\right) + e_t \tag{5.27}$$

where ω_{ij} ($i = 0, 1, 2, \ldots, P, j = 0, 1, 2, \ldots, Q$) and $\omega_j(j = 0, 1, 2, \ldots, Q)$ are model parameters often called connection weights; P is the number of input nodes; and Q is the number of hidden nodes. The logistic function is often used as the hidden layer transfer function, which includes a sigmoid function and a tan-sigmoid function. The mathematical expressions are given as Equations 5.28 and 5.29, and the shape curves are shown in Figures 5.8 and 5.9.

$$y = \frac{1}{1 + e^{-x}} \tag{5.28}$$

$$y = \frac{2}{1 + e^{-2x}} - 1 \tag{5.29}$$

Hence, the ANN model of Equation 5.27, in fact, performs a non-linear functional mapping from the past observations to the future value y_t, that is,

$$y_t = f(y_{t-1}, \ldots, y_{t-p}, W) + e_t \tag{5.30}$$

where W is a vector of all parameters and $f(\cdot)$ is a function determined by the network structure and connection weights. Thus, the neural network is equivalent to a non-linear autoregressive model. Note that Equation 5.30 implies one output node in the output layer, which is typically used for one-step-ahead forecasting. The simple network given by Equation 5.30 is surprisingly powerful in that it is able to

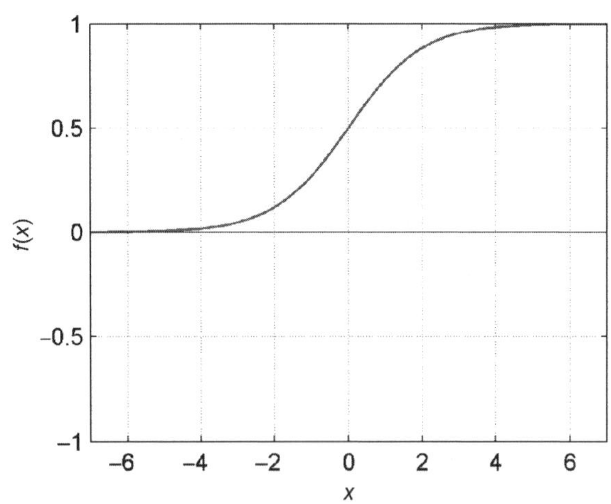

Figure 5.8 Sigmoid function plot

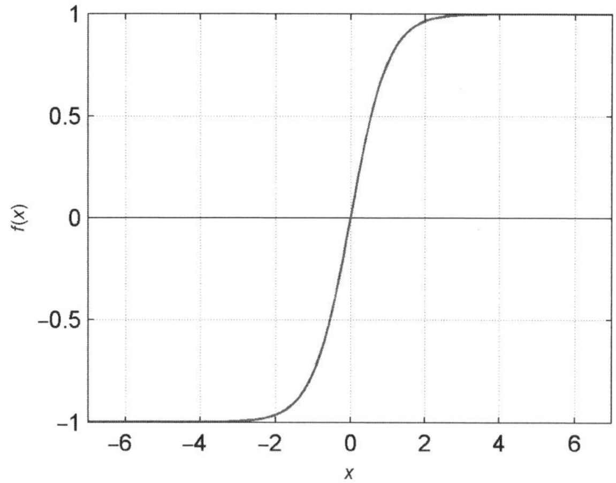

Figure 5.9 A tan-sigmoid function

approximate an arbitrary function as the number of hidden nodes Q is sufficiently large. In practice, a simple network structure that has a small number of hidden nodes often works well in out-of-sample forecasting. This may be due to the over-fitting effect typically found in a neural network modeling process. It occurs when the network has too many free parameters, which allow the network to fit the training data well, but typically lead to poor generalization. In addition, it has been shown experimentally that the generalization ability begins to deteriorate when the network has been trained more than necessary, that is when it begins to fit the noise of the training data.

Although ANN models have been widely used in many fields, several problems still need to be solved when the ANN models are utilized. The current existing problems of model optimization and their solutions are described as follows:

1. *Number of Hidden Nodes Identification*: The number of hidden neural nodes determine the structure of the network and the distribution of the error surface directly, unfortunately, there is not a mature method to instruct how to choose the proper hidden nodes. Based on experience, the hidden layer neural nodes range can be decided according to

$$N_{\mathrm{H}} = \sqrt{N_{\mathrm{O}} + N_{\mathrm{I}}} + \alpha \tag{5.31}$$

   where N_{H} is the number of hidden neural nodes, N_{O} is the number of neural nodes of the output layer, N_{I} is the number of neural nodes of the input layer and α is a constant between 1 and 10. Then, based on the nodes range, build the model of each network. Finally, compare each model's MSE (mean square error) to choose the smallest one as the optimal model.
2. *Initial Values of Weights and Biases Selection*: The initial values of the weights and biases directly determine the beginning optimize point in the error surface;

therefore, the initial value has a significant influence on the network's training time and training error. Here, we build a bunch of neural networks (the number is N_C) by initializing each network's weights and biases randomly, and then average the N_C trained network's output values, finally, we compare each model's MSE to choose the one with the smallest MSE as the optimal model for performance evaluation, M_E.

3. *Iteration Algorithm Selection*: The iteration algorithm has an impact on the running time of the network training process, for example, the gradient method has powerful local searching ability, but it is easy to fall into local minimum points; in contrast, the conjugate-gradient method has fast convergence speed and it is not easy to fall into local minimum points. Here, the conjugate-gradient method was employed as the iteration algorithm to perform optimization.
4. *Transfer Function Selection*: The transfer function contributes to convergence time and accuracy. For example, the sigmoid transfer function is defined as Equation 5.28. The range of y is between 0 and 1, when x is close to 0, the optimization speed of iteration is good, however, the optimization speed slows when x is away from 0. In contrast, for the tan-sigmoid transfer function defined as Equation 5.29, the range of y is between -1 and 1, its gradient is larger than that of the sigmoid function, which results in the optimization speed being faster than with the sigmoid function. Therefore the tan-sigmoid function was employed as the hidden layer transfer function and the output layer function relies on its output range: if the output range is between 0 and 1, then we choose the sigmoid transfer function or its improved transfer function; if the range is between -1 and 1, then we choose the tan-sigmoid transfer function to meet the mapping requirements

In order to predict the future performance value based upon a time-series value at an earlier point in time, the performance assessment results are used as inputs to the life prediction model M_P. The specific implementation procedures are described as follows: N-point time series sliding window. So, as the predicting time t increases, we can decompose one sample into a multi-group training datum to build one sample performance degradation prediction model, similarly, set up the other sample's training data. Eventually choose the network's proper transfer function, iterative algorithm, learning rate, and other parameters to train the model.

After the prediction model is obtained, use the trained model to carry out single-step continuous prediction, the specific implementation procedures are described as follows:

With the well trained network, we can get the remaining life prediction curve through single-step prediction. The evaluation standard of an optimal life prediction model is to compare the error calculated by Equation 5.32

$$\overline{E} = \frac{\sum_{i=1}^{n} |\hat{y}_i - y_i|}{n} \tag{5.32}$$

where $\hat{y}_i$ is the predicted remaining life from the predicted time point to the actual failure time point ($i = 1,2,3 \ldots \ldots n$); y_i is the actual remaining life from the predicted time point to the actual failure time point; n is the total predicted time from the first predicted time point to the last predicted time point.

In the above we introduce the procedure of using an ANN model to perform RUL prediction with input updating but the ANN model does not change once it has been trained. However, because the actual equipment/components have differences between samples, if we use the static life prediction model M_P to predict the remaining life this will lead to great error, therefore, in order to improve the model's robustness and accuracy of prediction we update the M_P's weights and biases at each predicting time point to get a new life prediction model M_P', and then use M_P' to carry out the RUL prediction. The specific implementation procedures are described as follows:

Get the K-point ($K > N$) time-series performance value before the prediction time $t = T$ as the sample to adjust the life prediction model M_P's weights and biases, and then, as shown in Figure 5.10, decompose the K-point time series into several N-point time series, such as $\{d_{T-K}, d_{T-K+1}, \ldots\ldots d_{T-K+N-1}\}$, $\{d_{T-K+1}, d_{T-K+2}, \ldots\ldots d_{T-K+N}\}, \ldots,$ $\{d_{T-N+2}, d_{T-N+3}, \ldots\ldots d_{T-1}\}$, so we can get $K - N + 1$ samples to adjust the model's weights and biases, see Figure 5.10. As the number of samples is limited, therefore, during the process of model adjusting, it is easy to generate a large error as a result of overtraining. Here, we adopt a slower iterative algorithm, a small learning rate, and short times of training epochs to avoid overtraining.

In order to evaluate the accuracy of prediction we employ the mean error and certainty factor as the criterion shown below:

$$\mu = \frac{1}{n}\sum(x_i - \hat{x}_i) \tag{5.33}$$

$$r^2 = 1 - \frac{\frac{1}{n}\sum(x_i - \hat{x}_i)^2}{\frac{1}{n}\sum(x_i - \bar{x})^2} \tag{5.34}$$

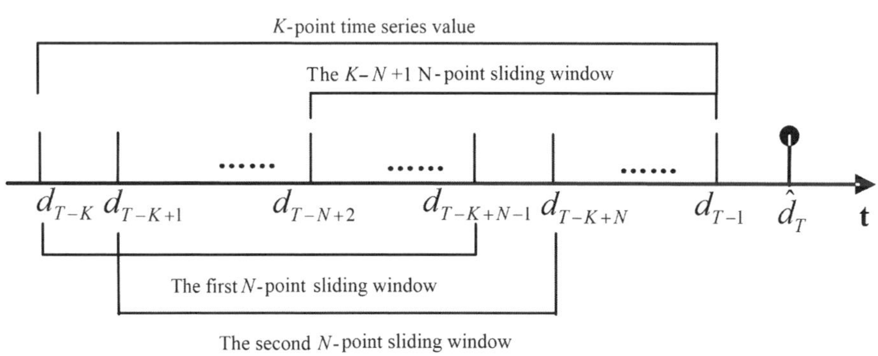

Figure 5.10 Dynamic weights and biases adjustment

where x_i is the actual value, $\widehat{x}_i$ is the predictive value and $\overline{x}$ is the average value of $\widehat{x}_i$ $(i=1 \ldots n)$. μ is used to evaluate the degree of predictive value deviation from the actual value and r^2 is a certainty factor, the predictive result is best with $r^2=1$.

5.3.2.5 SVM Regression Model

The learning process of a SVM regression model is essentially a problem in quadratic programing. Given a set of data points $(x_1, y_1) \cdots (x_k, y_k)$ such that $x_i \in R^n$ is the input and $y_i \in R^n$ the target output, the regression problem is to find a function such as Equation 5.35.

$$f(x) = (\omega \ \ldots \ x) + b \tag{5.35}$$

where $\omega, x \in R^n, b \in R$.

After training, the corresponding y can be found through $f(x)$ for the x outside the sample. The e-support vector regression (e-SVR) by Vapnik controls the precision of the algorithm through a specified tolerance error ϵ. The error of the sample is ζ, regardless of the loss, when $|\zeta| \leq \epsilon$; else consider the loss as $|\zeta| - \epsilon$. First, map the sample into a high dimensional feature space by a non-linear mapping function and convert the problem of the non-linear function estimates into a linear regression problem in a high dimensional feature space. If we let $\varphi(x)$ be the conversion function from the sample-space into the high dimension feature space, then the problem of solving the parameters of $f(x)$ is converted to solving an optimization problem Equation 5.36 with the constraints in Equation 5.37.

$$\min \frac{1}{2}\|\omega\|^2 = \frac{1}{2}(\omega \cdot \omega) \tag{5.36}$$

$$\text{subject to} \begin{cases} y_i - (\omega \cdot \phi(x) + b) \leq \epsilon \\ (\omega \cdot \phi(x) + b) - y_i \leq \epsilon \end{cases} \quad i = 1, 2, \cdots l \tag{5.37}$$

The feature space is one of high dimensionality and the target function is non-differentiable. In general, the SVM regression problem is solved by establishing a Lagrange function, converting this problem to a dual optimization problem, that is, Equation 5.38 with the constraint of Equation 5.39 in order to determine the Lagrange multiplier $\widehat{\alpha}_i, \alpha_i$.

$$\max -\frac{1}{2}\sum_{i,j=1}^{l}(\alpha_i - \widehat{\alpha}_i)(\alpha_j - \widehat{\alpha}_j)(x_i, x_j) - \epsilon\sum_{i=1}^{l}(\alpha_i + \widehat{\alpha}_i) + \sum_{i=1}^{l}(\alpha_i - \widehat{\alpha}_i) \tag{5.38}$$

$$\text{subject to} \begin{cases} \sum_{i=1}^{l} \left(\alpha_i - \widehat{\alpha}_i\right) = 0 \\ \alpha_i, \widehat{\alpha}_i \in [0, c] \end{cases} \tag{5.39}$$

where $\widehat{\alpha}_i$, α_i are Lagrange multipliers and $\alpha_i, \widehat{\alpha}_i \geq 0,\ \alpha_i \times \widehat{\alpha}_i = 0$.

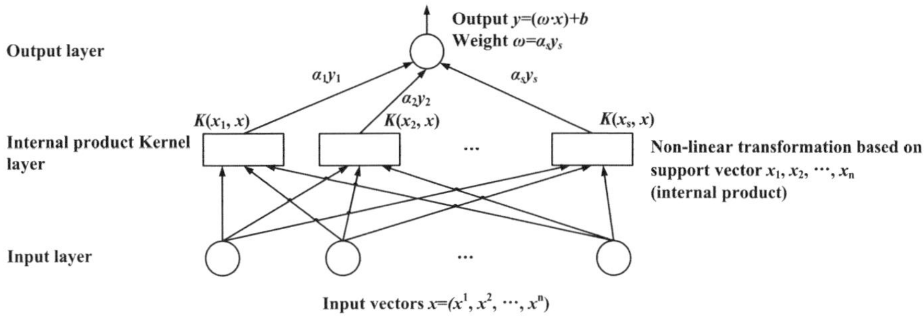

Figure 5.11 Abridged general view of SVM structure

The SVM regression problem has therefore been transformed into a quadratic programing problem. The regression equation can be obtained by solving this problem. With the kernel function $K(x_i, x_j)$, the corresponding regression function is provided by Equation 5.40.

$$f(x) = \sum_{i=1}^{N}(\alpha_i - \hat{\alpha}_i)(\alpha_j - \hat{\alpha}_j)K(x_i, x_j) + b \tag{5.40}$$

where the kernel function $K(x_i, x_j)$ is an internal product of vectors x_i and x_j in feature spaces $\varphi(x_i)$ and $\varphi(x_j)$. Only small parts of α_i and $\widehat{\alpha}_i$ are determined by solving the quadratic programing problem (Equation 5.38). The corresponding data points form the support vectors, as shown in Figure 5.11, which decide the regression function of SVM.

5.3.3 Applications

Suppose we have estimated the selected feature and obtained the degradation indicator for a cracked rotor as the crack propagates. 10 samples have been given and one of their profiles is shown in Figure 5.12. The index represents the health condition of the cracked rotor. It can be seen, as time elapses, that the index drops from almost "1" to "0". In Section 5.3.3.1 we will use the ARMA model and in Section 5.3.3.2 the ANN model to perform the RUL prediction based on these samples.

5.3.3.1 ARMA Model-Based Prediction Method

Here, we follow the procedure of the ARMA prediction method described previously. Given the input number of the ARMA model as 20, and selecting the best order as $p = 2$, $q = 3$: at time $t = 30$, the input vector of the model is the index values from $t = 10$ to $t = 29$. Considering the index drops very fast at the end of the time range, especially when the index value is smaller than 0.6, the RUL is very short. Therefore the threshold is set as 0.6. The prediction result can be seen in Figure 5.13.

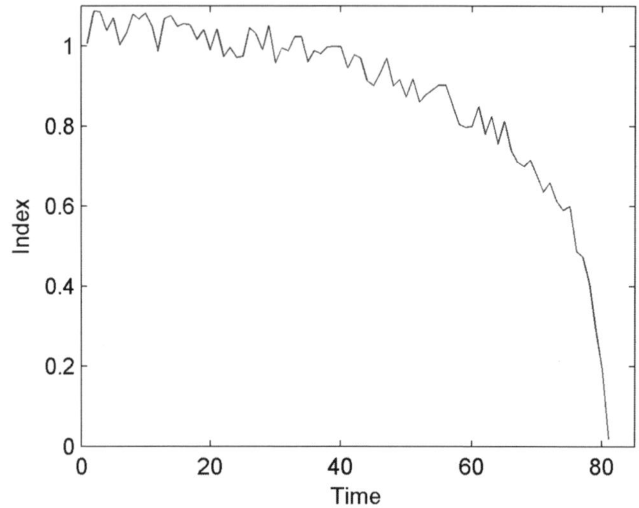

Figure 5.12 Degradation index curve

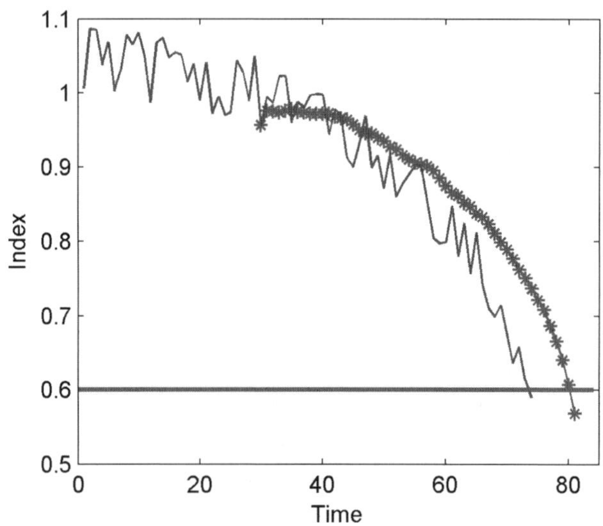

Figure 5.13 Prediction curve at $t = 30$

In Figure 5.13, the solid curve represents the actual index values of the system, the asterisk curve represents the predicted values, and the solid heavy line represents the threshold we set. We can see that the ARMA model gets the general trend of the index curve. At time $t = 81$, the predicted value, which is 0.56, becomes smaller than the threshold value 0.6, therefore we stop the prediction and we consider the prediction life to be $80 - 30 = 50$ time units. But actually, the true index value goes

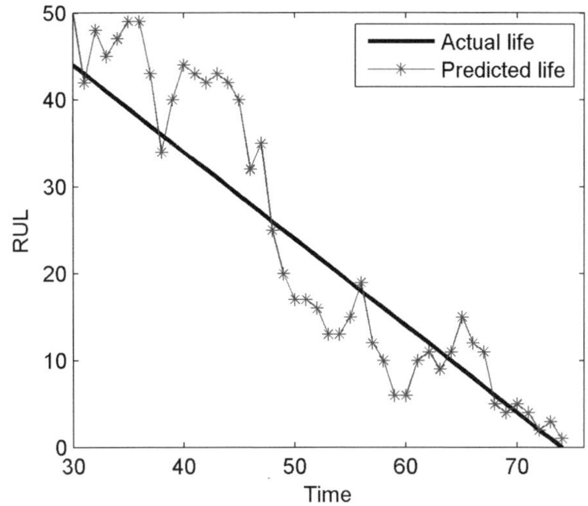

Figure 5.14 Remaining useful life prediction results by ARMA model

below threshold at $t = 73$, indicating the true life is 43 time units. Obviously the error between the predicted life and the true life is equal to 7 at this time moment. Then we calculate the RUL at other time moments and plot all the predicted life values and true life values together as in Figure 5.14.

Figure 5.14 shows that the predicted life values fluctuate around the actual life values. However, the results are acceptable since in the zone of end moments the errors get smaller. The mean absolute error of the whole predicted series is 5.244 units.

5.3.3.2 ANN-Based Prediction Method

Based on the introduction of an ANN-based prediction procedure, the first step of using ANN is to decide the structure of the network, mainly meaning the numbers of the hidden layers and the neuron numbers in each layer. Since usually an ANN contains one hidden layer that can approximate to any non-linear function, we construct a back propagation neural network (BPNN) with one hidden layer, one input layer, and one output layer. The next step is to decide the neuron numbers. Here we choose the index value at the current moment and its former four values as the input variables. The output value is the index value at the next moment which is actually the target value as the supervisor information in the training process and the prediction value in the testing process. Hence, according to Equation 5.31, the range of neuron numbers is from 3 to 13. For each neuron number of the hidden layer, 10 networks were built and the average prediction value is considered the final predicted result in order to eliminate the random influence of the initial connection weights between the neurons. For the total 10 index samples, 6 samples were randomly selected as the training samples

Table 5.1 Training error for different hidden neuron numbers

Hidden node	3	4	5	6	7	8	9	10	11	12	13
Prediction error	2.5	1.8	2.1	1.8	2.0	1.9	2.0	1.9	1.9	2.0	2.1
$\overline{E}$	54	68	41	26	39	99	53	03	52	58	82

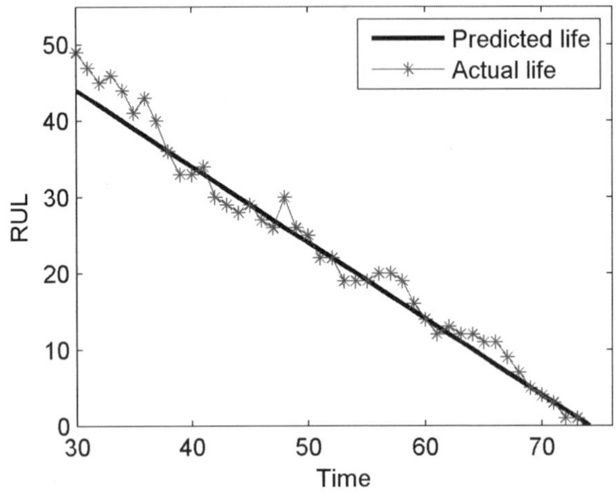

Figure 5.15 Remaining useful life prediction results by ANN model

and the remainder were regarded as the testing samples. Therefore the 6 training samples were used to train the BPNNs for each neuron number of the hidden layer with 10 random initial weights. After the training process, the final mean absolute errors for the BPNNs with different numbers of hidden neurons are listed in Table 5.1.

From Table 5.1, it can be seen that the best hidden node number is 6. Therefore we finally decide the structure of the BPNN and perform the RUL prediction for the testing samples. The RUL prediction results for the same sample as used with the ARMA model are shown in Figure 5.15.

Compared with Figure 5.15, it can be concluded that the BPNN model shows better prediction performance than the ARMA model for this case. The mean absolute error is 1.865 which is much smaller than with the ARMA model. The reason for this is the excellent non-linear mapping capability.

5.4 Remaining Life Prediction by the Crack-Growth Criterion

Since the end of the Second World War, the problem of brittle facture has been studied extensively. Because fractures caused by low stress, which is much smaller than the yield stress of the material, always originate at flaws or cracks of various types, the fracture mechanics approach has proved useful in problems of material development, design, and failure analysis. Beden *et al.* [16] reviewed the development of

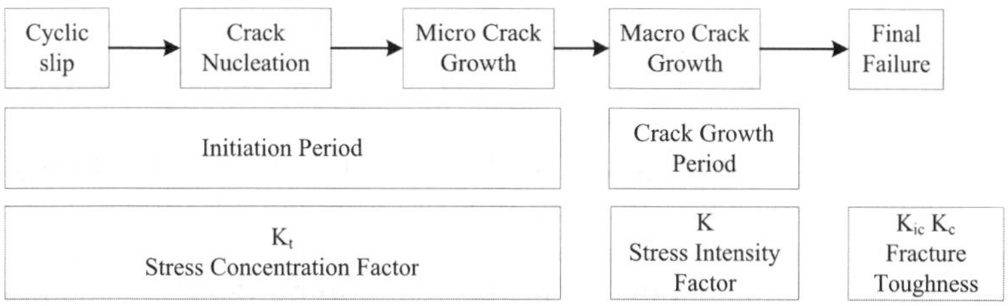

Figure 5.16 Different phase of the fatigue life and relevant factors

crack growth models for both constant amplitude and variable amplitude. Here we will provide the description of the analysis of the crack development process and the propagation models. Then an example will be given to show how to use the Paris law for prediction of component remaining life.

In the 1950s, many investigators mentioned how early in the fatigue life they could observe microcracks. Since then it was clear that the fatigue life under cyclic loading consisted of two phases, the crack initiation life followed by a crack growth period until failure. This can be represented in a block diagram, see Figure 5.16.

The crack initiation period may cover a large percentage of the fatigue life under high-cycle fatigue, that is, under stress amplitudes just above the fatigue limit. But for larger stress amplitudes the crack growth period can be a substantial portion of the fatigue life. A special problem is how to define the transition from the initiation period to the crack growth period. It was in the early 1960s that the stress intensity factor was introduced for the correlation between the crack growth rate, da/dN, and the stress intensity factor range, ΔK. The first paper was published by Paris *et al.* [17], and it turned out to be a milestone publication. In this paper, they adopted the K-value from the analysis of the stress field around the tip of a crack as proposed by Irwin [18]. Another milestone of the application of fracture mechanics, the well-known general equation in polar coordinates for the stress distribution around the crack tip is:

$$\sigma_{ij} = \frac{K}{\sqrt{2\pi r}} f(\theta_{ij}) \tag{5.41}$$

with K as the stress intensity factor and the polar coordinates r and θ. The stress intensity factor is given by:

$$K = \beta S \sqrt{\pi a} \tag{5.42}$$

with β as the geometry factor. The results of the crack growth tests of Paris *et al.* [19] were expressed in terms of da/dN as a function of ΔK on a double log scale, which shows a linear relation between log(da/dN) and log(ΔK). Many more crack growth tests carried out later indicated the same trend which led to the well-known Paris equation:

$$\frac{\mathrm{d}a}{\mathrm{d}N} = C(\Delta K)^m \tag{5.43}$$

with C and m as experimentally obtained constants. The equation is a formal description of the results of a fatigue crack growth experiment. At the same time, it must be recognized that fatigue crack growth is subject to physical laws.

The common approach for fatigue crack growth analysis is to describe the data by a differential equation, which is referred to as a fatigue crack growth law or model. By integrating the equation one can obtain the crack length versus number of cycles (a–N curve) and predict the number of cycles required for the crack to grow from an initial to final size. The differential equation used to describe the data is often of the form

$$\frac{\mathrm{d}a}{\mathrm{d}N} = f(\Delta K,\ R) \tag{5.44}$$

Based on the propagation forms of fatigue cracks, numerous crack-growth models have been developed, especially for constant amplitude loading. A simple and well-known model for predicting fatigue crack propagation is a power law described by Paris and Erdogan [19], and known as the Paris Law which is shown in Equation 5.43. The limitation of the Paris law is that it can only work well when the length of the plastic zone ahead of the crack tip is long compared with the mean grain size but much smaller than the crack length. In addition, the Paris law does not consider the effect of the stress ratio and it depends upon the material used. Considering this, Walker [20] improved the Paris model by including the effect of the stress ratio. A parameter ΔK was proposed which was an equivalent zero to maximum ($R = 0$) stress intensity factor that causes the same growth rate as the actual $K_{\max}$ and R combination. It can be expressed as

$$\overline{\Delta K} = K_{\max}(1 - R)^{\gamma_W} \tag{5.45}$$

where $K_{\max} = \Delta K/(1 - R)$. The above equation becomes

$$\overline{\Delta K} = \frac{\Delta K}{(1 - R)^{1-\gamma_W}} \tag{5.46}$$

Therefore, the Walker law can be represented by

$$\frac{\mathrm{d}a}{\mathrm{d}N} = C_{\mathrm{W}}(\overline{\Delta K})^{m_{\mathrm{W}}} = C_{\mathrm{W}}\left(\frac{\Delta K}{(1 - R)^{1-\gamma_{\mathrm{W}}}}\right)^{m_{\mathrm{W}}} \tag{5.47}$$

The significance of the Walker law is that a log–log plot of $\mathrm{d}a/\mathrm{d}N$ versus ΔK should result in a single straight line regardless of the stress ratio for which the data was obtained.

Forman [21] improved the Walker model by suggesting a new model given by the mathematical relationship as below

$$\frac{\mathrm{d}a}{\mathrm{d}N} = \frac{C_{\mathrm{F}}(\Delta K)^{m_y}}{(1 - R)(K_{\mathrm{C}} - K_{\max})} \tag{5.48}$$

where K_c is the fracture toughness for the material and thickness of interest.

Based on the previous study, other researchers proposed many different models to extend the applications on the crack propagation prediction.

Collipriest model:

$$\frac{\mathrm{d}a}{\mathrm{d}N} = C(K_c \Delta K)^{m/2} EXP\left[\ln\left(\frac{K_c}{\Delta K_o}\right)\operatorname{arctanh}\left(\frac{\ln\left[\frac{\Delta K^2}{(1-R)\,K_c \Delta K_o}\right]}{\ln\left[\frac{(1-R)K_c}{\Delta K_o}\right]}\right)\right] \tag{5.49}$$

McEvily Model:

$$\frac{\mathrm{d}a}{\mathrm{d}N} = \frac{4A}{\pi \sigma_\gamma E}(\Delta K^2 - \Delta K_{\mathrm{th}}^2) \tag{5.50}$$

Frost and Pook *M*odel:

$$\frac{\mathrm{d}a}{\mathrm{d}N} = \frac{9}{\pi}\left(\frac{\Delta K}{E}\right)^2 \quad \text{for plane stress} \tag{5.51}$$

$$\frac{\mathrm{d}a}{\mathrm{d}N} = \frac{7}{\pi}\left(\frac{\Delta K}{E}\right)^2 \quad \text{for plane strain} \tag{5.52}$$

The remaining fatigue life can be obtained by integrating the above crack propagating models for different cases. For the general differential equation (5.43), from a current measured crack a_0 to the final crack length a_{f}, the relationship between the remaining fatigue life N and the crack depth can be represented as

$$N = \int_{a_0}^{a_{\mathrm{f}}} f(\Delta K,\, R)\mathrm{d}a \tag{5.53}$$

For example, suppose the crack propagation of a steel rotor follows the Paris law and all the parameters have been tested in the experiments. By adopting Equation 5.53 we can obtain the relationship curve of the remaining life N and relative crack depth $\mu = a/R$ from 0.1 to 0.7 in Figure 5.17, where a is the crack depth and R is the rotor radius.

One critical step is to establish the parameters in these models. Usually these parameters are estimated from experimental data. For some commonly used materials, the parameters can be found in handbooks. Here is an example to show how to estimate the parameters [22].

For metallic components, the Paris law is the basis of other crack propagation models. It can be written as

$$da/\mathrm{d}N = D(\Delta K)^m \tag{5.54}$$

where D is a material constant of the crack growth equation, ΔK is the range of K during a fatigue cycle, m is the exponent.

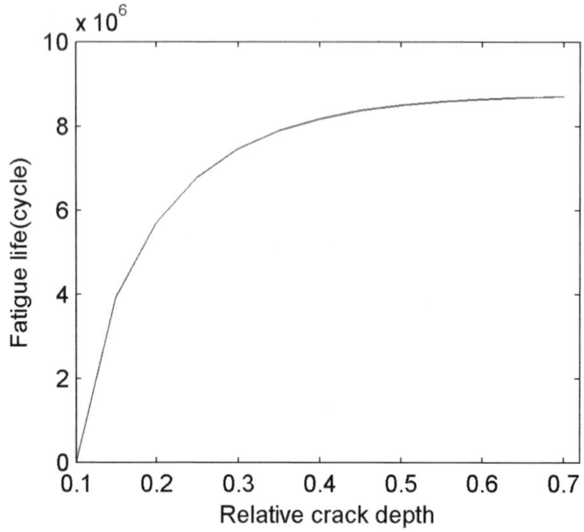

Figure 5.17 Fatigue life versus relative crack depth calculated by Paris law

The range of strain ΔK is given as

$$\Delta K = 2\sigma\alpha(\pi a)^{1/2} \tag{5.55}$$

where σ is gross strain, α is a geometric correction factor, a is the half crack length. Most of these variables are specific to a given material and test article. Usually some simplifying assumptions can be made. For many materials, the crack growth exponent is 2, which will be used as a default value. The geometric correction factor α is set to 1. The Equation 5.54 reduces to

$$\mathrm{d}a/\mathrm{d}N = D(4\sigma^2\pi a) \tag{5.56}$$

The goal is to determine the number of cycles N, remaining until a crack length a is reached. Taking the reciprocal of Equation 5.56, we obtain

$$\mathrm{d}N/\mathrm{d}a = 1/D(4\sigma^2\pi a) \tag{5.57}$$

Then we can integrate the above equation to get the remaining life from a current measured crack a_0 to the final crack length a_f. The relationship can be shown as

$$\begin{aligned} N &= \int_{a_0}^{a_\mathrm{f}} \mathrm{d}N/\mathrm{d}a \\ &= \int_{a_0}^{a_\mathrm{f}} \frac{1}{D(4\sigma^2\pi a)}\mathrm{d}a \\ &= \frac{1}{D(4\sigma^2\pi a)}(\ln(a_\mathrm{f}) - \ln(a_0)) \end{aligned} \tag{5.58}$$

In the above equation, the only unknown parameter is D. A Kalman filter is used to estimate the unknown parameter from observed data. Two Kalman filters are built: one to filter the measured health indicator (HI) and calculate the rate of crack growth; and one to estimate the unknown parameter D. An estimation of the HI and strain σ is derived from the current estimate of D. The state predictions of σ and a are:

$$\frown{a} = \frac{\mathrm{d}a/\mathrm{d}N}{\frown{D}(4\sigma^2\pi a)} \tag{5.59}$$

and

$$\frown{\sigma} = \sqrt{\frac{\mathrm{d}a/\mathrm{d}N}{\frown{D}(4\pi a)}} \tag{5.60}$$

where $\frown{D}$ is the state estimator for D.

The measurement matrix H, which is now the Jacobian of Equations 5.59 and 5.60 is given by

$$H = \begin{bmatrix} -\dfrac{\mathrm{d}a/\mathrm{d}N}{4D^2\pi a\sqrt{\mathrm{d}a/\mathrm{d}N/\frown{D}(4\pi a)}} & 0 \\ -\dfrac{\mathrm{d}a/\mathrm{d}N}{4D^2\pi\sigma^2} & 0 \end{bmatrix} \tag{5.61}$$

A crack growth data set of austenitic steel was used to validate the proposed method. A sequential extended Kalman filter was used to filter the crack length and to calculate $\mathrm{d}a/\mathrm{d}N$. Equations 5.59–5.61 were used to estimate D. The cycles remaining were calculated by using Equation 5.58.

References

1. Jardine, A.K.S., Lin, D. and Banjevic, D. (2006) A review on machinery diagnostics and prognostics implementing condition-based maintenance. *Mechanical Systems and Signal Processing*, **20**, 1483–1510.
2. Zio, E. and Maio, F.D. (2010) A data-driven fuzzy approach for predicting the remaining useful life in dynamic failure scenarios of a nuclear system. *Reliability Engineering and System Safety*, **95**, 49–57.
3. Naderi, M., Hoseini, S.H. and Khonsari, M.M. (2013) Probabilistic simulation of fatigue damage and life scatter of metallic components. *International Journal of Plasticity*, **43**, 101–115.
4. Myötyri, E., Pulkkinen, U. and Simola, K. (2006) Application of stochastic filtering for lifetime prediction. *Reliability Engineering & System Safety*, **91** (2), 200–208.
5. Si, X., Wang, W., Hu, C. and Zhou, D. (2011) Remaining useful life estimation – A review on the statistical data driven approaches. *European Journal of Operational Research*, **213**, 1–14.
6. Coble, J. and Hines, J.W. (2011) Applying the general path model to estimation of remaining useful life. *International Journal of Prognostics and Health Management*, **7**, 1–13.
7. Armstrong, N. and Hibbert, D.B. (2009) An introduction to Bayesian methods for analyzing chemistry data part 1: an introduction to Bayesian theory and methods. *Chemometrics and Intelligent Laboratory Systems*, **97**, 194–210.

8. Minakhi, R., Babita, M., Ritanjali, M. and Ganapati, P. (2014) Forecasting of currency exchange rates using an adaptive ARMA model with differential evolution based training. *Journal of King Saud University – Computer and Information Sciences*, **26**, 7–18.
9. Samuel, P.D. and Darryll, J.P. (2005) A review of vibration-based techniques for helicopter transmission diagnostics. *Journal of Sound and Vibration*, **282** (1), 475–508.
10. Yan, J., Muammer, K. and Lee, J. (2004) A prognostic algorithm for machine performance assessment and its application. *Production Planning and Control*, **15** (08), 796–801.
11. Peng, Y., Dong, M. and Zuo, M. (2010) Current status of machine prognostics in condition-based maintenance: a review. *International Journal of Advanced Manufacturing Technology*, **50**, 297–313.
12. Kayacan, E., Ulutas, B. and Kaynak, O. (2010) Grey system theory-based models in time series prediction. *Expert Systems with Applications*, **37** (2), 1784–1789.
13. Li, J., Mu, X., and Zheng, S. (2009) Research on lifetime grey prediction of electronic equipment based on improved genetic algorithm. International Conference on Advanced Computer Control, pp. 493–496.
14. Uang, W. and Liao, H. (2007) Application of improved GM(1,1) in the expenses forecasting of special equipments maintenance. *Journal of WUT*, **6**, 100–102.
15. Khashei, M., Bijari, M. and Ardali, G.A. (2009) Improvement of auto-regressive integrated moving average models using Fuzzy logic and Artificial Neural Networks (ANNs). *Neurocomputing*, **72** (4), 956–967.
16. Beden, S.M., Abdullah, S. and Ariffin, A.K. (2009) Review of fatigue crack propagation models for metallic components. *European Journal of Scientific Research*, **28**, 364–397.
17. Paris, P.C., Gomez, M.P. and Anderson, W.E. (1961) A rational analytic theory of fatigue. *The Trend in Engineering*, **13** (1), 9–14.
18. Irwin, G.R. (1957) Analysis of stresses and strains near the end of a crack traversing a plate. *Transactions of the ASME Journal Applied Mechanics*, **24**, 361–364.
19. Paris, P.C. and Erdogan, F. (1963) A critical analysis of crack propagation laws. *Journal of Basic Engineering*, **85**, 528–534.
20. Walker, E.K. (1970) The effect of stress ratio during crack propagation and fatigue for 2024-T3 and 7076-T6 aluminum, in *Effect of Environment and Complex Load History on Fatigue Life*, vol. **462**, American Society for Testing and Materials, Philadelphia, PA, pp. 1–14.
21. Forman, R.G. (1972) Study of fatigue crack initiation from flaws using fracture mechanics theory. *Engineering Fracture Mechanics*, **4** (2), 333–345.
22. Bechhoefer, E., Bernhard, A., and He, D. (2008) Use of Paris law for prediction of component remaining life. 2008 IEEE Aerospace Conference, March 2008, pp. 1–9.

6

Maintenance Planning and Scheduling

6.1 Strategic Planning in Maintenance

Historically, maintenance has been regarded as necessary activities which have a detrimental effect on management functions in an organization. However, in recent years this attitude has increasingly been replaced by one in which maintenance is recognized as a strategic issue in the organization.

6.1.1 Definition of Maintenance

6.1.1.1 Maintenance

A maintenance concept can be defined as the set of various maintenance interventions, which can be classified into four categories: corrective or breakdown maintenance, scheduled maintenance, preventive maintenance, and condition-based or predictive maintenance. Under maintenance interventions, facilities can be repaired, overhauled or replaced in a timely manner in order to guarantee their performanceand increase the availability of a system.

Corrective or Breakdown maintenance implies that repairs are made after the equipment has failed and can no longer perform its normal function. It is quite justified in small factories where downtimes are not critical and repair costs are less than other types of maintenance or there is not felt to be a financial justification for scheduling maintenance. However, corrective maintenance results generally in breakdown at inappropriate times, leading to poor and hurried maintenance, excessive delay in production, loss of output and profit, more accidents, and less safety for both workers and machines.

Scheduled maintenance is a stitch-in-time procedure and incorporates inspection, lubrication, repair, and overhaul of equipment. It is generally followed for overhauling machines, changing heavy equipment oils, or cleaning water and other tanks.

Machinery Prognostics and Prognosis Oriented Maintenance Management, First Edition. Jihong Yan.

Preventive maintenance locates the weak spots of machinery and equipment and provides them with periodic inspections and minor repairs to reduce the danger of unanticipated breakdowns. It can reduce breakdown and thereby downtime, it reduces odd-time repair and overtime for maintenance crews. It can also increase the safety of workers, decrease the maintenance and repair costs, and increase the chances to get production incentive bonuses.

Condition-based or predictive maintenance provides machinery with periodic monitoring of condition so that the maintenance crews can take timely actions, such as machine adjustment, repair, or overhaul. It makes use of human sense and other sensitive instruments, such as audio gages, vibration analyzers, amplitude meters, and pressure and resistance strain gages to know the current operating status of equipment and forecast incipient failures.

However, according to the viewpoint of Geert Waeyenbergh [1], the concepts described in the literature are often very time-consuming to implement or only valid for a special class of equipment or a specific industry. Most of the concepts from the literature, however, offer interesting and useful ideas. In this light, a few of the most important maintenance concepts are described by him briefly.

Reliability centered maintenance (RCM) was originally designed for the aircraft industry [2]. Moubray [3] described an extension to RCM, RCM II, designed for use in general industry. The first step in a RCM II analysis is gathering information. RCM II interprets and then defines the primary and secondary functions of the technical system. Next, the possible functional failures of both the primary and secondary functions are reviewed and listed in the RCM II information worksheet. Failure modes and causes are linked to these failures and their effects are determined. Based on this worksheet, the most critical items can be located. In other words, an RCM analysis starts with a failure modes effects and criticality analysis (FMECA). The RCM II decision diagram is used. This diagram integrates all the decision processes into a single strategic framework. With the aid of this decision diagram and the information worksheet, the following points are recorded in the RCM II decision worksheet: (i) What routine maintenance has to be done, how often it has to be done and who has to do it? (ii) Which failures are serious enough to warrant redesign? (iii) In which cases can failures happen deliberately (run to failure)? One of the biggest disadvantages of RCM II is its complexity and, as a consequence, its price. Reliability, rather than maintainability and availability is the main object. Such an approach is justifiable in aircraft/airline industries and in hightech/high-risk industries, but is often too expensive for general industries, where maintenance is rather an economic than a reliability problem.

Business centered maintenance (BCM) is a maintenance concept developed by Kelly [4, 5]. It consists of a framework based on the identification of the business objectives, which are then translated into maintenance objectives. The concept requires excessive data about the production process, production plan, forecast, workload, life plan, expected availability of the technical system, and so on (Figure 6.1). Kelly concentrated on the establishment of a ready-to-use maintenance concept for a plant. He provides guidelines to carry out maintenance activities, and aims at the best

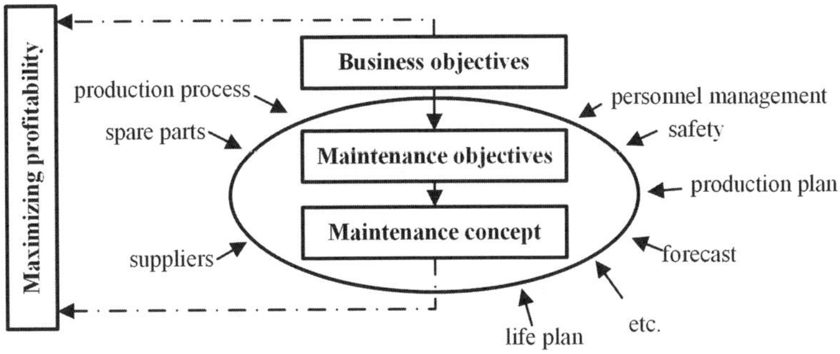

Figure 6.1 BCM approach, maximizing profitability

combination of maintenance activities for the various plant items. The main thrust of BCM is towards maximizing the contribution of maintenance to profitability.

Total productive maintenance (TPM) is based on productive maintenance, which was introduced in the 1950s at the General Electric Corporation. Later, it was further developed in Japan and re-imported into the West. Although maintenance is a key component in TPM, TPM is not really a maintenance concept. On the one hand, TPM goes much further than maintenance only, but on the other hand TPM is incomplete as a maintenance concept because it does not provide clear rules to decide which basic maintenance policy should be used (failure-based maintenance, design-out maintenance, detection-based maintenance, condition-based maintenance (CBM), or use-based maintenance). In fact, TPM is more and more translated as total productive manufacturing or total productive management. In this light, TPM is more like a management strategy. TPM is an approach to continuously improve the performance – effectiveness as well as efficiency – of certain industrial activities, and in the first place, maintenance. To do so, the overall equipment effectiveness (OEE) is used, which is the product of availability, speed, and quality performance. This OEE is computed by systematically reducing the theoretical availability of 100% by measuring the "six big losses": the downtime losses: (i) equipment failure and (ii) set-up and adjustment; and the speed losses: (iii) idling and minor stoppages and (iv) reduced speed; and the quality losses: (v) defects in the process and (vi) reduced yield. The goal of TPM is maximum equipment effectiveness and the OEE is used as a measure. To achieve an overall workshop improvement, TPM strives for the development of optimal human–machine conditions. To achieve this, the TPM model is based on five pillars: (i) individual equipment improvements to eliminate the six big losses, (ii) autonomous maintenance, (iii) planned preventive maintenance, (iv) maintenance/operations skills training, and (v) maintenance plan design and early equipment management (EEM). In contrast with some other maintenance concepts, TPM contains nothing that is wrong or detrimental to company economics. The calculation of the OEE as the product of availability, speed, and quality performance, however, is not really a complete analysis. Cost and profits are not taken into account and so it is not a complete measure by which competitive machines or systems should be compared. This is another reason why TPM is incomplete as a maintenance concept.

"*Life-cycle cost*" (LCC) *approaches*. Terotechnology evolved in the UK in the 1970s and is a combination of management, finance, engineering, building, and other practices applied to physical assets in pursuit of an economic LCC. Terotechnology is concerned with the specification and design for reliability and maintainability of physical assets such as a plant, machinery, equipment, buildings, and structures. The application of terotechnology also takes into account the processes of installation, commissioning, operation, maintenance, modification, and replacement. Decisions are influenced by feedback of information on design, performance, and cost throughout the life-cycle of a project. It applies equally to both assets and products because the product of one organization often becomes the asset of another. Even if the product is a simple consumer item, its design and customer appeal will benefit from terotechnology, and this will reflect in improved market security for the product.

Table 6.1 gives a schematic overview of all these maintenance concepts with their respective advantages and disadvantages.

More importantly, the maintenance concept should be customized because of the high direct and indirect cost involved (for inhouse as well as for outsourcing maintenance) and the operational impact maintenance may have on the equipment's performance; that is, it should consider all relevant factors of the situation on-hand. As such, it will be really tailored to the needs of the company in question, and consequently the maintenance concept will be unique for each company. The underlying structure for developing such a concept may, however, be very comparable. Another important remark is that since industrial systems evolve rapidly (think, e.g., about the high-speed technological innovation), the maintenance concept will also have to be reviewed periodically in order to take into account the changing systems and the changing environment. This calls for not only a structured, but also a flexible maintenance concept, allowing feedback and improvement.

To summarize, the purpose of maintenance is to maximize performance of production equipment efficiently and regularly. It can also prevent breakdown or failures to minimize production loss and increase the reliability of systems.

6.1.1.2 The Maintenance Challenge

Business leaders increasingly realize the strategic importance of the maintenance function for organizations which have significant investments in physical assets, and so it is a necessary expense in the operating budget. In other words, maintenance has become a critical issue in capital-intensive operations.

Unfortunately, in many industries, effective maintenance is usually not a high priority and the consequent cost of failures, as a percentage of the total cost, has risen. Organizations should be changing from a repair-focused to a reliability-focused culture.

Table 6.1 An overview of maintenance concepts

Concept	RCM	BCM	TPM	LCC-approaches
Advantages	Traceability	Accuracy	Increased productivity improvement of operations and workplace	Improvement of the designer/user interface (engineering approach)
	Cost savings	Business centered approach	Increased quality (TQM-link)	Life-cycle cost is of central importance
	Rationalization	Integrated auditing possibilities	Cost reduction (reduction of the six big losses)	Correct adaptation brings considerable benefits in most cases
	Plant improvement	–	Increased morale, safety, and environmental care	Feedback of information on design
	Education	–	–	–
	Involves operators a maintainers	–	Involves the operators	Full integration (ILS/LSA)
Dis-advantages	Complexity	Complexity	Not really a maintenance concept	Rather theoretical management philosophies
	Extensive need of data	Extensive need of data	No decision rules for basic maintenance policies	Difficult implementation, life-cycle cost analysis is complex (cash constraints, time constraints, uncertainty of forecasting demand, and life-cycle)
	Focus on "reliability"	–	Cost and profits are not taken into account	–
	Does not fully recognize that proper maintenance is also an economic problem	–	–	Less structured (collection of procedures rather than unambiguous standard method)

6.1.1.3 Maintenance Contribution to Profitability

An important criterion for investment in a company is the financial return on its fixed assets (ROFA). Asset management focuses on achieving the lowest total LCC to produce the required product or to provide a sought-after service. The goal is to achieve a higher ROFA than one's competitors in order to be the lower-cost producer of a product or service. The maintenance management impacts on the ROFA because maintenance costs are a significant contributor to manufacturing costs. If the maintenance cost as a percentage of manufacturing cost fluctuates, then the effectiveness of maintenance should be examined to find if it is the cause of the variation.

Downtime increases the industry's financial expenditure because of the costs of:

- idle production/operations personnel,
- late deliveries,
- overtime to make up for lost production in order to meet promised deliveries on time,
- lost sales as result of products not being made on time.

However, Japanese studies relating to TPM have concluded that "inefficiency" losses tend to exceed downtime losses. In industries, most inefficiency losses are never measured and reported. Also, many chronic problems, that have a dramatic impact on equipment effectiveness, are never even comprehended. Only if accurate maintenance records are kept are these problems realized. Then, utilizing the maintenance data, combined with pertinent financial data, a worthwhile estimate of the resulting costs can be achieved. As maintenance is regarded as an expense, any maintenance saving will contribute directly to the profit achieved. As the effectiveness of maintenance improves and downtime is reduced, there is less need for investment in standby (but otherwise) redundant plant. This will contribute to an overall rise in the ROFA for any organization.

6.1.2 Maintenance Strategy Planning

As explained above, the maintenance concept forms the framework from which expected maintenance policies are developed. Maintenance has been regarded as a vital core strategic business activity crucial for business survival and success. As a consequence, it influences every part of the maintenance activities in the company.

6.1.2.1 Maintenance Criteria and Objectives

In order to define strategic planning in maintenance, what is most significant is to define all relevant maintenance criteria and objectives that possibly could be of any importance in the decision process [6].

A generic list of maintenance objectives and criteria for the strategic and tactical levels of the organization is as follows:

- *Maintenance budget*: maintenance costs, maintenance value.
- *Functional and technical aspects*: availability, reliability, maintainability,
- *OEE*: productivity, output quality, and maintenance quality.
- *Plant design life*: capital replacement decisions and life-cycle optimization.
- *Support*: inventory of spare parts and logistics.
- *People and environment*: environmental impact, safety/risk/health, and personnel management.

Further subdivision of maintenance objectives into the operational level of an organization is possible according to the objectives defined in Figure 6.2.

By summarizing several studies of a wide range of industries, five strategic aspects of maintenance management have been identified, namely: maintenance methodology, support processes, organization and work structuring, comparable culture, and general management policy [7].

6.1.2.2 Framework of Maintenance Strategic Planning

Based on the objectives and criteria of maintenance management explained above, we know that maintenance strategy planning is the supporting structure of maintenance management. Siener and Aurich [8] classified maintenance strategy planning as reactive, time-based, or condition-based. Within the reactive maintenance strategy, maintenance tasks are initiated when a negative impact of deteriorated process objects on the chosen maintenance objectives occurs. Generally, this strategy is used if the scheduling of proactive maintenance tasks is technically not feasible or not cost-effective. Otherwise process objects are maintained under the terms of proactive maintenance strategies. Process objects can proactively be maintained either by using a time-based or condition-based maintenance strategy. Marquez and Gupta [9] suggested that maintenance management must be aligned with actions at three levels of business activities – strategic, tactical, and operational (see Figure 6.3). Actions at the strategic level transform business priorities into maintenance priorities. To meet these priorities, this process will help craft mid-to-long-term strategies to address current and/or potential gaps in equipment maintenance performance. As a result, a generic maintenance plan will be obtained at this level.

Transformation of business priorities into maintenance priorities is done by establishing critical targets in current operations. Detailed analysis creates measures of items such as the incidence of plant equipment breakdowns as these would impact the plant's operational targets. Maintenance management would then develop a course of strategic actions to address specific issues for the critical items. Other actions would focus on the acquisition of the requisite skills and technologies (for instance, condition

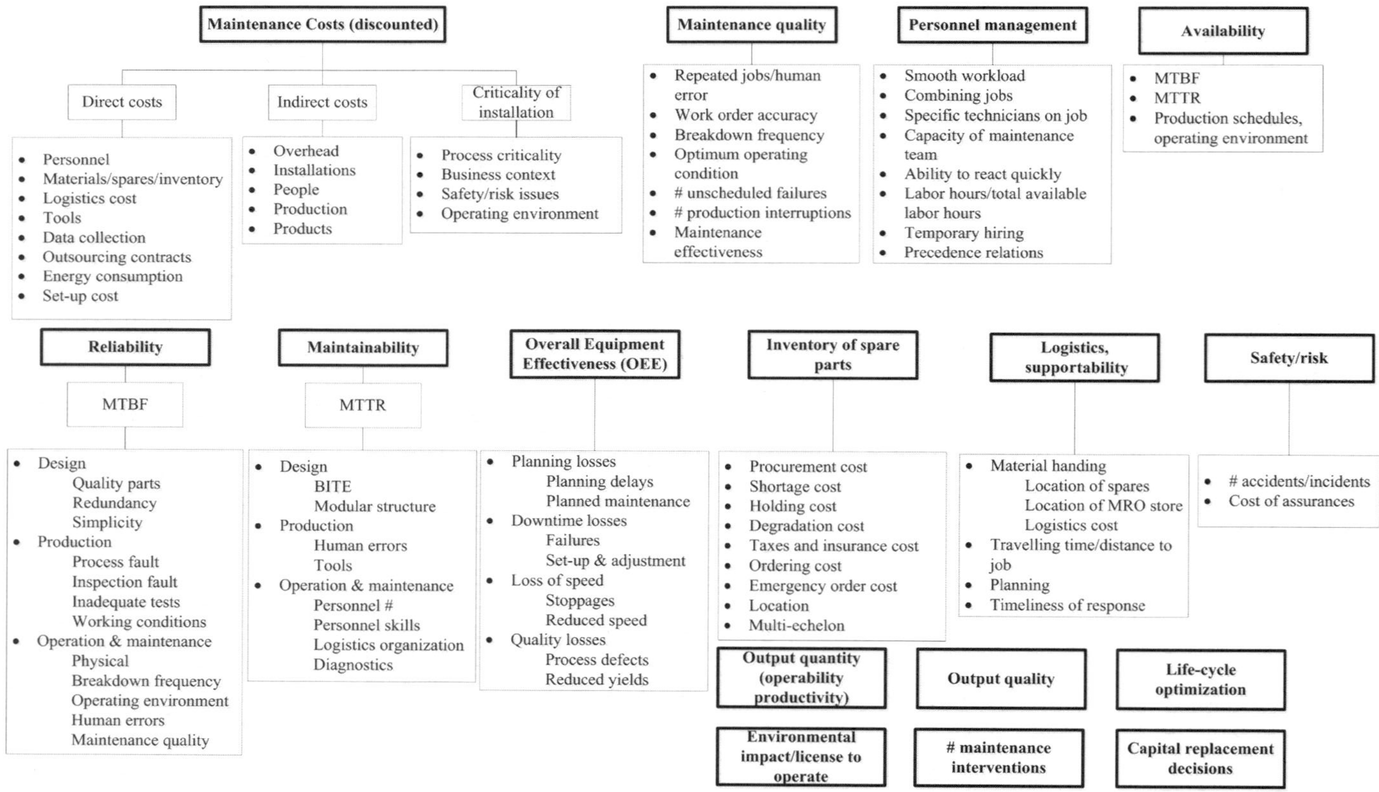

Figure 6.2 Tactical maintenance objectives further subdivided into operational maintenance objectives

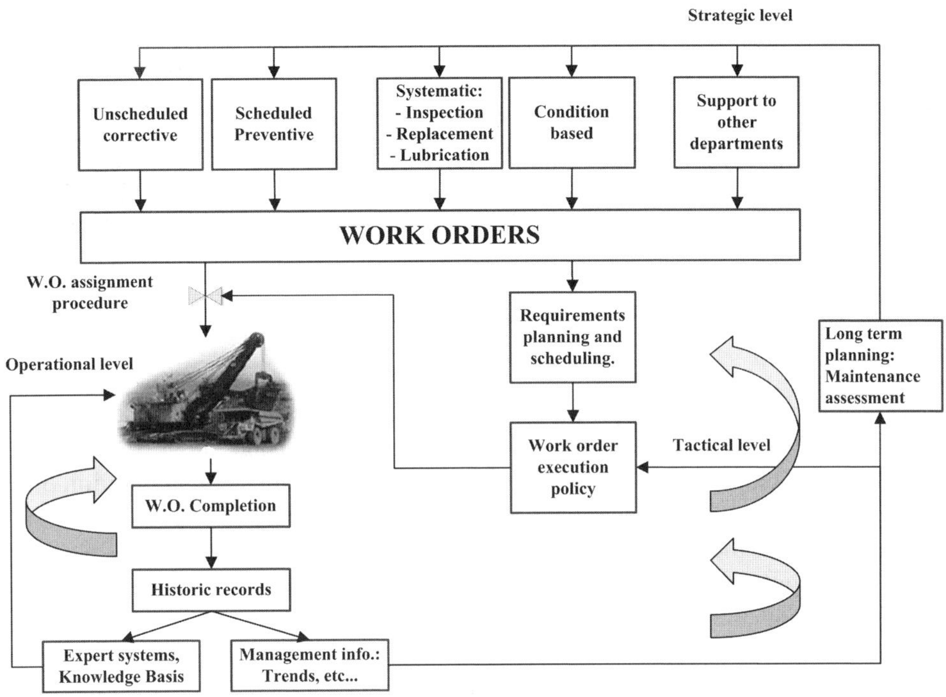

Figure 6.3 Maintenance process, course of action, and feedback operating at the three levels of business activities

monitoring technologies) for the micro-level improvement of maintenance effectiveness and efficiency.

The role of maintenance should be redefined as an essential means for life-cycle management [10]. Maintenance is the most efficient way to keep the functional level of a product above the level required from the viewpoint of environmental impact. Traditionally, the scope of maintenance activities has been limited to the operation phase. Three feedback loops for maintenance management are defined: for fulfilling the requirements of life-cycle maintenance, effective execution of a P–D–C–A (plan–do–check–action) cycle is essential. For this purpose, the framework for life-cycle maintenance shown in Figure 6.4 has been proposed. Then, a maintenance framework was proposed that shows management cycles of maintenance activities during the product life-cycle. In this framework, maintenance strategy planning plays a key role. This planning involves selecting the strategy of maintenance among various options based on the evaluation of potential problems that could occur during operation, as well as evaluation of failure effects and effectiveness of maintenance technologies. Maintenance strategy planning serves as a bridge between the product development phase and the operation phase. It obtains design data and production records from the development phase, and determines the maintenance strategy for each component of the product. These strategies are passed on to the operation phase,

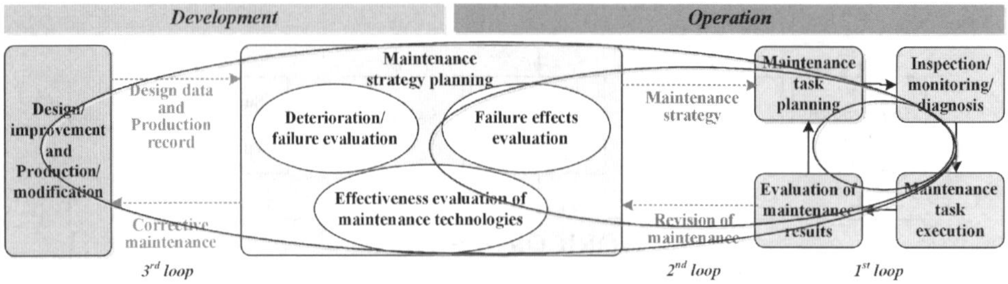

Figure 6.4 Framework for life-cycle maintenance

where maintenance tasks are planned in terms of procedures and schedules based on them. After maintenance tasks, such as inspection, monitoring, diagnosis, and treatment, are executed, the results are evaluated by comparing the actual condition of the product to what was anticipated when the maintenance strategy was selected. If there are discrepancies, the information is fed back to the maintenance strategy planning, where the maintenance strategies are revised based on re-evaluation of potential problems, taking the actual data into account. If corrective maintenance, that is, design improvement, is needed, the information is further fed back to the development phase, where improvements and modifications of product design are performed.

As shown in Figure 6.4, there are three feedback loops. The first is the loop of operational phase maintenance task management, which consists of maintenance task planning, task execution, and assessment of maintenance results. This is the loop for controlling routine maintenance work. The second loop includes maintenance strategy planning. By means of this loop, the maintenance strategies can be improved based on the observation of actual phenomena and knowledge accumulated during the product life-cycle. The third loop includes product development. This loop is essential for continuous improvement of the product during its life-cycle. These three loops provide effective mechanisms for adapting maintenance strategies to various changes, such as changes in operation conditions and environment, and also for continuously improving products.

As pointed out above, maintenance strategy planning plays a key role in life-cycle maintenance management. Maintenance strategies are categorized in terms of three factors: criteria for providing treatment, opportunity of maintenance task executions, and type of treatment, as shown in Figure 6.5. Among these options, a maintenance strategy is selected for each component based on two kinds of evaluations: technological evaluation and managerial evaluation, as shown in Figure 6.6.

Two major factors should be considered in the technological evaluation. The first involves the characteristics of deterioration and the resultant functional failures, which should be considered in the deterioration and failure analysis. The other is the applicability of maintenance technologies.

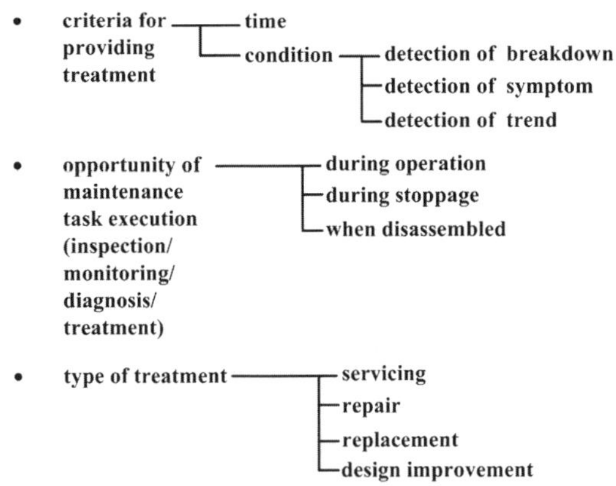

Figure 6.5 Categorizations of maintenance strategies

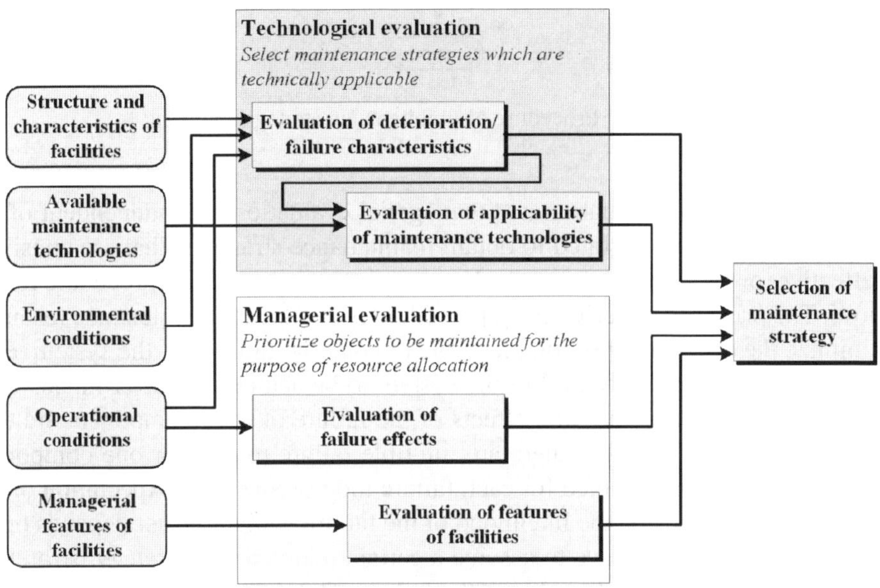

Figure 6.6 Factors for determining maintenance strategies

In the managerial evaluation, the severity of the failure is evaluated in terms of its effects outside the system concerned and in terms of its likelihood. The effects should be assessed from various perspectives. Typical examples are safety, operational, and economic factors. It is often difficult to make a quantitative evaluation of failure severity. In many practical cases, this severity is estimated qualitatively from various perspectives, and the results are combined to provide an overall rating.

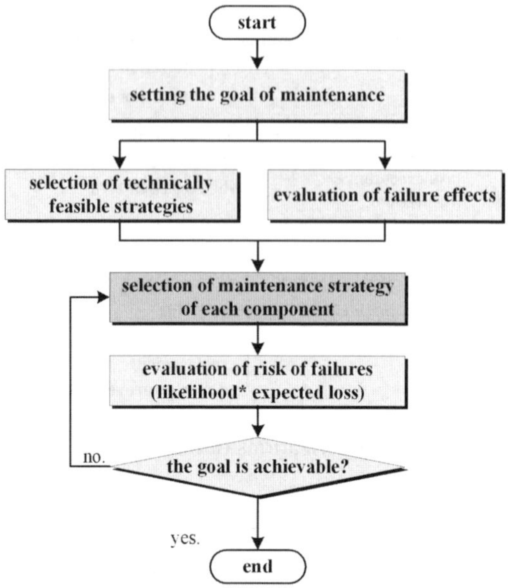

Figure 6.7 Procedure of maintenance strategy planning

While technological evaluation and managerial evaluation are independent of one another, they must be integrated to obtain maintenance strategies that are consistent and effective for the system as a whole. Figure 6.7 shows the general procedure for this purpose. The principle underlying the procedure is to allocate maintenance resources to minimize the expectation of total loss due to potential failures of the system. First, the goal of the maintenance level of the system to be achieved is determined. Then, technically feasible strategies and effects of the failure of each component are evaluated for each component. (If there are multiple failure modes for one component, evaluation should be performed for each failure mode.) Since the expectation of loss due to a failure depends on the likelihood of the failure, which further depends on the maintenance strategy, we have to assume a certain maintenance strategy beforehand for estimating the expected loss due to the failure. This assumption valuation loop is repeated until a proper maintenance strategy for the whole system is obtained, based upon which the expectation of the total loss can be kept below the acceptable level with affordable cost.

6.1.2.3 Computer-Aided Maintenance Planning

With the rapid development of Internet technology, there is more and more CNC (computer numerical control) equipment used in plants. In order to solve the maintenance problem of a high-tech CNC machine manufacturer, Ashayeri [11] presented a computer-aided integrated approach for the machine maintenance and repair business

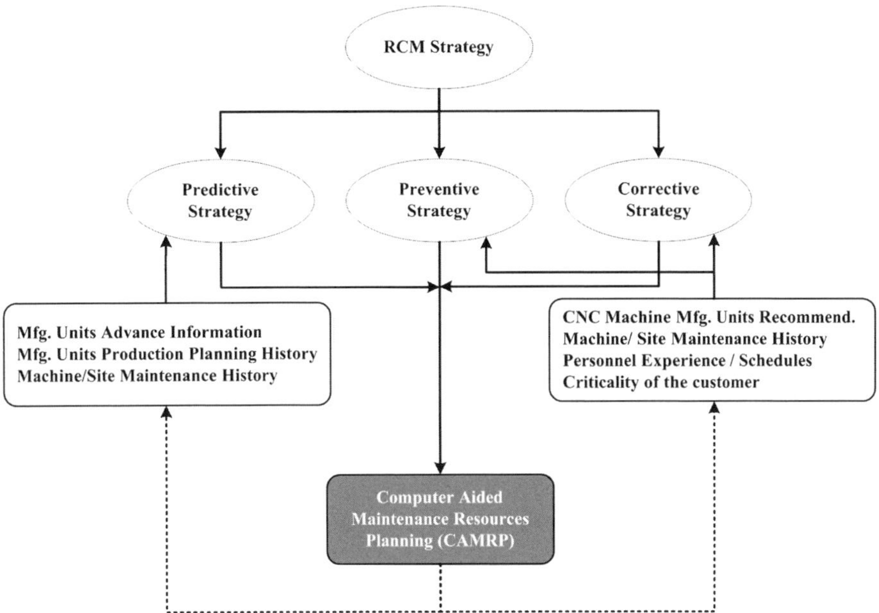

Figure 6.8 Computer-aided maintenance resources planning supporting blocks

unit (MMRBU) management system that would enhance and optimize the maintenance process, ensuring that the maintenance projects' load would receive a consistent level of maintenance resources, reducing overall delays and costs.

To establish a computer-aided maintenance resources planning system, the RCM is considered the driving point. Figure 6.8 shows different components of this approach, including the strategies required for maintenance resources planning optimization. The RCM approach considered here is very empirical, it is analysis of need and priorities. Using a series of classical quality control (QC) tools implemented in Delphi, it allows the MMRBU to properly articulate and adjust and balance preventive, predictive, and corrective maintenance strategies.

The most critical part of this approach is the planning of scarce maintenance resources, which affects the overall performance of the MMRBU. In other words, we need to determine a plan that measures the consequences of breakdown projects on the preventive maintenance projects, while critical customers and the machines leading to extra loads on resources are identified through predictive measures. All machines of different manufacturing units need to be analyzed, and the most critical parts of machines should be determined. We also need to understand the different manufacturing units (customers) needs in terms of reliability, service lead-times, cost, and so on. These attributes can then be weighted to determine the best maintenance policy to deal with each manufacturing unit.

In order to optimize the maintenance resources plan, all relevant information must be collected to most effectively initiate, schedule, track, record, and analyze maintenance tasks of different projects. An open communication protocol that enables various monitoring devices (of the internal as well as external manufacturing units) to talk with MMRBU would best suit the needs of such a computer-aided approach which uses various data sources from other software solutions.

6.2 Maintenance Scheduling

6.2.1 Fundamentals of Maintenance Scheduling

As explained in Section 6.1, within the strategic planning in maintenance, maintenance strategies for deteriorating systems are defined, including the object, framework, and process. Maintenance scheduling (MS) is the next important stage after maintenance strategic planning. In the past several decades, the MS problem has been extensively investigated.

6.2.1.1 Maintenance Scheduling Definition

The MS problem can be described as determining the optimal starting time for each preventive maintenance outage in a weekly period for one year in advance, while satisfying the system constraints and maintaining system reliability. Due to the nature of the problem formulation, high dimensionality and complexity characterize the MS problem [12]. It can be categorized into three levels, that is, decision-making on maintenance timing, facility grouping, and the sequencing of maintenance units.

Decision-making on maintenance timing is the first level of MS, it determines the best preventive maintenance periods for the production system as well as the most fitting maintenance actions in different periods. A reasonable maintenance timing decision allows maintenance to occur at the best time point. In addition, decision-making on maintenance timing is of great importance to ensure the reliability of the system, and reduce system energy consumption and maintenance cost. Zheng and Fard [13] presented a model for a system with several types of units. A unit is replaced at failure or when its hazard (failure) rate exceeds limit L, whichever occurs first. When a unit is replaced because its hazard rate reaches L, all the operating units with their hazard rate falling in the interval ($L - u$ to L) are replaced. This policy allows joint replacements and avoids the disadvantages resulting from the replacement of new units, downtime, and unrealistic assumptions for distributions of unit life. Optimal L and u are obtained to minimize the average total replacement cost rate. Li *et al.* [14] investigated the problem of integrating production scheduling and preventive maintenance in a flow shop composed of M different machines in series, aiming to minimize the total weighted system cost. They assume that for a multi-machine series manufacturing system, whenever one of the M machines is stopped to perform a preventive maintenance activity, the whole system must be stopped. This assumption leads to an increase in preventive maintenance opportunities for the other machines in the system.

Then, an integrated model is presented based on the opportunistic maintenance (OM) policy while taking into account the economic dependence of different machines. The model aims to search for an optimal combination of production and preventive maintenance planning. To facilitate the construction of the model, a judgment factor and a reason factor are introduced to describe the working state of the system and to explain the reasons for system downtime. The numerical example optimized with the Genetic Algorithm on Matlab indicates that the integrated model can reduce the total weighted system cost by nearly 11.72%. In addition, the optimal inspection and maintenance policy for the multi-unit series system with economic dependence is investigated in [15]. The system is composed of two kinds of units, which are subjected to the deterioration failure and the Poisson failure, respectively. Since costs can be saved when several units are repaired at the same time instead of separately, the optimal maintenance model for a multi-unit system should not limit itself to a simple juxtaposition of the mono-unit models and leads to a complex problem. To solve this problem, a classical OM policy is extended to coordinate the maintenance of the two kinds of units and minimize the maintenance cost of the system over the long term. To get the multi-threshold control-limit policy, the improved Markov decision approach is presented. Finally, a numerical example is put forward to illustrate the implementation of the model and iteration algorithm.

Facility grouping is an effective method to diminish the scale of scheduling problems, by maintaining facilities in groups under certain conditions. For large-scale production systems, there are usually a large number of facilities to be maintained in each maintenance activity. Therefore, it is necessary to divide maintenance facilities into different groups before sequencing the maintenance units. In [16], the group maintenance (GM) policy is introduced for the optimization of complex system RCM tasks, and mathematical models are established to minimize the whole maintenance cost per unit time. The costs of traditional periodic replacement and a functional check considering potential failure are analyzed. By integrating several types of preventive maintenance, the complex system GM cost model is obtained. By the joint execution of maintenance tasks, the times and loss of system shutdown are reduced with consequent reduction in maintenance costs. Finally, the effectiveness of the proposed models is illustrated through a numerical example. In [17] one methodology for identifying alternative cell designs is the use of clustering algorithms coupled with dissimilarity measures. The performance of seven hierarchical clustering techniques (six previously developed and one developed specifically for cell formation (CF)) and eight dissimilarity measures (three well-known measures and five versions of a recently developed parametric measure) were investigated. Twenty-four data sets, at close to 200 partition levels, and 10 measures of performance are used for this purpose. They first identify clustering techniques and dissimilarity measures which should not be used for CF when binary data are involved. From the remaining clustering techniques and dissimilarity measures, they then identify clustering technique/dissimilarity measure combinations which are consistently good or poor performers when cell characteristics are observed. High internal cell cohesiveness and low levels of machine duplication are shown to be conflicting goals. The dependence of the performance of clustering techniques on dissimilarity measures, data sets, stopping rules, and metrics is also clearly illustrated. Another result is that the choice of clustering technique is more critical than the choice of dissimilarity measure. However, differences among clustering techniques (due to chaining tendencies) can be sharply reduced by restricting the solution space for acceptable cell configurations. A cellular manufacturing system (CMS) is an application of group technology (GT) to the production environment. There are many advantages of CMS over traditional manufacturing systems, like reduction in set-up time, throughput time, and so on. The grouping of machine cells and their associated part families so as to minimize the cost of material handling is a major step in CMS and it is called the CF problem. CF is important for the effective performance of manufacturing. In [18], an attempt has been made to effectively apply the K-harmonic means (KHM) clustering technique to form machine cells and part families simultaneously, which we call KHM-CF. A set of 20 test problems of various sizes, taken from the literature, are used to test the performance of the proposed algorithm. Then, the results are compared with the optimal solution and the efficacy of the proposed algorithms is discussed. The comparative study shows that the proposed KHM-CF algorithm improves the grouping efficacy for 70% of the test problems, and gives the same results for 30% of the test problems.

Sequencing of maintenance units is the last but the most important level of the scheduling problem. After facility grouping, sequencing of maintenance units determines which units should be maintained before others. Some key factors that affect the costs will be considered in this level, including the facility's maintenance time, the maintenance resources required, and the system's productivity reduction caused by the facility's downtime. El-Sharkh and El-Keib [12] present an evolutionary programming (EP)-based technique for the unified model of the MS problem of power generation and transmission systems. In their paper, the hill-climbing technique (HCT) is used in conjunction with the EP to find a feasible solution in the neighborhood of the new infeasible solutions during the solution process. The EP search ability and the feasibility watch of the HCT motivate the sequential solution of the two interrelated subproblems of the MS problem. The paper reports test results of the proposed algorithm on the IEEE 30-bus system with 6 generating units and 41 transmission lines. Camci [19] presents a solution that optimizes system availability and cost with system-maintenance constraints using genetic algorithms. The proposed tool acquires the forecasted failure probability of individual components from the prognostics module, and their reliability expectations after maintenance. The trade-off between maintenance and failure is quantified in risk as the objective function to be minimized. The risk is minimized utilizing genetic algorithms for the whole system rather than individual components. The results of the proposed tool are compared with PM, CM, and CBM in which prognostics information of components is analyzed individually. In [20], a multi-objective hybrid genetic algorithm (MOHGA) is proposed to optimize a multi-objective imperfect preventive maintenance (MOIPM) model. The MOHGA proposed not only utilizes a Pareto-based technique to determine and retain the superior chromosomes as the GA chromosome evolutions are performed, but also guides their search direction. In order to obtain diverse non-dominated solutions that approach the optimized Pareto-efficient frontier, the closeness metric and diversity metric are employed to evaluate the superiority of the non-dominated solutions. Accordingly, decision makers can easily determine the most appropriate maintenance alternative to constitute a maintenance strategy from the optimized non-dominated solutions, given the practical requirements of system performance under the constraints of maintenance resources.

The primary objective of MS in manufacturing systems is to preserve equipment functions in a cost-effective manner. For many years, the relationship between production and maintenance has been considered as a conflict in management decisions. This situation is still the same because of the lack of communication regarding the scheduling requirements of each function [21]. The conflicts may result in an unsatisfied demand or machine breakdowns if the production and maintenance services do not respect each other's requirements. Berrichi *et al.* [22] suggested that the maintenance and production services must collaborate to achieve a common goal, that of maximizing system productivity. Therefore, both objectives of maintenance and production must be considered with the same importance level. Hence, a solution of the joint production and maintenance problem must be a trade-off between the objectives of the two services. In addition, the ultimate goal of the manager is to have a system which is the most available (or the least unavailable) possible, enabling him to execute the production jobs as soon as possible. An effective maintenance schedule should be able to balance all factors and provide a feasible and economical result to support the manager's decision.

Recently, with the increasing emphasis on sustainable manufacturing, MS is further complicated by introducing energy consumption to the objective function [23].

6.2.1.2 Maintenance Policies

Maintenance Policies for a Single Machine

Basically, one-unit systems have certain classes of maintenance policy, that is, age-dependent maintenance, periodic maintenance, failure limit maintenance, sequential maintenance, and repair limit [24].

Age-dependent maintenance is the common and popular maintenance policy. Under this policy, a unit is preventively maintained at some predetermined age T, or repaired at failure, until a perfect maintenance, preventive or corrective, is received.

Periodic maintenance is a preventive maintenance policy, in which a unit is preventively maintained at fixed time intervals kT ($k = 1, 2, \dots$) independent of the failures, here T is a constant.

Failure limit maintenance makes a unit work at or above the minimum acceptable level of reliability. Under this policy, preventive maintenance is performed only when the failure rate (FR) or other reliability indices of a unit reaches a predetermined level and intervening failures are corrected by repairs.

Sequential maintenance is different from a periodic maintenance policy. Under this policy, a unit is preventively maintained at unequal time intervals. Usually, the time intervals become shorter and shorter as time passes, considering that most units need more frequent maintenance with increased age.

Repair limit maintenance can be classified into two types: a repair cost limit policy and a repair time limit policy. When a unit fails, the repair cost is estimated and repair is undertaken if the estimated cost is less than a predetermined limit; otherwise, the unit is replaced. This is called the repair cost limit policy. The repair time limit policy, proposed by Nakagawa and Osaki [25], is one in which a unit is repaired at failure: if the repair is not completed within a specified time T, it is replaced by a new one; otherwise the repaired unit is put into operation again. T is called the repair time limit.

Basically, each maintenance policy for one-unit systems depends either on counting/recording the number of repairs, the preventive maintenance time, or the reference time. In practice, all are possible.

Maintenance Policies of Multi-Unit Systems

For multi-unit production systems, proper maintenance policies have great significance in saving maintenance cost, and reducing the time length of maintenance activity. Research on maintenance policy for multi-unit systems is mainly focused on OM and GM policy [24]. OM policy, in which the failure of one subsystem results in a possible opportunity to undertake maintenance on other subsystems, has been intensively studied and widely applied due to its advantage to obtain economies of scale in maintenance [26]. GM policy, under which facilities are maintained in groups under certain conditions, so that there is a smaller scheduling problem, more simplified maintenance management, and more reasonable logistics of spare parts, has great potential to facilitate maintenance by improving efficiency and saving time and cost, thus arousing the interest of researchers.

In terms of GM, Gertsbakh [27] proposed a GM policy that failed facilities should be renewed if the number of failed facilities reaches a certain prescribed threshold. Assaf and Shanthikumar [28] employed periodical inspection of facilities to check the number of failed ones. According to Assaf, failed facilities are left idling and are maintained when their number reaches a certain threshold. The maintenance policies proposed by Gertsbakh and Assaf are the so-called m-failure GM policy. Another two policies, namely T-age group and (m, T) maintenance policies share similar ideas with the m-failure policy [29]. According to the T-age GM policy, failed facilities are either repaired or replaced when the age of the system reaches T. According to (m, T) GM policy, failed facilities are maintained when either m facilities break down or the age of the system reaches T, whichever comes first. Sheu proposed a different GM policy with two different phases, $(0, T]$ and $(T, T + W]$, and two types of failures considering two kinds of maintenance actions, that is, minor repair and replacement [30]. According to Sheu and Jhang [30], group replacement is carried out at time

$(T + W)$ or when the number of idling facilities reaches a certain threshold. Bai *et al.* optimized the maintenance interval for complex systems by adjusting the time interval of single tasks so that they can be carried out as a group at common multiples of their intervals [31].

Under the policies mentioned above, facilities are maintained in groups according to either the age of the system or the number of failed facilities. However, under these policies, similarities between facilities, which have great potential to improve the maintenance efficiency, are not considered. For large-scale production systems, there are usually a large number of facilities to be maintained in each maintenance activity. The maintenance efficiency is a top consideration in order to reduce the production loss caused by suspension of production.

GT is a manufacturing philosophy that identifies and brings together related or similar parts and processes, to take advantage of the similarities which exist during all stages of design and manufacture [32]. By GT, facilities with high similarity are brought into one maintenance group [33] so that the time or resources needed to carry out maintenance actions for this group can be reduced. Clustering analysis methods, for example, HC methods [17], coupled with dissimilarity or similarity measures is one of the approaches often used in GT to form groups. Ünler and Güngör [18] study the application of the HC method by measuring the similarity in failure mode among facilities. Besides failure mode, some other maintenance-related similarities can be considered in grouping to improve maintenance efficiency and facilitate MS, which, however, have not yet been thoroughly studied. Due to the complexity of the systems, a comprehensive consideration of the similarities is necessary. Such similarities include the location of the facility, which is closely related to the logistics of maintenance resources, the facility type and maintenance type needed by the facility, which determine the maintenance process, the structural position of the facility, which affects its influence on the system's production, reasonable time length of a maintenance unit, and so on.

6.2.1.3 Production System Topology

In order to describe a production system more clearly and solve the MS problem effectively, it is necessary to build the topology of a production system. To do this, each facility in the system is assigned a facility number and a data unit, which records the facility numbers of the facility and its upstream and downstream facilities. It must be satisfied that the facility number of a facility should be bigger than those of its upstream facilities. The input and output of a production system are also considered as facilities and assigned facility numbers. The topology of one simple series-parallel production system is shown in Figure 6.9 where facility 5 has facilities 2, 3, and 4 as its upstream facilities, and facility 6, the output, as its downstream facility.

If multiple production lines exist in one production system, each facility has to be assigned a production line number. For example, in the production system shown in

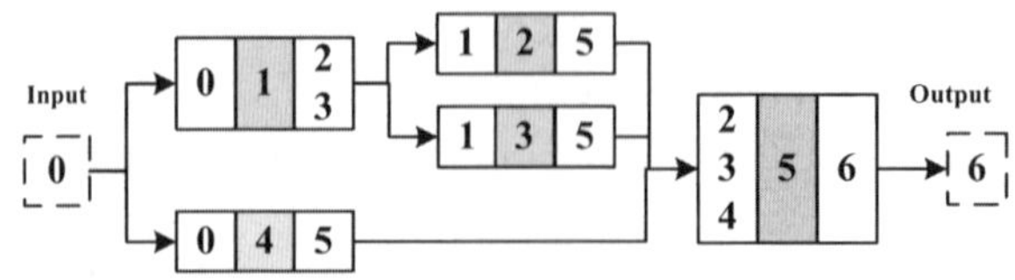

Figure 6.9 Topology of a simple series-parallel system

Figure 6.9, facilities 1, 2, and 3 compose production line 1 to manufacture part A; facility 4 itself composes production line 2 to manufacture part B; and facility 5 composes production line 3 to assemble parts A and B.

6.2.2 *Problem Formulation*

6.2.2.1 Objective and Constraints

The MS problem is to determine the period for which machines should be taken off line for planned maintenance and which types of maintenance should be carried out for each machine in order to minimize the operating cost, reduce the energy consumption, and increase the system reliability. In our study, minimal maintenance cost rate is set as the optimization objective of MS.

The constraints of MS problems are usually the maintenance resources needed to implement a maintenance activity, including spare parts, maintenance tools, maintainers, and consumables such as lubricant oil and electricity. In practice, the maintenance of facilities often calls for professional maintainers and tools, which are often very expensive and uneconomical for a company to possess. Usually, maintainers and maintenance tools in a single maintenance activity are assigned according to the resources needed for this activity. In this book, it is assumed that there are enough spare parts and consumables in reserve or available immediately for purchase, but maintenance tools and maintainers are assigned to a maintenance group according to the maximum numbers needed to maintain any one facility in this group.

6.2.2.2 Dependences in Production Systems

Dependences between facilities are important traits of multi-unit systems. Here, structural dependence and economic dependence are studied.

Structural dependence exists in most multi-unit systems. It means that the shutdown of one facility causes production reduction or suspension of other facilities. The structural dependence between facilities is determined by their structural position in the system. In this book, the structural model of production systems is established to describe the facilities' structural position. As shown in Figure 6.10, each facility is assigned a facility number and a three-digit code $[s_1, s_2, s_3]$ recording its structural position in the system. s_1 stands for the production line (each production line produces

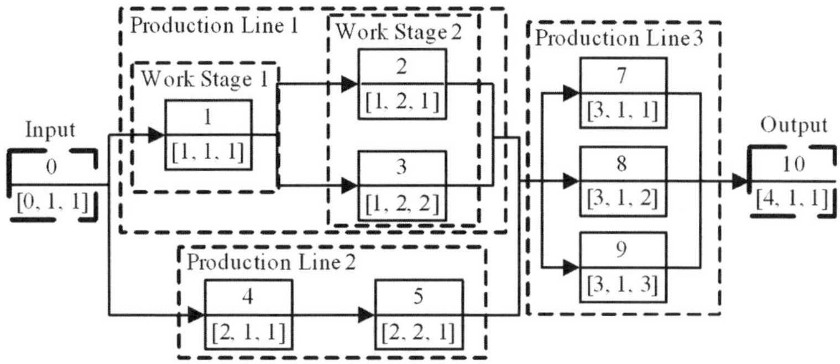

Figure 6.10 Structure dependence of a series-parallel system

different products); s_2 stands for the work stage (each work stage carries out a certain process); and s_3 stands for the label of the facility in the corresponding work stage.

For instance, in the system shown in Figure 6.10, there are three production lines. Production Line 1 and 2 produce components A and B, respectively, and production line 3 is the assembly line. Facility 3 in the system is the second parallel facility in Work Stage 2 of Production Line 1, whose structural code is [1, 2, 2].

Based on the structural model, the production loss during maintenance activity can be calculated. This will be presented in detail in Section 6.4.2.

Due to the structural dependence between facilities, conducting maintenance on several facilities jointly usually costs less money and/or time than treating each facility separately. This type of dependence is called economic dependence. In this book, OM policy is employed for the concern of economic dependence, which will be presented in Section 6.3.1.

6.2.3 Models for Maintenance Scheduling

6.2.3.1 Performance Degradation Modeling

The performance degradation of a facility is modeled by reliability, a two-parameter Weibull distribution is employed in this book. If t stands for the lifetime of a facility, its reliability, $R(t)$, can be calculated by Equation 6.1.

$$R(t) = \exp[-(t/\eta)^{\beta}] \tag{6.1}$$

where, η is the scale parameter, which is defined as the life of the product at which 63.2% of all facilities fail. β is the slope parameter, which is defined as the mode of failure.

6.2.3.2 Maintenance Effect Modeling

Four common types of maintenance actions are considered in this book: minor maintenance, medium maintenance, overhaul, and replacement.

- *Minor maintenance* is cleaning, adjusting, and lubricating a facility. It has a minor improvement effect on the reliability of the facility.
- *Medium maintenance* is repairing or replacing a few components that have been most seriously damaged. The reliability of a facility can be improved effectively after a medium maintenance.
- *Overhaul* is to inspect all the components of a facility and replace those which are likely to fail in the next operation period. It can improve the reliability of the facility significantly but not to "as good as new".
- *Replacement* is to replace a facility with a new one.

As shown in Figure 6.11, minor maintenance, medium maintenance, overhaul, and replacement are carried out at t_1, t_2, t_3, and t_4, respectively. No improvement in reliability is obtained after minor maintenance but reliability degradation is slowed; after medium maintenance and overhaul, the reliability is improved, and overhaul has a more significant effect; after replacement, the facility is as good as new. The first three types of maintenance are triggered by referring to three thresholds of reliability, T_{h}^1, T_{h}^2, and T_{h}^3. When improvement of reliability is below a certain level denoted as L_{R}, the reuse of the facility is no longer economic and replacement should be carried out.

To model the reliability improvement after the four types of maintenance actions, Malik's proportional age reduction (PAR) model [34] is introduced. Its basic form can be written as:

$$R_k(t) = \exp\{-[(t - t_k + T_k)/\eta]^{\beta}\} \tag{6.2}$$

$$T_k = \sum_{j=1}^{k}(1 - I_j) \cdot (t_j - t_{j-1}) \tag{6.3}$$

where, t_k denotes the time when the kth maintenance is carried out; T_k is the theoretical operation time of the facility when the kth maintenance is carried out, which indicates that the facility's condition after the kth maintenance equals that at time T_k

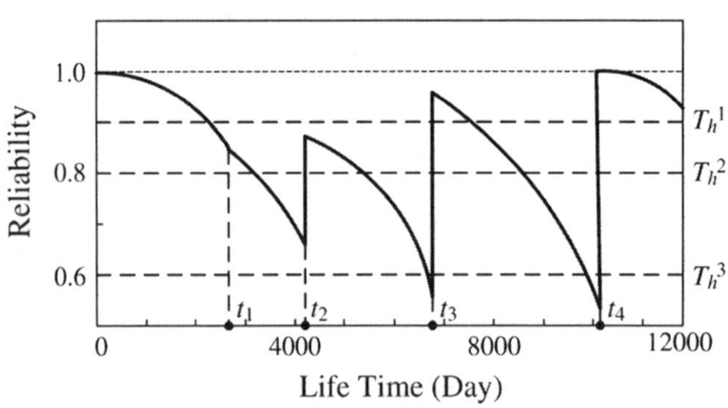

Figure 6.11 Reliability evolution of a facility with maintenance

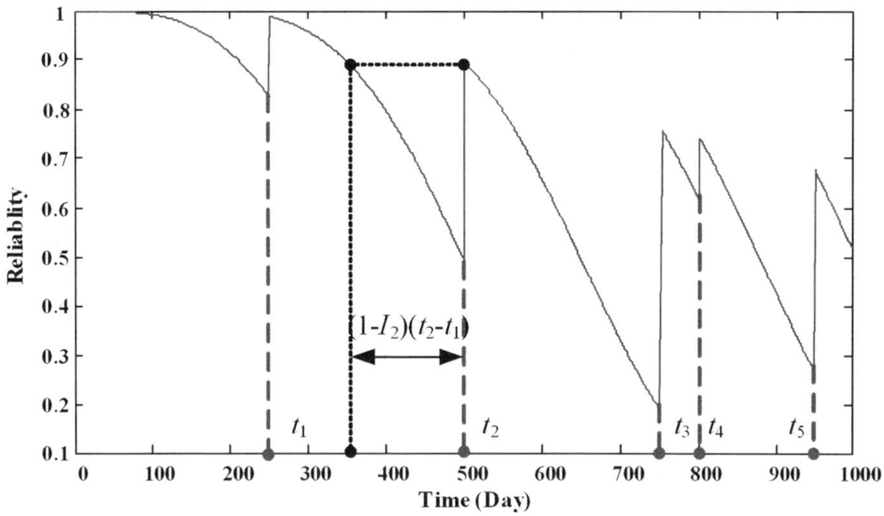

Figure 6.12 Illustration of PAR model

if no maintenance is conducted on the facility; I_k is the improvement factor after the kth maintenance is performed and is set between 0 and 1.

According to the PAR model, after the kth maintenance, the facility's reliability is improved to a certain level between the $(k-1)$th and kth maintenance, which is shown in Figure 6.12. This means that the maintenance cannot increase the reliability to a level higher than that after the previous maintenance. Due to this limitation, the PAR model is not suitable when different types of maintenance are considered.

In this book, the PAR model is adjusted, and Equation 6.3 is replaced with Equation 6.4.

$$T_k = \begin{cases} (1 - I_k) \cdot t_k, & k = 1 \\ (1 - I_k) \cdot (T_{k-1} + t_k - t_{k-1}), & k > 1 \end{cases} \quad (6.4)$$

According to Equation 6.4, after the kth maintenance, the theoretical operation time of the facility can be reduced to a certain value between 0 and $(t_k - t_{k-1} + T_{k-1})$. For example, as shown in Figure 6.13, the dashed line denotes the facility's reliability evolution in terms of the theoretical operation time, and the solid line demonstrates the actual reliability evolution of the facility; if the fourth preventive maintenance is carried out at t_4, before the maintenance, the theoretical operation time is $(t_4 - t_3 + T_3)$, and after the maintenance, the theoretical operation time is reduced to $(1 - I_4)(t_4 - t_3 + T_3)$, which is denoted as T_4.

In this model, the larger I_k, the higher the reliability improvement will be. By assigning a different value to I_k, the four types of maintenance actions can be modeled. Particularly, when I_k equals 1, the theoretical operation time of the facility is reduced

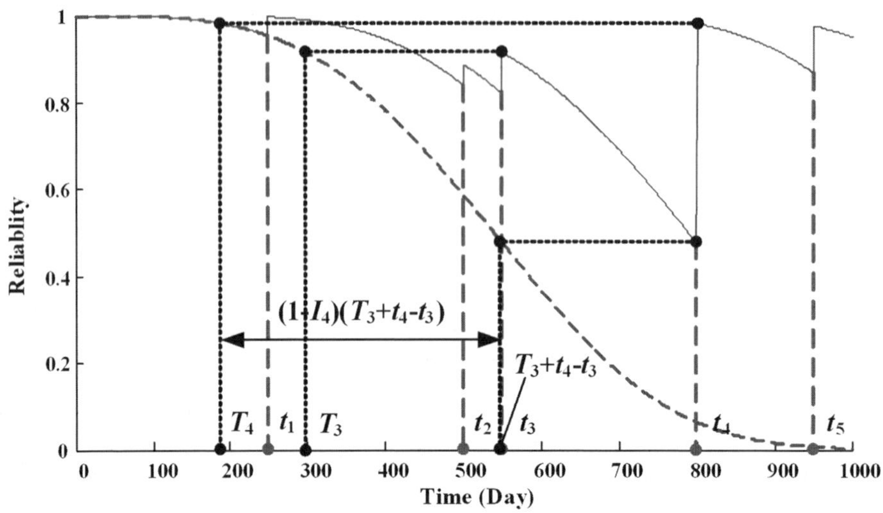

Figure 6.13 Illustration of adjusted PAR model

to 0, which means the facility is replaced with a new one. In practice, the improvement factor can be obtained by analyzing the historical maintenance records.

In this book, a facility's improvement factors of minor maintenance, medium maintenance, and overhaul are considered to be related to both the actual and theoretical operational time of the facility. The improvement factor can be calculated by Equation 6.5.

$$I_{j,k} = I_0^{j,k} - [w_o T_{j,k} + (1 - w_o)t_{j,k}] \cdot d_m^j / \eta_j \tag{6.5}$$

where, w_o is the weight for the consideration of the theoretical operational time; d_m^j is the impact factor of the operational time; and $I_0^{j,k}$ is the improvement base.

6.2.3.3 Maintenance Cost Modeling

In practice, minimal maintenance cost is usually set as the most important optimization object of the MS. Therefore, a maintenance cost model must be built in this section, helping the manager to analyze and calculate the cost during the maintenance activities and find a way to minimize it.

Traditionally, the maintenance cost can be categorized into two parts: direct maintenance cost and indirect maintenance cost.

Direct maintenance cost includes the set-up cost of the maintenance and the cost of maintenance actions for maintenance units, that is, the costs of maintainers, maintenance tools, spare parts, consumables for maintenance, and energy consumption during maintenance activities.

The costs of maintainers and maintenance tools are usually related to the unit price of using maintenance tools and maintainers, the numbers of maintenance tools and maintainers needed in every maintenance activity, and the time needed to carry out all the maintenance actions. The costs of spare parts and consumables depend on the unit price and the total number of the parts or consumables within the four common types of maintenance actions described previously. The costs of the energy consumption are caused by activities including lighting, ventilation, and heating.

Indirect maintenance cost, which consists mainly of production loss due to termination of machines under maintenance, can be calculated by the product of the value of one product and the productivity at the downtime of the machines.

Therefore, the maintenance cost for maintenance unit *i*, C^i_{total}, can be calculated by

$$C^i_{\text{total}} = C^i_{\text{d}} + C^i_{\text{I}} \tag{6.6}$$

where C^i_{d} and C^i_{I} are direct costs and indirect costs for maintenance unit *i*.

6.3 Scheduling Techniques

In order to solve the MS problem, which has become more and more complex with the expansion of multi-unit production systems, some mature scheduling techniques have to be presented in this chapter, including the maintenance timing decision-making method, maintenance grouping technology, and the MS method for maintenance units.

6.3.1 *Maintenance Timing Decision-Making Method Based on MOCLPSO*

The multi-objective comprehensive learning particle swarm optimization (MOCLPSO) presented by Liang *et al.* [35], uses a novel learning strategy whereby all other particles' historical best information is used to update a particle's velocity. The particle swarm optimization (PSO), which does not use evolution operators such as crossover and mutation, has been confirmed to be a convenient and practical method to solve many optimization problems. However, the PSO cannot perform well on complex multimodal problems due to its premature convergence.

Compared to conventional PSO, the MOCLPSO uses a learning strategy, which enables the MOCLPSO to make use of the information in a swarm more effectively, to generate better quality solutions frequently. Based on the results of the 9 algorithms on the 16 chosen test problems belonging to 4 classes, Liang *et al.* [35] have proved that MOCLPSO significantly improves the PSO's performance and gives the best performance on most multimodal problems, irrespective of whether they are unrotated or rotated when compared with eight other PSO versions.

A flow chart for the MOCLPSO is shown in Figure 6.14. The procedures of MOCLPSO are presented as follows.

Step 1: Generate population P_0 and initialize randomly the positions and associated velocities of P_0.

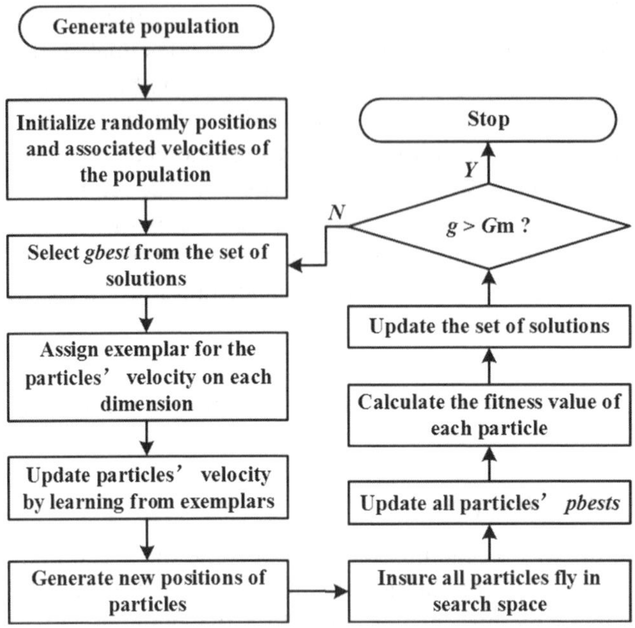

Figure 6.14 Flow chart of MOCLPSO

Step 2: Do the operations to each particle as follows.
1. Select *gbest* from the external archive.
2. Assign exemplar for the particle's velocity on each dimension.
3. Update particles' velocity by learning from exemplars.
4. Generate new positions of particles.
5. Insure all particles fly in search space.
6. Update all particles' *pbests*.
7. Calculate the fitness value of each particle.

Step 3: Use particles' *pbests* and *gbests* to update the external archive.

Step 4: The optimization process by MOCLPSO is stopped when the population has evolved for G_m generations. Return to Step 2 if iteration is not over.

When MOCLPSO is used to solve the problem of maintenance timing decision-making in this chapter, three major challenges are: solution encoding, the learning strategy of the particles, and updating the strategy for the external archive.

6.3.1.1 Solution Encoding

A preventive maintenance decision-making coefficient, $e_{i,j}$, which denotes the maintenance action for the *j*th facility in the *i*th maintenance activity, is presented in this section. It can be written as

$$e_{i,j} = \begin{cases} 0, & \text{if } j\text{th facility will not be maintained in } i\text{th maintenance activity} \\ 1, & \text{if } j\text{th facility will be maintained in } i\text{th maintenance activity} \end{cases} \tag{6.7}$$

The solution for MS can be stated as the following matrix, in which each element $e_{i,j}$ presents the preventive maintenance decision-making coefficient of activity.

$$x = \begin{bmatrix} e_{1,1} & e_{1,2} & \cdots & e_{1,n} \\ e_{2,1} & \cdots & & \vdots \\ \vdots & & \cdots & \vdots \\ e_{m,1} & \cdots & \cdots & e_{m,n} \end{bmatrix} \tag{6.8}$$

In the matrix, each row represents maintenance actions for all facilities in a maintenance activity, and each column represents one facility's maintenance actions in each maintenance activity.

Furthermore, according to the value of each element of the matrix we can, but do not have to, do maintenance for each facility when the production systems stop running. For instance, $e_{1,1} = 0$ means that we would not do maintenance for the first facility in the first maintenance activity, but we will maintain it because the first facility satisfies the conditions of preventive maintenance.

Therefore, the problem of preventive maintenance decision-making can be transformed to a 0–1 integer programing problem.

6.3.1.2 Comprehensive Learning Strategy

In the standard PSO, the velocity and position of the particle are updated by Equations 6.9 and 6.10.

$$v_{iD}^{k+1} = wv_{iD}^{k} + c_1\xi(pbest^k - x_{iD}^k) + c_2\varsigma(gbest^k - x_{iD}^k) \tag{6.9}$$

$$x_{iD}^{k+1} = x_{iD}^{k} + v_{iD}^{k+1} \tag{6.10}$$

where v_{iD}^k is the velocity of the kth dimension of the iDth particle and x_{iD}^k is the associated position of the kth dimension of the iDth particle, which is equal to a solution in the design space of Pareto (see Section 6.3.1.4); and w is the inertia weight, which is used to balance the global and local search abilities. A large inertia weight is more appropriate for global search, and a small inertia weight facilitates local search. c_1 and c_2 are the acceleration constants reflecting the weighting of stochastic acceleration terms that pull each particle toward "*pbests*" and "*gbests*" positions. The two random numbers ξ and ς are independently generated in the range [0, 1].

The MOCLPSO utilizes a new learning strategy, in which all particles' *pbests* are used to update the velocity of any one particle. For each dimension of particle, we generate a random number. If this random number is larger than the learning probability, the corresponding dimension will learn from its own *pbest*; otherwise it will learn from another particle's *pbest*.

The standard PSO performs well in solving continuous optimization problems, however, it can do nothing for discrete problems due to the conversion of the value of the particle's position and velocity from a discrete data to a continuous one. For instance, as presented in Equation 6.8, the value of each element in the matrix is either 0 or 1, which is a discrete data. When we update the velocity and position of the particle by Equations 6.9 and 6.10, the new velocity and position will be equal to their initial value if the particle learns from its own *pbest*. That will play the devil with evolution of populations. In addition, it may easily get trapped in a local optimum due to a single limitation of value. Therefore, in order to use MOCLPSO to solve the MS problem, the original PSO should be improved.

At present, there are very few studies on solving the 0–1 integer programing problem. In order to figure out maintenance timing decision-making, a mutation operation is added to a new variant learning strategy which is proposed in this section. The procedures of the learning strategy are presented as follows.

Step 1: Determines the number of particles which have to be refreshed by mutation operators, and the number of rows which will learn from *gbests* or *pbests*.

Calculate the inertia weight w_k of each particle. Then, n_r, the number of particles which have to be refreshed by mutation operators can be stated by Equation 6.11 according to w_k.

$$n_r = (1 - w_k) \times n \tag{6.11}$$

where n is the number of rows in the matrix.

Calculate m_r, which is the number of rows that will learn from *gbests*, by

$$m_r = m \cdot c_1/(c_1 + c_2) \tag{6.12}$$

where m is the number of particle's columns. Then the result of m_r should be rounded up.

Step 2: Mutation

For each row of P_1, a vector consists of $0 \sim n$ random integers is generated. Each element of the vector can be regarded as the ID numbers of the elements in particle P_1. The first n_r elements of the vector are taken out to generate a new vector X, which represents all the ID numbers of the elements that need mutation in particle P_1. Then the mutation operates according to vector X, after that a new particle P_2 is generated.

Step 3: Learn from gbest

A vector consisting of $0 \sim m$ random integers is generated. The first m_r elements of the vector are taken out to generate a new vector Y, which represents all the ID numbers of rows which will learn from *gbest* in particle P_2. The other rows of P_2 will learn from *pbest*.

For each particle of P_2, we select randomly one solution as a *gbest* from the Pareto-front of the external archive according to the sorting of it. Then, for each row which will learn from *gbest* in particle P_2, calculate the number of elements that require learning from *gbests* by

$$n_l = \xi \times m \tag{6.13}$$

The result of n_l should be rounded up.

A vector consisting of $0 \sim m$ random integers is generated. The first n_l elements of the vector are taken out to generate a new vector Z. According to vector Z, the corresponding dimension in each row will change value.

Step 4: Learn from pbest

First, a learning probability, t_p, is set. For each particle, a random number ς is generated to make the decision that the particle will learn from its own *pbest* or any particle's *pbest*. If ς is larger than t_p, the corresponding dimension of population will learn from its own *pbest*, otherwise it will learn from another particle's *pbest*. Then the number of elements, which need to learn from *pbest* in each row, can be calculated by Equation 6.13 with a different value of ξ. Then, a vector consisting of $0 \sim m$ random integers is generated. The first n_l elements of the vector are taken out to generate a new vector Z'. According to vector Z', the corresponding dimension in each row will change value.

After that, a new population will be generated.

6.3.1.3 Parameter Settings for MOCLPSO

The balance of the global and local search abilities, which is dependent on the inertia weight and acceleration constants, has a great effect on the performance of MOCLPSO.

For different stages of optimization, there should be different balances between the local and global search abilities. The bigger the inertia weight, the less dependent on initial population the solution, and the more capable the PSO is to exploit new areas. For MOCLPSO, a large inertia weight will be needed to possess more exploitation ability at the beginning, then a small one will be needed to have more exploration ability to fine search the local area around the seed. Therefore, instead of a fixed constant, the inertia weight is defined as a decreasing function of time as in Equation 6.14.

$$w_k = w_{max} - \frac{k(w_{max} - w_{min})}{N_{max}} \tag{6.14}$$

where w_{min} and w_{max} are the minimum and maximum of the inertia weight, respectively, N_{max} represents the maximum of iteration, and k is the number of iterations.

Similarly, a large c_1 but a small c_2 will be needed to possess more exploitation ability at the beginning, therefore their variable functions of time are as shown in

Equations 6.15 and 6.16, respectively.

$$c_1 = (c_{1f} - c_{1i})k/N_{max} + c_{1i} \tag{6.15}$$

$$c_2 = (c_{2f} - c_{2i})k/N_{max} + c_{2i} \tag{6.16}$$

Generally, the algorithm performs well with the parameters set as $c_{1i} = 2.5$, $c_{1f} = 0.5$, $c_{2i} = 0.5$, $c_{2f} = 2.5$.

6.3.1.4 Updating the External Archive

In each iteration, the external archive is updated by comparing to the new population. Then the particle's *gbest* will be taken out from the external archive. The procedures of updating the external archive are as follows:

Step 1: Merge new population into the external archive.
Step 2: Have all the particles sorted by their fitness values.
Step 3: Update the external archive by keeping the high quality particles and eliminating redundant inferior particles.

A major challenge consists in particle sorting, which is now addressed in detail.

Generally, a multi-objective optimization problem consists of n decision variables, M objective functions, and K constraints, which are presented as Equations 6.17–6.19.

$$\min y = f(x) = [f_1(x), f_2(x), \cdots, f_M(x)] \tag{6.17}$$

$$\text{s. t. } g_i(x) \le 0, \; i = 1, 2, \cdots, p \tag{6.18}$$

$$h_i(x) = 0, \; i = 1, 2, \cdots, q \tag{6.19}$$

where $x = (x_1, x_2, \cdots, x_n) \in X$ is the decision vector. $y = (y_1, y_2, \cdots, y_M) \in Y$ is the objective vector. X is the decision space consisting of decision vectors and Y is the objective space consisting of objective vectors.

In the multi-objective problem, due to having more than one objective, there is a set of non-dominated solutions instead of only one best solution. Optimization of one objective may cause deterioration of another one. Therefore, it is important to balance all objectives during optimization. For instance, during decision-making of maintenance timing, the minimized energy consumption, maintenance cost, and maximized reliability of the system are set as three goals of the optimization. Increasing the number of maintenance activities will improve the reliability of the system but will also result in an increase in the cost. Therefore, conversion and processing have to be done to all objectives of the optimization. In the next section, a method for multi-objective particles is presented, called Pareto space comparison.

6.3.1.5 Implementation of Pareto Space Comparison

In the design space of Pareto, x^0 is said to dominate x^1 if and only if they satisfy the following conditions, which can be denoted by $x^0 \succ x^1$.

$$f_i(x^0) \le f_i(x^1), \qquad i = 1, 2, \cdots, M$$
$$f_i(x^0) < f_i(x^1), \qquad \exists i \in \{1, 2, \cdots, M\}$$

x^0 that cannot be dominated by other solutions, is called a Pareto-optimal solution. The set of all Pareto-optimal solutions is called the Pareto-optimal set, which can be denoted by $P_S = \{x^0 | \neg\exists x^1 \succ x^0\}$. The corresponding images of the Pareto-optimal set in the objective space are called the Pareto-optimal frontier denoted as $F_1 = \{f(x) = (f_1(x), f_2(x), \cdots, f_M(x)) | x \in P_S\}$.

The Pareto space comparison consists of two steps, namely non-dominated sorting selection and crowding distance comparison.

Non-dominated Sorting Selection

In the non-dominated sorting procedure, individuals characterized as a Pareto solution are assigned with front number 1. Other individuals only dominated by those with front number 1 are assigned with front number 2. Similarly, other individuals only dominated by those with front number 2 are assigned with front number 3, and so on.

For a bi-objective optimization problem, an example of Pareto design space is shown in Figure 6.15. All circles in the figure represent the positions of solutions in the Pareto design space. In Figure 6.15a, a hollow circle represents a solution dominated by at least one non-dominated solution represented by a solid circle. All of the non-dominated solutions represented by a solid circle make up the Pareto-optimal

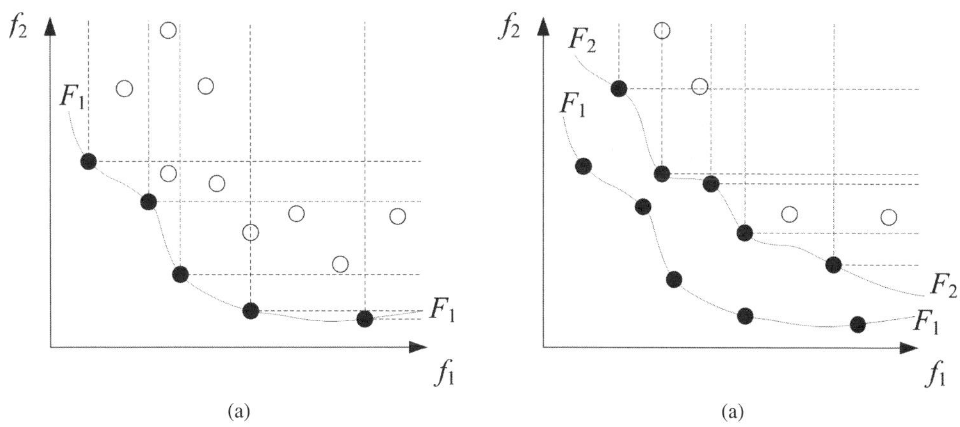

Figure 6.15 An example of Pareto design space. (a) The formation of Pareto-optimal frontier F_1 and (b) the formation of Pareto-optimal frontier F_2

frontier F_1. In Figure 6.15b, other solutions only dominated by the solutions of the Pareto-optimal frontier F_1 format the Pareto-optimal frontier F_2.

Crowding Distance Comparison

Within the multi-objectives optimization, in order to update the population, there are a certain amount of solutions that are selected from the whole set of visited solutions to be as near to the Pareto-optimal front as possible. For individuals belong to the same Pareto front, crowding distance comparison is utilized in non-dominated sorting selection.

The crowding distance gives an indication of the gap between the non-dominated solution members in the same Pareto front. There are three objectives in decision-making of maintenance timing, so that a method for calculating crowding distance based on three-dimensional Pareto space is presented.

Definition 1. In the three-dimensional Pareto space, there are three points, namely A (a_1, a_2, a_3), B (b_1, b_2, b_3), and C (c_1, c_2, c_3), which are inconsistent with each other. B is said to be surrounded by A and C if and only if: $\forall i \in \{1, 2, 3\}$, $a_i \leq b_i \leq c_i$, or $a_i \geq b_i \geq c_i$.

The position of any point in the three-dimensional Pareto space can be stated as its coordinate (x, y, z). For two points A (a_1, a_2, a_3) and C (c_1, c_2, c_3) that are inconsistent with each other, a closed space can be formatted.

Definition 2. A point is called a boundary point if it is surrounded by nothing in the Pareto space.

Definition 3. Every two points in the same Pareto front with point C will format a closed space. Two points, whose closed space has the minimal summation of side lengths, are called neighbors of point C.

Definition 4. For any point C in the Pareto space, if it is a boundary point, the value of its crowding distance is infinity. Otherwise, its crowding distance is the summation of the side lengths of the closed space, which is formatted by neighbors of point C.

In the multi-optimization of maintenance timing decision-making, there are a certain amount of solutions that are selected from the whole set of visited solutions to be as near to the Pareto-optimal front as possible. For individuals belong to the same Pareto front, the individuals with larger crowding distance will be retained as exemplars to avoid getting trapped in a local optimum. Thereby, MOCLPSO will be more capable to exploit new areas MOCLPSO.

In order to verify the validity of the MOCLPSO to solve maintenance timing decision-making, a case study is addressed in Chapter 8.

6.3.2 Grouping Methods for Maintenance

After the decision-making for maintenance timing, another major challenge of MS is to decide how to group different machines together in each maintenance activity. In this section, the clustering-based group maintenance (CGM) method is presented.

6.3.2.1 Clustering-Based Group Maintenance Method

Based on GT, products or processes with high similarity can be grouped together to achieve higher efficiency. For instance, cellular manufacturing based on GT can bring not only reduction in set-up time, throughput time and work-in-process inventories, but also enhanced quality and lower costs [18]. In this book, GT is employed to group facilities into maintenance units by measuring the similarities that are related to maintenance among them. Similarities in location, facility type, type of maintenance needed, structural position, and maintenance time needed are considered. The HC method is utilized to form maintenance groups.

As maintenance is conducted on groups of facilities, by clustering facilities that are close to each other into the same group, time can be saved and better logistics of maintenance resources can be achieved. Therefore, we consider the facilities' similarity in location in grouping, which is determined by the distance between any two facilities. According to a relative coordinate system on the shop floor, facility i is assigned two coordinate values, that is, x_i and y_i, to describe its layout and location on the shop floor. Thus the distance $D_{\text{dis}}^{i,j}$ between facilities i and j can be calculated by Equation 6.20.

$$D_{\text{dis}}^{i,j} = \sqrt{(x_i - x_j)^2 + (y_i - y_j)^2} \tag{6.20}$$

And the similarity of facilities i and j in location is calculated by normalizing the distance between them, as in Equation 6.21.

$$S_l^{i,j} = (D_{\text{dis}}^{\max} - D_{\text{dis}}^{i,j})/(D_{\text{dis}}^{\max} - D_{\text{dis}}^{\min}) \tag{6.21}$$

where, $D_{\text{dis}}^{\min}$ and $D_{\text{dis}}^{\max}$ are the minimum and maximum distances between any two facilities considered in clustering.

High similarities in structure, failure mode, and performance degradation among facilities of the same or similar type can be utilized to improve the maintenance efficiency. To measure the similarity of facility type, the types of facilities are encoded with two digits. The first digit stands for the function of the facility, and the second stands for its sub-type. For instance, if there are lathes, milling machines, and grinding machines on one shop floor, then the first digits for the three types of machine tools are L, M, and G. Suppose there are five different types of milling machines, then for these milling machines, the second digits of their codes are the numbers 1–5. Denote the first and second digits of facility i as d_1^i and d_2^i, and the similarity in facility type $S_{\text{p}}^{i,j}$ between facilities i and j is defined by Equation 6.22.

$$S_{\text{p}}^{i,j} = \begin{cases} 0, \text{ if } d_1^i \neq d_1^j \text{ and } d_2^i \neq d_2^j \\ 1, \text{ if } d_1^i = d_1^j \text{ and } d_2^i = d_2^j \\ 0.5, \text{ else} \end{cases} \tag{6.22}$$

Usually, the maintenance type determines the process of the maintenance action, as well as the maintenance resources needed. By grouping facilities that require the same type of maintenance, the preparation work before maintenance can be simplified and the efficiency of the maintenance can be improved. To measure the similarity of facilities in their type of maintenance action, a one-digit code is assigned to each facility. Particularly, in this book, maintenance actions are categorized into M (minor maintenance), D (medium maintenance), O (overhaul), and R (replacement). Denote the code digit of facility i as d^i, the similarity between facilities i and j in the type of maintenance action needed, $S_n^{i,j}$, is defined by Equation 6.23.

$$S_a^{i,j} = \begin{cases} 0, & \text{if } d^i \neq d^j \\ 1, & \text{if } d^i = d^j \end{cases} \tag{6.23}$$

In GM, maintenance actions of facilities in the same group start and end simultaneously. Facilities at a different work stage should be assigned to the same group to accelerate the recovery of productivity of the system. For example, assume that in a maintenance activity, Facility 1, 2, and 3 in the system shown in Figure 6.14 need maintenance, and all of them should be divided into two groups, which cannot be maintained simultaneously. If Facilities 1 and 2 are clustered in Group 1, Facility 3 in Group 2, and Group 1 is maintained first, the productivity can be recovered to half of normal once Group 1's maintenance ends. However, if Facility 2 and 3 are clustered in Group 1, and Facility 1 in Group 2, the productivity of Production Line 1 will remain suspended until both groups are maintained. The similarity between facilities i and j in their structural position, $S_s^{i,j}$, is defined by Equation 6.24.

$$S_s^{i,j} = \begin{cases} 0, & \text{if } s_1^i = s_1^j \,\&\, s_2^i = s_2^j \,\&\, s_3^i = s_3^j \\ 1, & \text{else} \end{cases} \tag{6.24}$$

To avoid too much maintenance time for one group, the maintenance time needed for each facility should be considered. As longer maintenance time increases the risk of improper clustering, the sum of maintenance times for two facilities is used to measure their similarity $S_t^{i,j}$, which can be calculated by Equations 6.25 and 6.26.

$$\overset{\frown}{t}{}_{\mathrm{t}}^{i,j} = t_{\mathrm{m}}^i + t_{\mathrm{m}}^j \tag{6.25}$$

$$S_{\mathrm{t}}^{i,j} = (\overset{\frown}{t}{}_{\mathrm{t}}^{i,j} - \overset{\frown}{t}{}_{\mathrm{t}}^{\mathrm{min}})/(\overset{\frown}{t}{}_{\mathrm{t}}^{\mathrm{max}} - \overset{\frown}{t}{}_{\mathrm{t}}^{\mathrm{min}}) \tag{6.26}$$

where, $\overset{\frown}{t}{}_{\mathrm{t}}^{\mathrm{min}}$ and $\overset{\frown}{t}{}_{\mathrm{t}}^{\mathrm{max}}$ are the minimal and maximal time needed to maintain any two facilities considered in clustering.

Therefore, the similarity between facility i and j can be calculated by Equation 6.27.

$$S^{i,j} = W_{\mathrm{l}} \cdot S_{\mathrm{l}}^{i,j} + W_{\mathrm{p}} \cdot S_{\mathrm{p}}^{i,j} + W_{\mathrm{a}} \cdot S_{\mathrm{a}}^{i,j} + W_{\mathrm{s}} \cdot S_{\mathrm{s}}^{i,j} + W_{\mathrm{t}} \cdot S_{\mathrm{t}}^{i,j} \tag{6.27}$$

where W_{l}, W_{p}, W_{a}, W_{s}, and W_{t} are the corresponding weights for the five similarity measurements.

With the similarity between any two facilities, clustering analysis can be carried out to divide the facilities into maintenance groups. In this book, the weighted average linkage method is employed due to its ability to measure the similarity between two clusters comprehensively. The similarity between clusters P and Q, denoted as $S_C^{P,Q}$, can be calculated by Equation 6.28.

$$S_C^{P,Q} = \sum_{i \in G_P, j \in G_Q} S^{i,j}/(n_P \cdot n_Q) \tag{6.28}$$

where, G_P and G_Q are clusters P and Q, n_P and n_Q are the numbers of facilities in clusters P and Q, respectively. If clusters P and Q are merged into a new cluster R, then the similarity between cluster R and the other clusters can be calculated by Equation 6.29 where K stands for any a pre-existing cluster except clusters P and Q.

$$S_C^{K,R} = (n_P \cdot S_C^{K,P} + n_Q \cdot S_C^{K,Q})/n_R \tag{6.29}$$

As all the facilities are merged into one cluster, the agglomerative clustering process stops and a dendrogram can be plotted. Figure 6.16 shows an example of dendrogram. Each upside-down U-shape line in the dendrogram is called a "link" between two objects (clusters or facilities). The height of a link is the similarity between two objects.

The last but the most important step is to decide where to partition the complete cluster into several smaller ones. In this book, the partition process is conducted by measuring the inconsistency coefficient of each link. If the inconsistency values of one link and all the links below it are smaller than a prescribed threshold T_{h}^d, then all the objects connected by these links are clustered into one group. Links that join distinct clusters have a large inconsistency value. The inconsistency value can be calculated using the similarity presented in the dendrogram. As is shown in Figure 6.16, the three links, L_1, L_2, and L_3, have similarities S_1, S_2, and S_3. The inconsistency value I_{con} of L_1 can be calculated by Equation 6.30.

$$I_{\mathrm{con}} = |S_1 - \mathrm{avg}(S_1, S_2, S_3)|/\mathrm{std}(S_1, S_2, S_3) \tag{6.30}$$

where $\mathrm{avg}(S_1, S_2, S_3)$ and $\mathrm{std}(S_1, S_2, S_3)$ are the average and standard deviation of S_1, S_2, and S_3. In this context only one level of links below link L_1, that is, links L_2 and L_3, have been used to calculate its inconsistency value. The depth of levels, d_{L}, can

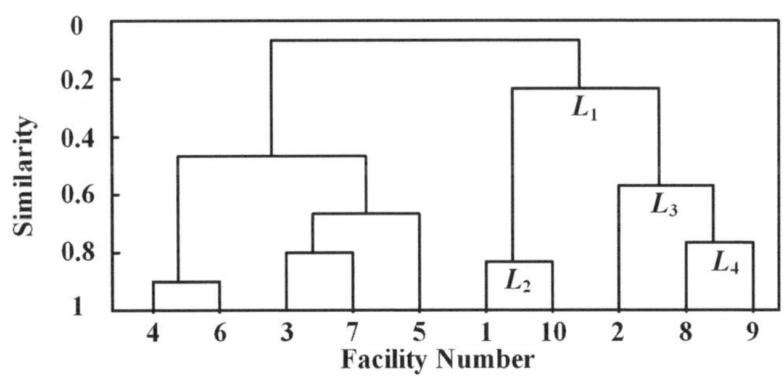

Figure 6.16 An example of a dendrogram

also be adjusted so that more levels of links below can be included in the calculation. For instance, if the depth of levels is set as 3, then 2 or less than 2 levels of links below one link should be considered to calculate its inconsistency value. For links that have no other links below them, their inconsistency values are set as zero.

In this book, the depth of levels d_L is set as 3, and the threshold T_h^d is set as 0.8. Thus, the facilities in Figure 6.16 can be divided into four groups: the first group includes facilities 4 and 6; the second group includes 1 and 10; the third group includes facilities 3, 5, and 7; and the fourth group includes facilities 2, 8, and 9.

6.3.2.2 Rule-Based Group Maintenance Method

To verify the effectiveness of the CGM policy, RGM the (rule-based group maintenance) policy proposed in previous research is employed to carry out a comparison.

According to the RGM policy, facilities are maintained by groups that are formed following a set of rules. First, static groups are formed according to the structure dependence of a production system, which will not change once formed. Five rules should be followed to form static groups:

Rule 1 – According to the layout of a workshop, only facilities that are closely located should be included in one static group.

Rule 2 – Facilities that carry out similar production processes should be included in one static group, preferably under Rule 1.

Rule 3 – According to the logistics of a workshop, only facilities that are in the same flow of work-in-progress should be included in one static group.

Rule 4 – The production capacity in one static group should be balanced.

Rule 5 – The number of facilities in one static group should be neither less than 2 nor more than 5.

In addition, when the facilities in one static group all need minor maintenance, they are not maintained in the present maintenance activity.

After all the possible static groups are formed, there may be some facilities not included in any static groups. Moreover, in a maintenance activity, it is possible that not all the facilities in one static group will need maintenance. Therefore, dynamic groups are formed according to the similarities among facilities. Three rules should be followed to form dynamic groups:

Rule 6 – Only facilities of the same type can be included in one dynamic group.

Rule 7 – Only facilities in the same production line can be included in one dynamic group.

Rule 8 – The number of facilities in one dynamic group should be neither less than 2 nor more than 5.

6.3.2.3 Dynamic Grouping Maintenance Method

A major challenge of the maintenance optimization consists in joining the stochastic processes regarding the components (time-dependent probabilities of failure) with the combinatorial problems regarding the grouping of maintenance activities. While a long term or infinite planning horizon can be assumed to solve this problem for stable situations, dynamic models have been introduced in order to change the planning rules according to short-term information (e.g., failures and varying deterioration of components), using a rolling (finite) horizon approach which seems to be a very powerful method in the framework of dynamic maintenance optimization. However, the approach developed is applicable only when maintenance durations are neglected. From a practical point of view, the system may be stopped during maintenance execution of components, maintenance durations should therefore be taken into account, especially when the system unavailability cost rate is high. Furthermore, each component is assumed to be preventively maintained only one time within a scheduling interval. However, a system may be composed of different components with different lifetime cycles so the maintenance frequencies of the components will be different. For example, the engine oil has to be changed more frequently than the driving belt on a heavy vehicle. The first objective of this research is to develop the rolling horizon approach by taking into account both the preventive maintenance durations and the multiple occurrences of maintenance operations in the scheduling interval.

In the framework of dynamic situations, inactivity periods of the system may occur with time for whatever reason, for example, due to production/commercial planning. They can be considered as interesting opportunities to perform preventive or/and corrective maintenance operations since the maintenance costs may thus be reduced. This is especially true for series systems, where a single failure results in a system downtime. Preventive maintenance at opportunities with restricted duration, which can occur randomly, is proposed. The optimal components for each opportunity are chosen according to their importance ranking. The second objective of this research (and one of its original contributions) is to propose a new algorithm taking into account random maintenance opportunities in the grouping maintenance optimization procedure. This second contribution can help to update online the grouped maintenance plan when maintenance opportunities become available.

Grouping of several maintenance activities could reduce the maintenance cost as the set-up cost can be shared when performing maintenance by group. We are therefore interested in constructing a grouped maintenance plan in which at each maintenance occasion several maintenance activities to be optimized are carried out. It must be noted, however, that when several maintenance activities are performed in the same maintenance occasion, the maintenance cost could be indirectly penalized with:

1. Reduction of the component's useful life, which is represented by its nominal maintenance periodicity, if the maintenance dates are advanced.
2. Increasing probability of components failure if the maintenance dates are postponed, which could lead to system immobilization.

In order to find the optimal groups which could balance to minimize the system maintenance cost on the scheduling horizon, the rolling horizon approach introduced recently will be developed by taking into account the preventive maintenance durations and the multiple occurrences of maintenance operations.

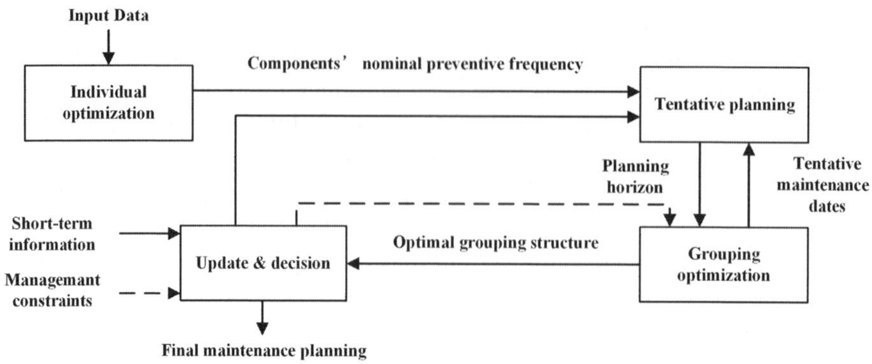

Figure 6.17 Dynamic grouping maintenance approach

Moreover, it is assumed in this work that the system may be randomly stopped in specific time intervals during which several preventive activities could be performed with reduced maintenance cost. The information concerning these inactivity periods of the system is assumed to occur randomly with time. In this way, when an opportunity occurs, the current grouped maintenance plan might no longer be the optimal one. To take into account the maintenance opportunity, a new grouped maintenance plan is needed.

The dynamic grouping maintenance approach is illustrated in Figure 6.17. The developed approach is divided into four steps:

Step 1: Individual optimization
Step 2: Tentative planning
Step 3: Grouping optimization and
Step 4: Update and decision.

Step 1: Individual optimization

The objective is to find the optimal individual preventive maintenance interval for each component using an infinite-horizon maintenance model in which we assume an average use of component i and in which the interactions between components are neglected.

Let $M_i(x)$ denote the expected deterioration cost for component i, that is, the expected costs incurred in x time units since the latest execution of activity i. According to a minimal repair policy, $M_i(x)$ can be written as

$$M_i(x) = C_i^c \cdot \int_0^x r_i(y)\mathrm{d}y$$

where $r_i(.)$ is the rate of occurrence of failure of component i. $r_i(y)$ represents the expected failure numbers of component i within interval $[0,x]$. The expected deterioration cost for component i can be expressed as

$$M_i(x) = c_i^c \cdot \left(\frac{x}{\lambda_\iota}\right) \beta_i$$

If component i is preventively maintained at x, the expected cost within interval $[0, x + d_i]$ is determined. By using the renewal theory [36], the long-term average cost of component i can be determined. The optimal interval length for the preventive maintenances of the component i can be obtained when it leads to the minimum value of the long-term average cost.

Step 2: Tentative planning

In order to evaluate the performance of the dynamic grouping, a finite planning horizon is usually defined according to the current date, denoted t_{begin}, and the ending date t_{end} that guarantees that all components are preventively maintained at least one time in this horizon interval $[t_{\text{begin}}, t_{\text{end}}]$.

Step 3: Grouping optimization

The main idea of this step is to find all optimal maintenance occasions in order to minimize the expected maintenance cost in the considered scheduling horizon. In each maintenance occasion, several optimal maintenance operations can be sequentially performed. Here, we develop and extend the application possibilities of the algorithm by taking into account:

- duration of maintenance activities
- dependences between multiple occurrence dates of a maintenance activity
- grouping two or more maintenance occurrences of the same maintenance activity is forbidden.

A maintenance occasion (or a group) is defined by three parameters: the execution date, the maintenance operations, and the duration. The first two parameters are optimally identified in order to minimize the expected maintenance cost. The latter is the sum of the duration of all maintenance operations that are in the group.

Step 4: Update and decision

Due to the previous step, we have an optimal grouping structure within the finite planning horizon $[t_{\text{begin}}, t_{\text{end}}]$. The maintenance manager can change the plan in case he/she is not satisfied with it and then go back to step 3 or he/she can carry out one or more groups of activities according to the generated grouping structure and start with step 3.

Furthermore, short-term information or maintenance opportunities may become available with time. In the presence of opportunities, the current maintenance plan may no longer be an optimal one. To update the maintenance plan, a new optimal grouping structure within a new period must be identified. To this end, we simply go back to step 2. A new maintenance plan can then be established without losing the optimality of the previous one.

6.3.3 Maintenance Scheduling Based on a Tabu Search

In terms of solving MS problems, common methods include traditional optimization algorithms such as dynamic programing, and intelligent algorithms such as GA [12]. Traditional optimization algorithms are becoming unsatisfactory as MS problems become increasingly complex. GA is widely used in solving MS problems due to its strong global searching ability, whereas its disadvantage is also obvious – its fast initial convergence followed by progressive slower improvements. It is suggested that GA should be combined with other algorithms such as SA, which form HGA, to overcome the disadvantage. Esbensen and Mazumder [37] combined GA with SA and this algorithm is verified to be more effective than simple GA.

In addition, most of the research mentioned above is based on the assumption that facilities are independent ones in the production system, however, in most cases, connections between facilities and their process assignment should be considered, especially for complex production systems.

In this section, a MS method for a complex series-parallel system is proposed under GM policy combined with OM policy utilizing a TS (Tabu search). In addition, HGA, which combines GA with SA, will be presented in Chapter 7 to support prognosis oriented maintenance decision-making.

A flow chart for TS is shown in Figure 6.18 where S is the maximum iteration time. The initial population is created after initialization of the parameters. A neighbor of x is created by swapping two randomly selected integers in its solution string. Tabulist keeps a record of the swap moves by which x is created. In terms of an aspiration criterion, a solution created by a swap move in the Tabulist is accepted if the solution is better than the best solution x^* obtained so far. The size of the neighbor is set as V, and the length of the Tabulist is set as $V/2$.

6.3.3.1 Solution Encoding

In this section, either a single facility that does not belong to any groups or a maintenance group is considered as a maintenance unit, which is assigned with an integer unit number. Hence integer encoding is utilized. In addition, the string that contains an individual's encoding is referred to as a chromosome, and each integer is referred to as a gene. If there are M units in one maintenance activity, feasible chromosomes are obtained by putting integers from 1 to M in random orders.

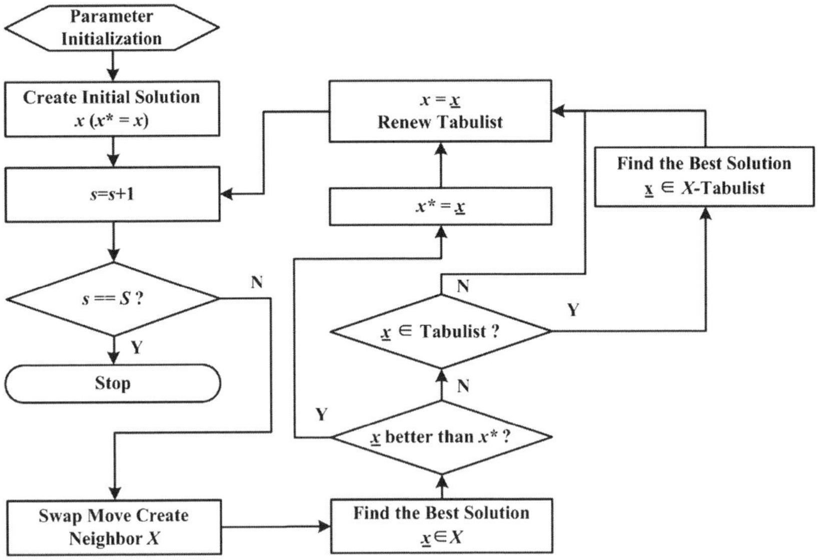

Figure 6.18 Flow chart of TS

6.3.3.2 Fitness Function

For a number of maintenance schedules, once their maintenance cost and production lost are obtained, their fitness values can be calculated. Suppose there are Q maintenance schedules, for the qth schedule, its fitness value f_q can be calculated by Equation 6.31.

$$f_q = 1/\left[\left(C_{m,q}^{k} + L_{p,q}^{k}\right) / \sum_{r=1}^{Q}(C_{m,r}^{k} + L_{p,r}^{k})\right] \tag{6.31}$$

where C_m^k and L_p^k are the maintenance cost and production in the kth maintenance activity, respectively.

6.3.4 *Dynamic Scheduling of Maintenance Measure*

In complex production systems, the unplanned failure of even a single machine can have significant consequences (e.g., loss of production) for the upstream and downstream process steps and equipment.

In order to enhancc thc planning process, condition monitoring systems are increasingly applied. These systems allow monitoring of the condition of particular components susceptible to wear during operation (e.g., for feed drives, spindle bearings, monorail guidance systems). Thereby, it is possible to detect maintenance needs long before the components fail (CBM strategy). This results in a surplus of planning lead time which can be used to systematically integrate planned maintenance measures (scheduled and condition-based maintenance) in the production planning process and to avoid the mentioned loss of production.

However, experience shows that, for various production systems, planned maintenance measures are predominantly scheduled on the basis of the availability of qualified personnel and the existence of production-free periods. This is because, especially for complex production systems, it is hardly possible for the production planner to predict the impact of planned maintenance measures on the productivity of the whole system. As a consequence, high energy consumption and maintenance costs tend to occur.

A static prediction of the system's behavior with average values (e.g., for transport time) is not sufficient. Consequently, a novel approach which allows the dynamic scheduling of maintenance measures in production systems is being developed. This planning approach has been conceptualized as a model-based coordination where the production structures and procedures of complex, stochastic, and dynamic production systems (multi-level process chain) have been represented by means of event-driven simulation. The required means of planned maintenance of machine tool components and their effects on the original production planning have been similarly characterized. As a result, an integration of planned maintenance measures in the production programs has been enabled. In order to introduce the approach properly, an overview of the state of research on short- and long-term scheduling of maintenance tasks is provided and the necessary further course of action is illustrated. Afterwards, a general procedure for the dynamic scheduling approach is introduced. Taking into consideration a real application scenario of a company, this approach is evaluated and key findings are generalized.

6.3.4.1 Short- and Long-Term Scheduling of Maintenance

Approaches to condition-based, energy-effective maintenance planning (M-planning) with a long-term time horizon focus on the life-cycle of machine components (e.g., spindles, ball screws). The life-cycle usually includes the initial installation to the moment when the component is to be dismantled, either because of a failure or in order to prevent one.

A variety of approaches focuses on the one-machine-component case or the one-machine-system case. They include two main steps: the modeling of the stochastic wear of the machine component over a given period of time and the development of suitable procedures for maintenance planning. Each of these predominantly analytical approaches aims to derive an efficient inspection plan or to identify suitable parameters for the optimal preventive replacement of components, for example, in the form of a replacement limit. Classical representatives of these approaches focus on minimizing the production and maintenance costs. Approaches which aim at minimizing the energy consumption are included in some cases.

Castanier *et al.* [38] and Maksoud *et al.* [39] extend the previously-mentioned approaches by developing maintenance planning for a two-machine-component and two-machine-system, respectively. Maksoud *et al.* [39] model the second machine as a replacement machine in order to secure the overall availability if the first machine is to be maintained. Castanier *et al.* [38] analyze the advantages of a simultaneous maintenance of both components on the assumption that the costs for the combined maintenance, including the associated set-up costs are incurred only once.

Further approaches consider multi-machine-components or multi-machines-systems. Lu and Sy [40] implement a fuzzy logic approach which enhances the maintenance planning process by providing maintenance requirements in real time. Marseguerra and Zio [41] as well as Camci [19] develop an approach to maintenance planning based on genetic algorithms. Thereby, Marseguerra and Zio [46] focus on the determination of an optimal wear limit for the implementation of preventive maintenance measures while Camci [19] proposes a maintenance plan minimizing the risk of an unplanned standstill. Wang [42] combines maintenance planning with an appropriate inventory policy.

The above-presented approaches with a long-term time horizon fail to integrate the maintenance measure into the existing production processes. Typically, they focus on one or multiple machine(s) or machine-component(s) and their condition and schedule a cost- and energy-minimal maintenance time point without taking the underlying production system into consideration. Therefore, these approaches are not qualified for scheduling of maintenance measures in complex production systems.

Research approaches focusing on cost-optimal scheduling of the required maintenance measures for the affected resources in the operative production process (start and end date of the maintenance measures) are summarized as maintenance planning with a short-term time horizon. Moore and Starr [43] develop an approach to short-term maintenance planning, which prioritizes the present maintenance tasks in addition to evaluating the technical failure risk. In his cost-based criticality (CBC) methodology, Moore and Starr [43] analyze not only the costs and the risk of failure, but also other factors, such as resource utilization, environment impact, and quality losses. Cheung *et al.* [44] propose an analytical model for scheduling of necessary maintenance measures for a chemical production plant.

The described approaches for short-term maintenance planning take into account the existing production structures and processes, but they fail to accurately represent the complexity of real production systems (restrictive assumptions). For various analytic, statistic and numeric methods it is often required (due to performance issues) to make simplified assumptions, since the adequacy of these approaches for supporting the decision-making in today's complex production systems is limited. Furthermore, these methods quickly meet their limits when it comes to integrating the time dynamics of a production process in the calculation. Thus, a dynamic assessment of the impact of a maintenance measure on the production (indirect maintenance costs, such as failure and failure-related costs), in particular on complex production systems, is hardly possible.

In conclusion, we see that the described approaches are rarely tailored to the analysis of the dynamic behavior of complex production systems.

6.3.4.2 Approach to Dynamic Scheduling of Maintenance Measures

Parameters and Control Variables of the Planning Approach

The parameters, which are part of this planning approach and of the considered production system, are summarized in Table 6.2.

In order to exemplify and concretize the planning problem, a two-stage production system consisting of five machines and four buffer areas has been used (Figure 6.19). Scheduling the maintenance measure MA_1 and the production orders $A_1 - A_4$ in such a way that the resulting production and maintenance costs are as low as possible is a major objective of a coordinated production and maintenance planning approach. For this purpose, it is assumed that the starting time of the maintenance action MA_1 on

Table 6.2 Parameters of the planning approach to dynamic scheduling of maintenance measures

Planning data	Data of the production system	
Production planning	Organizational data	Technical data
Production orders	Product data (e.g., variants geometry)	Capacity of buffers/storages
Batch sizes/reserved capacity for production orders	Structural organization (e.g., layout of machines, conveyors, buffers, and storage)	Capacity of machine
Sequences	Operational organization (e.g., process steps)	Machine processing times for product variants
Machine assignment	Strategies (e.g., for material flow, set-up changeover)	Set-up times
Quantity demanded	Breaks	Availability of machines (MTBF-mean time between failures, MTTR-mean time to repair)
Maintenance planning	Shift calendar	Scrap rate
Maintenance measure	Restrictions	Material flow data
Maintenance object	–	Capacity of conveyors
Maintenance time	–	Speed of conveyors
Starting point of maintenance measure	–	–

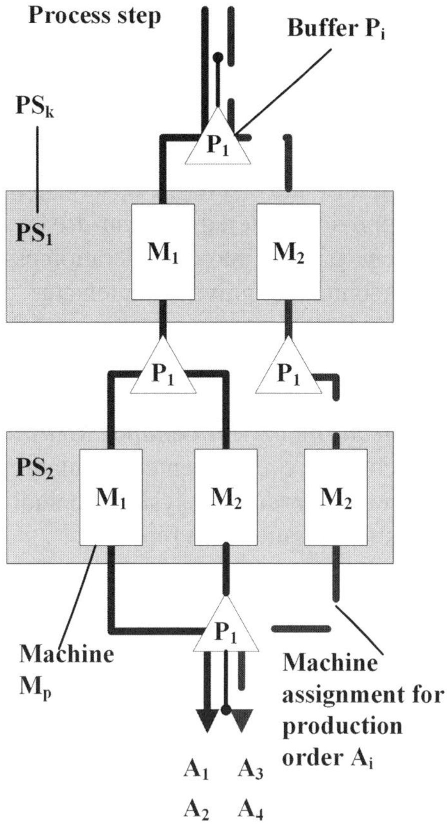

Figure 6.19 Approach to scheduling planned maintenance measures

machine M_3 can be varied. The control variable of the approach is thus the starting point t_{S1} of the maintenance measure MA_1.

Ane ssential prerequisite for determining the most cost-effective starting point is to estimate the impact of the intended maintenance measure on the production system. The implementation of the maintenance measure on machine M_3, for example, can have different effects on the production process:

1. The number of intermediate products in the preceding buffer area P_2 for the duration of the standstill of the machine M_3 will probably be increased. This can be explained by the fact that the given resource (in this case M_3) is temporarily unavailable for the processing of the production order.
2. For the same reason, the level in the following buffer area P_4 is expected to decrease.
3. Depending on the initial state of the system (e.g., machine processing times, current buffer level, etc.) and on the duration of the maintenance measure MA_1, this might result in disruption of supply in the subsequent production areas.

Assuming that the consequences of this scenario can be quantified with dynamic methods, it can be used for an efficient scheduling of the maintenance measure MA_1. In the case discussed above, the implementation of the maintenance measure during the production can be considered economically viable if the entire, reserved capacity of the redundant machine M_4 is not fully utilized and if the resulting short-term loss of production can be reversed until the end of the observation period.

A model-based planning approach centered on event-driven simulation will enhance the depicted planning problem. It takes into consideration essential limitations (e.g., availability of qualified personnel, required maintenance time) and dynamically determines the point of time for maintenance. This approach is described in the following.

Procedure for Dynamic Scheduling of Maintenance Measures

A central step of the approach is the event-oriented simulation which is used to accurately represent the real, complex production system, including its production structures, processes, and stochastics (Figure 6.20) [45].

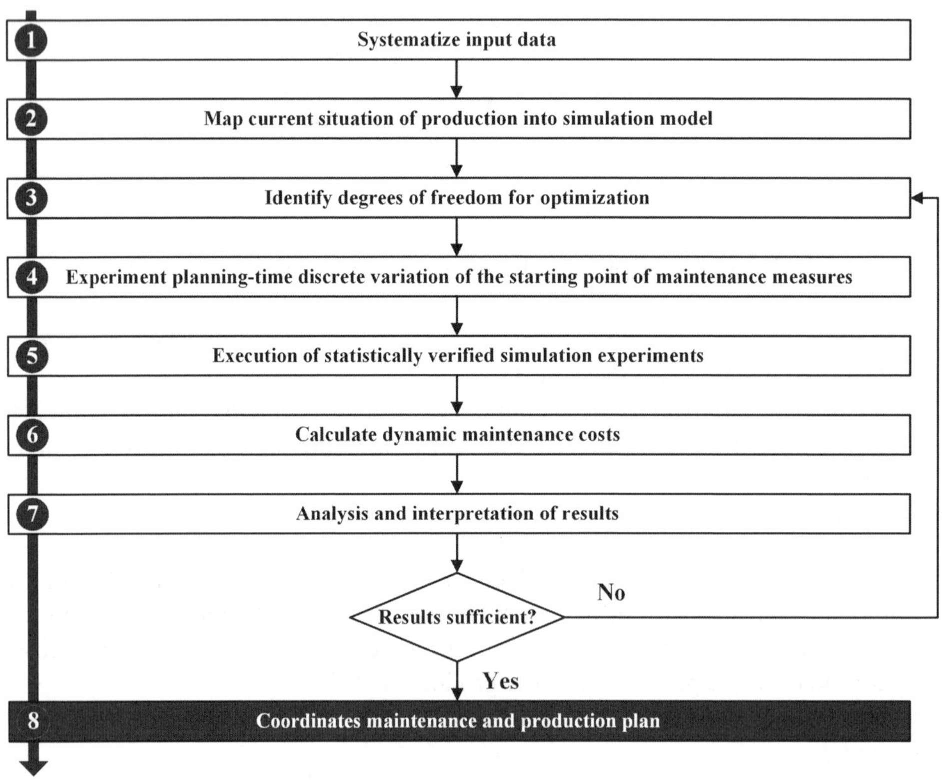

Figure 6.20 Procedure for dynamic scheduling of maintenance measures

At the beginning of the planning period, it is necessary to transfer essential parameters of the real production (e.g., processing times, current buffer levels) into the simulation model (steps 1 and 2). The existing production plan (including batch size, machine assignment, sequences, etc.) serves as a basis for the integrated production and maintenance planning. Maintenance requirements (e.g., maintenance objects, maintenance times, etc.) which are often based on the expert knowledge of experienced employees are also mapped in the model. In addition, the optimization parameters (e.g., for statistically verified simulation results, see Section 3.3.4) concerning the model-based coordination and the degrees of freedom of its optimization (e.g., possible periods for scheduling the maintenance measure) are also taken into consideration (step 3).

An automated, simulation-based assessment of potential starting points of maintenance measures is carried out based on the initial data. It comprises the two stages: experiment planning (step 4) and its subsequent evaluation (steps 5 and 6).

All possible planning alternatives are systematized as part of the experiment planning; the ensuing simulation experiments are assembled into the experimental design. Then, the experimental design is implemented with the help of statistically verified simulation experiments. Based on so-called "what if" scenarios, the control variable t_{sj} is varied for the different experiments, and the resulting target variable (dynamic maintenance costs) is determined with the help of the simulation (step 6).

In order to ensure the time-efficient execution of the simulation experiments, a procedure based on statistical methods has been developed. This procedure solves the conflict between statistically verified outcome data derived from all simulation experiments and the minimum number of necessary simulation observations.

After execution of the simulation study, the resulting values are linked to each other, whereas the dynamic maintenance costs are calculated and displayed graphically. The selection of the most cost-effective start time (optimization) of the maintenance measure is carried out by the user at the end of the procedure (step 7).

6.3.5 Case Study

6.3.5.1 Case Description

Here, a case study of the MS of a bearing production workshop is presented. The production system has 45 facilities, as shown in Figure 6.21. Facilities 0, 46, and 17 are input, output, and heat treatment, respectively, and it is assumed that their performances do not degrade with time. Arrows on the left-hand side connect production lines for the outer race, those on the right-hand side connect the lines for the inner race. The horizontal arrows at the bottom connect the assembly line of the bearings. The layout of the workshop is also as presented in Figure 6.21. Facilities 1 to 16 carry out lathing processes, 18 to 35 milling, 36 and 37 grinding, 38 and 39 demagnetizing, 40 and 41 cleaning, 42 and 43 sizing, 44 assembling, and 45 riveting. Based on

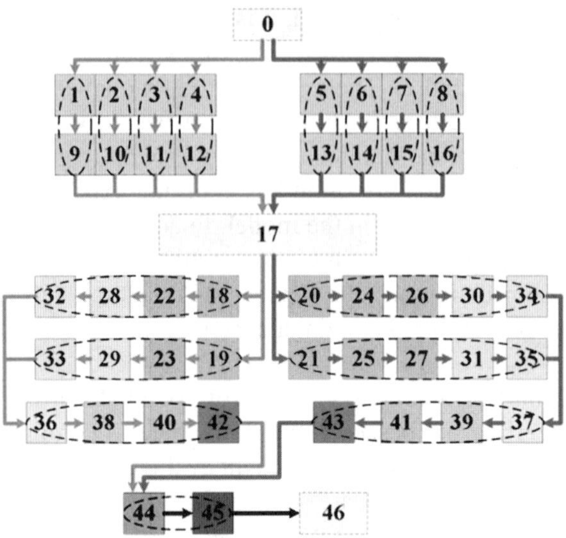

Figure 6.21 Production system for bearings

the above information, the topology of the system is built, and accordingly 15 static groups are formed, which are marked with dashed ellipses in Figure 6.21.

6.3.5.2 Parameter Settings

The two parameters in reliability modeling, η and β, are given to represent the endurance and aging rate of each facility. In this research, the three thresholds, T_{h}^{1}, T_{h}^{2}, and T_{h}^{3}, are set as 0.9, 0.75, and 0.6, respectively; and L_{R} is set as 0.2; improvement factors for minor maintenance, medium maintenance, and overhaul are set as 0.2, 0.6, and 0.7; the compensation factor F is calculated by Equation 6.32 where O_n is the number of overhauls for a single facility.

$$F = 0.1^{(1/(1+O_n))} \tag{6.32}$$

The set-up cost C_{s} of each maintenance activity is set as 1000; the unit prices for four types of maintenance resources, that is, spare parts, tools, maintainers, and energy, are set as 100, 50, 50, and 10, respectively; the initial value of the production lost rate r_0 is set as 1000.

For the TS, the maximum iteration time S is set as 100, the size of the neighbor V is set as $(M-1)\cdot M/2$.

6.3.5.3 Simulation and Result Analysis

To verify the effectiveness of the proposed method, MS of the production system from the 1st to the 3000th day of operation is carried out with maintenance resource constraints.

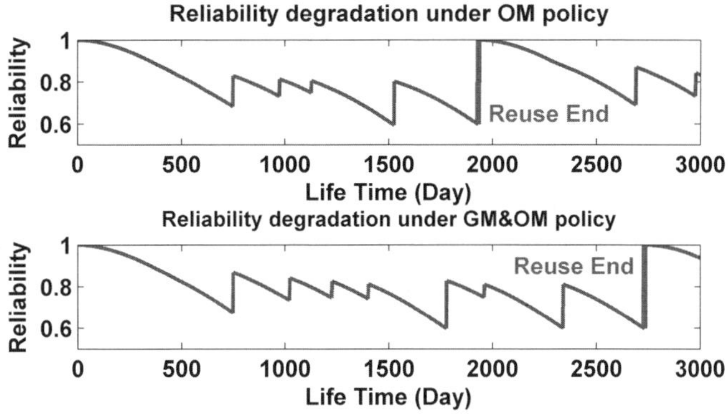

Figure 6.22 Reuse situation of facility 2 under two maintenance policies

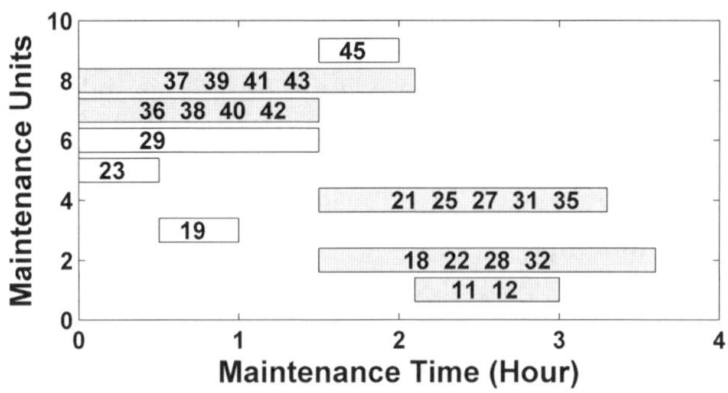

Figure 6.23 Gantt chart of maintenance scheduling under GM&OM policy

During the 3000 days, 84 maintenance activities are carried out if the group maintenance combined with opportunistic maintenance (GM&OM) policy is followed, and 85 maintenance activities are carried out if only the OM policy is followed. In addition, about 74% of the facilities have longer reuse periods under the GM&OM policy. For instance, the reuse period of facility 2 was extended from 1932 to 2730 days if the GM&OM policy was followed, as shown in Figure 6.22.

In each maintenance activity, the maintenance tasks are scheduled using TS. Figure 6.23 is an example of a Gantt chart under GM&OM policy, where the filled bars stand for GM.

In addition, it can also be concluded that the maintenance cost rate under the GM&OM policy is approximately 12% less than that under the OM policy.

6.4 Heuristic Methodology for Multi-unit System Maintenance Scheduling

The maintenance decision is an essential issue for production systems and has been researched for decades. Researchers have proposed hundreds of models from different perspectives. Statistical approaches have been developed for maintenance decision-making. However, most of the existing models [46–48] are established for a single unit or system which is not applicable to practical production systems consisting of multi-units or multiple systems.

So far few of the existing models for multi-unit systems take a proper consideration of the topology connection of hybrid multi-unit systems. In addition, for complex multi-unit systems, the need arises for more efficient search engines to effectively span the search space in a reasonable computing time. This section focuses on multi-unit systems with any topology (series, parallel, hybrid structures, etc.) and attempts to give a heuristic-based AI approach to schedule maintenance activities considering three kinds of maintenance actions, such as minor repair, imperfect overhaul, and replacement.

6.4.1 Models or Multi-Unit System Maintenance Decision

It is assumed that the performance degradation of units is independent. The corresponding models for decision-making are discussed as follows.

6.4.1.1 Topology Modeling

The topology connection can be described by three definitions:

Definition 1: Layer number ($L_{i,\mathrm{N}}$). Each unit i is assigned a layer number starting from the upstream activity.

Definition 2: Number of direct connections ($N_{i,\mathrm{dc}}$). This describes the number of units that connect to the current unit directly, both backward and forward.

Definition 3: Number of units to be shut down ($N_{i,\mathrm{ts}}$): This term indicates how many units must be shut down (stopped) when the current unit fails.

6.4.1.2 Imperfect Maintenance Modeling

In this work, three kinds of maintenance actions are considered: minor repair, imperfect overhaul, and replacement. The relations between deterioration of the unit and maintenance actions are shown in Figure 6.24. For example, in a minor repair, the FR turns out to be smaller after maintenance, see interval (t_M, t_I).

The FR curve can be acquired from historical data and approximately simulated by a Weibull function curve. A Weibull function with two parameters is defined as follows [49]:

$$F(t) = 1 - \mathrm{e}^{-\left(\frac{t}{\eta}\right)^{\beta}} \tag{6.33}$$

where $\eta > 0$ and $\beta > 0$.

For each unit i, three kinds of maintenance actions (minor repair, imperfect overhaul, and replacement) correspond to a set of parameters, $\eta_{i,\mathrm{M}}$, $\beta_{\mathrm{i,M}}$, $\eta_{\mathrm{i,I}}$, $\beta_{\mathrm{i,I}}$, $\eta_{i,\mathrm{R}}$, $\beta_{\mathrm{i,R}}$,

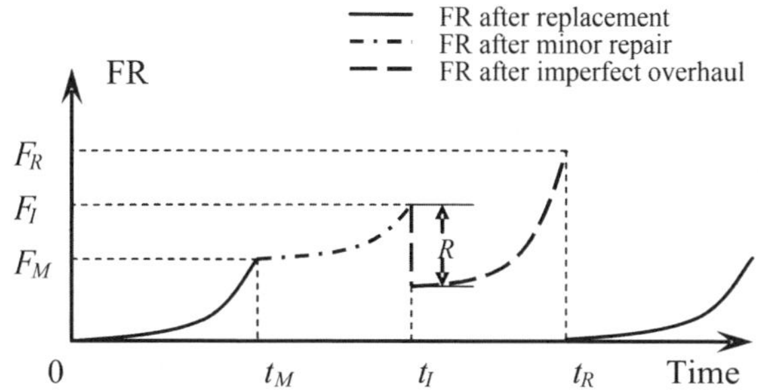

Figure 6.24 Schematics of FR after maintenance actions

respectively. In this context, three thresholds are considered: F_{R} (replacement threshold), F_{I} (imperfect overhaul threshold), and F_{M} (minor repair threshold).

6.4.1.3 Cost Modeling of One Maintenance Activity

In each maintenance activity, there are a number of minor repairs, imperfect overhauls, and replacements which, in this context, are called maintenance actions . Cost is the objective of the maintenance decision in this work. Two kinds of cost are considered: maintenance cost C_{m} and downtime cost C_{d} , which are estimated by

$$C_{\mathrm{m}} = \sum_{i=1}^{k_{\mathrm{M}}} c_{i,M} + \sum_{i=1}^{k_{\mathrm{I}}} c_{i,\mathrm{I}} + \sum_{i=1}^{k_{\mathrm{R}}} c_{i,\mathrm{R}} \tag{6.34}$$

$$C_{\mathrm{d}} = c_{\mathrm{d}} \sum_{i=1}^{k} (T_i(1 + N_{i,\mathrm{ts}}) - t_{\mathrm{o}i}) \tag{6.35}$$

In Equation 6.34, k_{M}, k_{I}, k_{R}, $c_{i,\mathrm{M}}$, $c_{i,\mathrm{I}}$, and $c_{i,\mathrm{R}}$ denote the number of minor repairs, the number of imperfect overhauls, the number of replacements, the minor repair cost of unit *i,* the imperfect overhaul cost of unit *i* and the replacement cost of unit *i*. In Equation 6.35, c_{d}, k, T_i, and $t_{\mathrm{o}i}$ denote the average downtime cost per unit time, the number of units needed to be maintained, the executive time to maintain the *i*th unit and the time saved by OM of the *i*th unit.

Therefore, the total cost of one maintenance activity is:

$$C_{\mathrm{T}} = C_{\mathrm{m}} + C_{\mathrm{d}} \tag{6.36}$$

6.4.2 Heuristic Maintenance Scheduling Algorithm

Four kinds of available resources are considered in this work: spare parts, tradesmen, energy resources, and maintenance tools. Supposing that the resources needed by each unit on any kind of maintenance action are given, the maintenance actions are scheduled according to heuristic rules.

Here, an integrated criterion function is proposed to evaluate the priority of each unit for MS under limited resources. The priority function is defined as

$$P_j = w_{\mathrm{t}}(1 - n_{j,\mathrm{t}}) + w_{\mathrm{l}}(1 - n_{j,\mathrm{l}}) + w_{\mathrm{f}}n_{j,\mathrm{f}} + w_{\mathrm{d}}n_{j,\mathrm{d}} + w_{\mathrm{r}}(1 - n_{j,\mathrm{r}}) \tag{6.37}$$

In Equation 6.37, $n_{j,\mathrm{t}}$ is the normalized executive time of the jth unit; $n_{j,\mathrm{l}}$ is the normalized layer number of the jth unit, $n_{j,\mathrm{f}}$ is the normalized number of forward connections of the jth unit; $n_{j,\mathrm{d}}$ is the normalized number of units to be shut down when the jth unit stops, $n_{j,\mathrm{r}}$ is the normalized resources of the jth unit, w_{t} is the weight of executive time, w_{l} is the weight of the layer number, w_{f} is the weight of the number of forward connections, w_{d} is the weight of number of units to be shut down, and w_{r} is the weight of resources needs.

Tasks with a larger magnitude of P_j are given higher priority during the resource allocation process. The scheduling procedure is as follows: (i) Updating available resources at time t. (ii) Finding all the schedulable units and calculating the priority function P_j of each action. (iii) Choosing the schedulable actions under the limited resources according to the priority. (iv) Applying/waiting for resources if the available resources are inadequate. (v) resource is released immediately when a maintenance action is accomplished. Return to (i).

6.4.3 *Case Study*

A case is studied to illustrate how the methods described in Section 6.3 are applied. Considering a system which is described in Figure 6.25, which is a typical multi-unit system consisting of five machines, the processes are simplified to six units, as shown in Figure 6.26.

Taking machine 1 as an example, the available maintenance resources and the resources needed by each kind of maintenance action of machine 1 are shown in

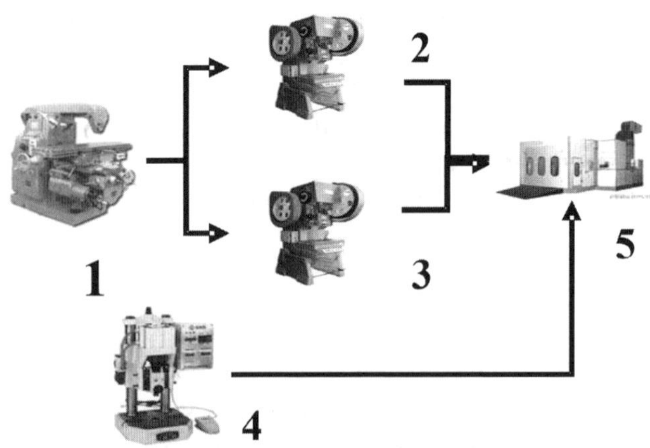

Figure 6.25 System structure

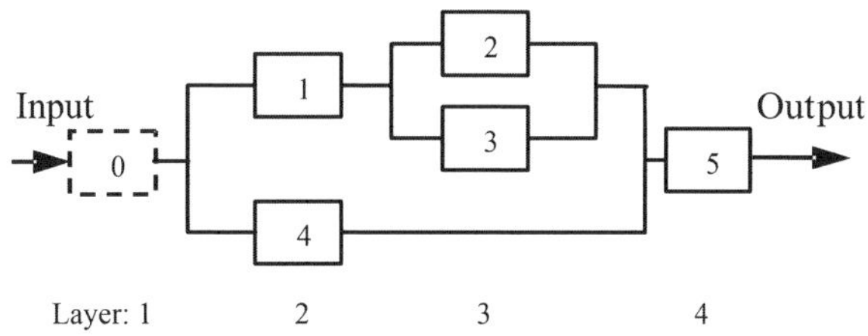

Figure 6.26 Topology of a system

Table 6.3 Resources list

Resources		I	II	III	IV
Total available resources		9	10	8	10
Resources needed for minor repair	Unit 1	1	4	2	3
Resources needed for imperfect overhaul	Unit 1	2	5	3	4
Resources needed for replacement	Unit 1	3	7	5	6

Table 6.4 Maintenance time (hours)

Units	Minor repair	Imperfect overhaul	Replacement
Unit 1	5	12	20

Table 6.5 Weibull parameters list

Parameters	$\eta_{i,\mathrm{M}}$	$\eta_{i,\mathrm{I}}$	$\eta_{i,\mathrm{R}}$	$\beta_{i,\mathrm{M}}$	$\beta_{i,\mathrm{I}}$	$\beta_{i,\mathrm{R}}$
Unit 1	3.91	2.92	3.81	5.15	2.55	4.24

Table 6.3, the corresponding maintenance time is listed in Table 6.4, the deteriorations of the units over time are simulated by Equation 6.33 using the corresponding parameters shown in Table 6.5.

The scheduling process and the GA optimization are carried out in MATLAB. Considering a period of $D = 1800$ days $= 1800 \times 24$ hours, common cost $c_{\mathrm{c}} = 1000$. Presetting thresholds: $F_{\mathrm{M}} = 0.3$; $F_{\mathrm{I}} = 0.5$; $F_{\mathrm{R}} = 0.7$, and weights: $\mathrm{w}_{\mathrm{t}} = 0.3$; $w_{\mathrm{l}} = 0.2$; $w_{\mathrm{f}} = 0.15$; $w_{\mathrm{d}} = 0.2$; $w_{\mathrm{r}} = 0.15$ according to experience, an overall scheduling result is shown in Figure 6.27, in which the FR curves of the 5 units are shown corresponding to schedules.

By the heuristic rules proposed in this section, the maintenance activities are scheduled under the constraints successfully. However, the thresholds and weights are set subjectively. In order to reduce the overall cost rate and maximize the utilization of

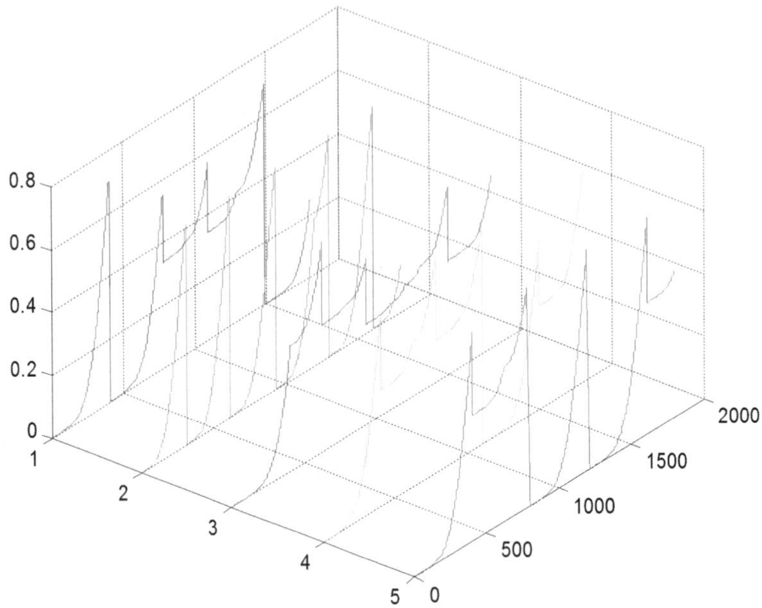

Figure 6.27 Overall scheduling results of units

Table 6.6 Optimization results

	Rule based	Rule with optimized thresholds	Rule with optimized thresholds and weights
Cost rate	21.3467	17.6739	17.2483
Maintenance time (h)	556	486	471
Number of maintenance activities	10	7	7

resources, GA is employed to optimize the thresholds of the maintenance actions and the weights of the heuristic rules.

Through GA optimization, the thresholds are: $F_M = 0.2792$; $F_I = 0.4397$; $F_R = 0.7825$. Based on the optimal thresholds the optimized weights were achieved by GA as: $w_t = 0.0791$; $w_l = 0.0135$; $w_f = 0.0637$; $w_d = 0.3752$; $w_r = 0.4733$. Note that the summation of the weights is 1.

Consequently, we obtain an optimized scheduling based on the optimized threshold and weights. The results of scheduling are shown in Table 6.6, and indicate that the overall cost rate has been optimized effectively. Table 6.6 implies that optimization of maintenance thresholds has great impact on reducing the overall cost rate.

6.4.4 Conclusions and Discussions

A framework for maintenance decision-making for a multi-unit system has been established. The topology model for hybrid connected systems has been proposed to give a proper consideration of its influence on decision-making. The maintenance activities have been scheduled under resource constraints by a heuristic algorithm developed in this work, and then extended to multi-stage maintenance activities scheduling which is further optimized by GA.

References

1. Geert, W. and Liliane, P. (2002) A framework for maintenance concept development. *International Journal of Production Economics*, **3** (77), 299–313.
2. Nowlan, F.S. and Heap, H.F. (1978) *Reliability Centered Maintenance*, United Airlines Publications, San Fransisco, CA.
3. Moubray, J. (1997) *Reliability Centered Maintenance*, Butterworth-Heineman, Oxford.
4. Kelly, A. (1984) *Maintenance Planning and Control*, Butterworths, London.
5. Kelly, A. (1997) *Maintenance Organizations a Systems: Business-Centred Maintenance*, Butterworth-Heinemann, Oxford.
6. Van Horenbeek, A. and Pintelon, L. (2014) Development of a maintenance performance measurement framework–using the analytic network process (ANP) for maintenance performance indicator selection. *Omega*, **42** (1), 33–46.
7. Eti, M.C., Ogaji, S.O.T. and Probert, S.D. (2006) Strategic maintenance-management in Nigerian industries. *Applied Energy*, **83** (3), 211–227.
8. Siener, M. and Aurich, J.C. (2011) Quality oriented maintenance scheduling. *CIRP Journal of Manufacturing Science and Technology*, **4** (1), 15–23.
9. Marquez, A.C. and Gupta, J.N. (2006) Contemporary maintenance management: process, framework and supporting pillars. *Omega*, **34** (3), 313–326.
10. Takata, S., Kirnura, F., Van Houten, F.J.A.M. *et al.* (2004) Maintenance: changing role in life-cycle management. *CIRP Annals-Manufacturing Technology*, **53** (2), 643–655.
11. Ashayeri, J. (2007) Development of computer-aided maintenance resources planning (CAMRP): a case of multiple CNC machining centers. *Robotics and Computer-Integrated Manufacturing*, **23** (6), 614–623.
12. El-Sharkh, M.Y. and El-Keib, A.A. (2003) An evolutionary programming-based solution methodology for power generation and transmission maintenance scheduling. *Electric Power Systems Research*, **65** (1), 35–40.
13. Zheng, X. and Fard, N. (2009) Hazard-rate tolerance method for an opportunistic replacement policy. *International Journal of Production Economics*, **118** (2), 361–366.
14. Li, M., Li H., and Liu, Q. (2010) Integrated production scheduling and opportunistic preventive maintenance in the flowshop manufacturing system. 2010 2nd International Conference on Information Science and Engineering, pp. 294–298.
15. Cheng, Z., Yang, Z., Tan, L. *et al.* (2011) Optimal inspection and maintenance policy for the multi-unit series system. 2011 9th International Conference on Reliability, Maintainability and Safety, pp. 811–814.
16. Bai, Y. (2009) Cost model based optimization of RCM group maintenance interval. Industrial Engineering and Engineering Management, pp. 1174–1178.

17. Vakharia, A.J. and Wemmerlöv, U. (1995) A comparative investigation of hierarchical clustering techniques and dissimilarity measures applied to the cell formation problem. *Journal of Operations Management*, **13**, 117–138.
18. Ünler, A. and Güngör, Z. (2009) Applying K-harmonic means clustering to the part-machine classification problem. *Expert Systems with Applications*, **36**, 1179–1194.
19. Camci, F. (2009) System maintenance scheduling with prognostics information using genetic algorithm. *IEEE Transactions on Reliability*, **58**, 539–552.
20. Wang, C.H and Tsai, S.W. (2011) Multi-objective optimization using genetic algorithm: applications to imperfect preventive maintenance model. International Conference on Computer and Education, pp. 1355–1360.
21. Weinstein, L. and Chung, C.H. (1999) Integrating maintenance and production decisions in a hierarchical production planning environment. *Computers & Operations Research*, **26** (10), 1059–1074.
22. Berrichi, A., Yalaoui, F., Amodeo, L. *et al.* (2010) Bi-Objective Ant Colony Optimization approach to optimize production and maintenance scheduling. *Computers & Operations Research*, **37** (9), 1584–1596.
23. Li, X. (2013) Research on methodology of intelligent maintenance scheduling with energy consumption considered for parallel-serial production systems. Master thesis. Harbin Institute of Technology, Harbin, China.
24. Wang, H. (2002) A survey of maintenance policies of deteriorating systems. *European Journal of Operational Research*, **139** (3), 469–489.
25. Nakagawa, T. and Osaki, S. (1974) The optimum repair limit replacement policies. *Operational Research Quarterly*, **25** (2), 311–317.
26. Radner, R. and Jorgenson, D.W. (1963) Opportunistic replacement of a single part in the presence of several monitored parts. *Management Science*, **10** (1), 70–84.
27. Gertsbakh, I.B. (1984) Optimal group preventive maintenance of a system with observable state parameter. *Advances in Applied Probability*, **16**, 923–925.
28. Assaf, D. and Shanthikumar, J.G. (1987) Optimal group maintenance policies with continuous and periodic inspections. *Management Science*, **33** (11), 1440–1452.
29. Ritchken, P. and Wilson, J.G. (1990) (m, T) group maintenance policies. *Management Science*, **36** (5), 632–639.
30. Sheu, S.H. and Jhang, J.P. (1997) A generalized group maintenance policy. *European Journal of Operational Research*, **96** (2), 232–247.
31. Yongsheng, B., Xisheng, J., and Feng, L. (2009) Cost model based optimization of RCM group maintenance interval. 16th International Conference on Industrial Engineering and Engineering Management, 2009, IEEE. IE&EM'09, October, 2009, pp. 1174–1178.
32. Gallagher, C.C. and Knight, W.A. (1986) *Group Technology Production Methods in Manufacture*, 1st edn, Ellis Horwood Limited, West Sussex.
33. Abdelhadi, A. (2010) Preventive maintenance grouping using similarity coefficient methodology. Unpublished Dissertation. University of Wisconsin – Milwaukee, Milwaukee.
34. Malik, M.A.K. (1979) Reliable preventive maintenance scheduling. *AIIE Transactions*, **11** (3), 221–228.
35. Liang, J.J., Qin, A.K., Suganthan, P.N. *et al.* (2004) Evaluation of comprehensive learning particle swarm optimizer, in *Neural Information Processing*, Springer, Berlin, Heidelberg, pp. 230–235, January 2004.
36. Ross, S. (1996) *Stochastic Processes*, Wiley Series in Probability and Statistics, John Wiley & Sons, Inc., NewYork.
37. Esbensen, H. and Mazumder, P. (1994). SAGA: a unification of the genetic algorithm with simulated annealing and its application to macro-cell placement. Proceedings of the Seventh International Conference on VLSI Design, IEEE, January, 1994, pp. 211–214.

38. Castanier, B., Grall, A. and Bérenguer, C. (2005) A condition-based maintenance policy with non-periodic inspections for a two-unit series system. *Reliability Engineering & System Safety*, **87** (1), 109–120.
39. Maksoud, M.A., Hänel, D. and Lantermann, U. (2010) Modeling and computation of cavitation in vortical flow. *International Journal of Heat and Fluid Flow*, **31**, 1065–1074.
40. Lu, K.Y. and Sy, C.C. (2009) A real-time decision-making of maintenance using fuzzy agent. *Expert Systems with Applications*, **36**, 2691–2698.
41. Marseguerra, M. Zio, E. (2000). System design optimization by genetic algorithms. Reliability and Maintainability Symposium, Los Angeles, CA, pp. 222-227.
42. Wang, H. (2002) A survey of maintenance policies of deteriorating systems. *European Journal of Operational Research*, **139**, 469–489.
43. Moore, W.J. and Starr, A.G. (2006) An intelligent maintenance system for continuous cost-based prioritisation of maintenance activities. *Computers in Industry*, **57**, 595–606.
44. Cheung, K.Y., Hui, C.W., Sakamoto, H. *et al.* (2004) Short-term site-wide maintenance scheduling. *Computers and Chemical Engineering*, **28**, 91–102.
45. Kroning, S. and Denkena, B. (2013) Dynamic scheduling of maintenance measures in complex production systems. *CIRP Journal of Manufacturing Science and Technology*, **6**, 292–300.
46. Apeland, S. and Scarf, P.A. (2003) A fully subjective approach to modeling inspection maintenance. *European Journal of Operational Research*, **148**, 410–425.
47. Lu, K.Y. and Sy, C.C. (2008) A real-time decision-making of maintenance using fuzzy agent. *Expert Systems with Applications*. doi: 10.1016/j.eswa.2008.01.087
48. Zhou, X., Xi, L. and Lee, J. (2008) Opportunistic preventive maintenance scheduling for a multi-unit series system based on dynamic programming. *International Journal of Production Economics*. doi: 10.1016/j.ijpe.2008.09.012
49. Rachaniotis, N.P. and Pappis, C.P. (2008) Preventive maintenance and upgrade system: optimizing the whole performance system by components' replacement or rearrangement. *International Journal of Production Economics*, **112**, 236–244.

7

Prognosis Incorporating Maintenance Decision-Making

7.1 The Changing Role of Maintenance

Maintenance concepts and methodologies have advanced significantly over the past several decades, although maintenance still has a negative image because it is regarded as merely a measure against trouble. A maintenance department is usually regarded as a cost-center, which does not create profits.

However, if we look at the role of maintenance from the perspective of life-cycle management, which is important for a sustainable manufacturing system, we realize that the picture is completely different. The purpose of life-cycle management is to control the conditions of products to provide the functionality required by customers or by society, while keeping the environmental load to a minimum and maintaining appropriate corporate profits. There are two reasons why it is necessary to control the condition of products. One is the change in product conditions due to deterioration. Another is the changing needs of customers or of society. The former is referred to as the product's physical life and the latter as its functional life. In both cases, the measure that should be considered first is maintenance including upgrade, because maintenance generates a lesser environmental load. If maintenance does not work well, other measures should then be considered, such as remanufacturing. Production of new products should be the last measure taken. In this context, the priority relationship between production and maintenance has been completely reversed. What we need to consider from the perspective of life-cycle management is the notion of "*production-free*" rather than "*maintenance-free*."

The perspective of life-cycle management for closed-loop manufacturing has brought about transformation of the business models of manufacturing companies from product providers to service providers [1]. Maintenance could be one of the major services associated with life-cycle management. If this business transformation goes further, companies will sell utilization and customers will pay only for

Machinery Prognostics and Prognosis Oriented Maintenance Management, First Edition. Jihong Yan.

utilization. In this context, achieving effective maintenance could be of benefit to companies, increasing their profits by reducing maintenance costs, as well as to customers who can enjoy improved service quality [2].

As the paradigm of manufacturing shifts toward realizing a sustainable society, we should begin to recognize the changing role of maintenance. The goal of manufacturing is no longer to produce products in an efficient way, but rather to provide the functions needed by society while minimizing material and energy consumption. Life-cycle management is becoming a crucial issue in order to achieve this goal. The role of maintenance should be redefined as an essential means for sustainable development within a manufacturing system. Maintenance is the most efficient way to keep the functional level of a product above the level required from the viewpoint of environmental impact.

To realize sustainable manufacturing, it is crucial to analyze the whole life-cycle of a product. One of the most significant stages, which has great influence on the environment, is evaluating the product's potential for reuse (i.e., reusability) and reusing the product as far as possible [3]. Additionally, the legislation mandates that manufacturers bear the economic burden of collection and disposal of products at the end of their useful lives, which means that reuse of some components might be more cost-effective than disposal and provide an opportunity for recovery of their economic value [4].

According to the Organization for Economic Cooperation and Development (OECD)/Euro stat Joint Questionnaire on waste, reuse shall mean any operation by which end-of-life products and equipment (e.g., electrical and electronic equipment) or its components are used for the same purpose for which they were conceived. RREUSE (the network for Reuse and Recycling European Union Social Enterprises) argues that reuse is also a set of activities including reconditioning and repair, without entailing the remanufacturing or upgrade of the product or its components.

Although reuse without repair and remanufacturing are environmentally and economically superior to other methods such as recycling, the uncertain quality and reliability of used products at the end of the first lifetime tend to reduce the attractiveness of reuse and hence it is commonly agreed that the reliability of facilities is the main concern when they are reused [5–7]. Technically, reliability is often defined as the probability that a system, vehicle, machine, device, and so on perform their intended functions under operating conditions, for a specified period [8]. Researchers focus their interests on the reuse strategy: Anityasari and Kaebernick [6] proposed that in the reuse strategy, reliability of a used facility must be assessed based on the probability of its survival during the second life and only facilities that fall within an "acceptable" reliability are worth being reused. A mathematical model of reusability was defined by Murayama *et al.* [7] based on reliability theory. Ohta and Sato [9] proposed a method for reliability prediction for a reused electronic circuit board to realize its reuse.

In this chapter, we present prognosis-incorporating maintenance that facilitates maintenance to save routine maintenance costs and to enhance the reuse of a facility.

7.2 Development of Maintenance

In the past, maintenance was regarded as repair work. Machines were operated until they broke down, and there was no way to predict failures. With development of reliability engineering in the 1950s, the concept of preventive maintenance (PM) was advocated, and time-based maintenance (TBM) was introduced. TBM was based on the so-called bathtub curve, which represents the increase in the failure rate of products after a certain period of operation. However, in many cases, product condition cannot be identified from the extent of the operational period, since the rate of deterioration depends not only on elapsed time but also on various other factors, including operational and environmental conditions. Therefore, TBM sometimes imposes unnecessary treatments, which often disrupt normal operations and induce malfunctions due to missed operations [10]. After the limitations of TBM as a means of PM were recognized, the concept of condition-based maintenance (CBM) was proposed, based on the development of machine diagnostic techniques in the 1970s.

CBM is a maintenance program that recommends maintenance actions based on the information collected through condition monitoring. It attempts to avoid unnecessary maintenance tasks by taking maintenance actions only when there is evidence of abnormal behavior of a physical asset. A properly established and effectively implemented CBM program can significantly reduce maintenance cost by reducing the number of unnecessary scheduled PM operations [11]. Therefore, CBM enables taking the proper actions at the right timing to prevent failures, if there is a proper diagnostic technique.

Traditional approaches of reliability estimation are based on the distribution of historical time-to-failure data of a population of identical facilities obtained from in-house tests. Many parametric failure models, such as Poisson, exponential, Weibull, and log-normal distributions have been used to model machine reliability. However, these approaches only provide overall estimates for the entire population of identical facilities, which is of less value to an end user of a facility [12]. In other words, reliability reflects only the statistical quality of a facility, which means it is likely that this certain facility will not necessarily obey the distribution that is determined by a population of tested facilities of the same type.

Therefore, it is recommended that condition-monitoring data should also be used to reflect the quality and degradation severity of this particular facility so that the reusability of the used facility can be estimated more specifically.

Prognosis, which is defined as a systematic approach that can continuously track health indicators to predict reliability over time [13], can serve the purpose of assessing the degradation of a facility's quality based on acquired online condition-monitoring data. The most widely used prognosis is to predict the time left before failure, namely remaining useful life (RUL). It generates the lifetime of the facility which would indicate the time interval until the next maintenance activity.

Using sufficient data, efficient prognosis methods, which could generate results of a health indicator, can be considered as one decision-making tool to support decisions of maintenance actions. As such, it is natural to include maintenance policies in the consideration of the machine prognostic process. Maintenance in this situation is the so-called CBM. The main idea of prognosis-incorporating maintenance policies is to optimize the maintenance actions according to certain criteria, such as cost, reliability, and availability.

Most of the existing prognostics models can be divided into two main categories, mechanism-based models and data-driven models, though the real-life system mechanism is often too stochastic and complex to model and hence a physics-based model might not be the most practical solution. An artificial neural network (ANN) is currently the most commonly found data-driven technique in prognostics researches [14]. Yan and Wang [14] developed two Elman neural networks for fatigue severity assessment and trend prediction, respectively. Satish and Sarma [15] have made an attempt to combine neural networks and fuzzy logic in order to form a fuzzy back-propagation network for identifying the present condition of the bearing and estimating the remaining life of the motor.

The objective of this chapter is to illustrate the prognostic methodology that could be applied for supporting decision-making on maintenance. An efficient methodology of ANN-based prognosis combined with reliability methods is presented in later sections. The prognosis could support a scheduling methodology which schedules the maintenance actions during the life-cycle of a manufacturing system.

7.3 Maintenance Effects Modeling

The objective of maintenance is to preserve the condition of a facility to fulfill its required functions throughout its life-cycle. Maintenance is an important part of life-cycle management within the manufacturing system, whose main purpose is to enhance reuse throughout the life-cycle. To fulfill the requirements of reuse-oriented maintenance, effective strategies for maintenance, modeling of reliability, and methodologies of maintenance scheduling decision-making are essential. This involves the strategy of maintenance among various options, such as TBM and CBM, based on the evaluation of potential problems that could occur during operation as well as evaluation of the effects of failure and the effectiveness of maintenance technologies.

Therefore, we use the term “life-cycle maintenance” to stress its role in life-cycle management. As previously mentioned, there are several reasons why it is necessary to control the conditions of products: changes in the condition of products due to deterioration, and the need to enhance the sustainability of products.

The degradation of a facility would generate gaps between the required function and the realized function. Maintenance is executed to compensate for these gaps by means of treatment or upgrading and this action enhances reuse due to prolonged functional life-time, as shown in Figure 7.1.

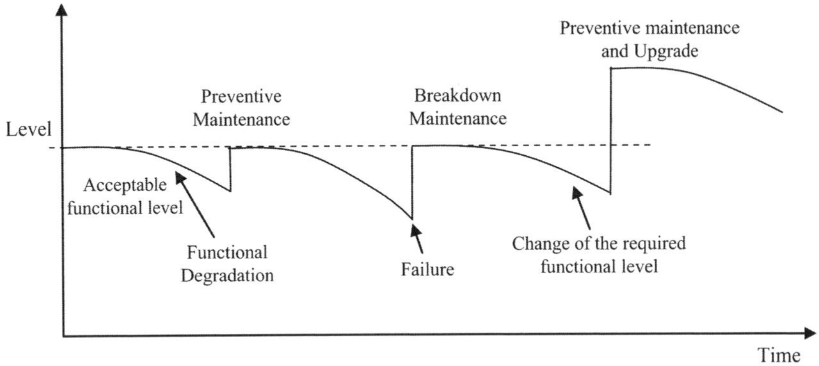

Figure 7.1 Model of maintenance activities

For effective maintenance management, all information associated with maintenance should be integrated in such a way that it is available from any phase of the life cycle. In the development phase, for example, it is essential to know the real operating situations and the problems encountered during past operations. On the other hand, it is necessary to have exact design data for maintenance strategy planning and maintenance task control.

After the maintenance activities are taken into consideration, then the modeling procedure for reliability and reliability improvement should be presented.

The reliability modeling contains the following steps: reliability estimation and reliability improvement modeling.

7.3.1 Reliability Estimation

To estimate the reliability of a facility, a collection of time-to-failure data of a population of identical facilities should be available. The estimation is conducted by fitting the data to a suitable life distribution.

Reliability can be modeled utilizing widely used distributions in their standard forms. Among these distributions, normal, exponential, gamma, and Weibull distributions are most commonly applied in reliability engineering. Sometimes, the researchers select one of these distributions so that the deterioration process can be modeled satisfactorily. To do so, different distributions should be fit to the in-house test data, and analysis and comparison of the fitting result are also carried out to select the optimal distribution.

Additionally, methods for estimation of the parameters for fitting a statistical model to data are multiple, of which the maximum likelihood estimation method (MLE) is a popular one and is employed to illustrate the procedure of estimation for the model's parameters.

The principle of MLE, originally developed by Fisher in the 1920s, states that the desired probability distribution is the one that makes the observed data "most likely" [16].

Given the observed data set D and a distribution of interest, the parameters, θ, of the distribution can be estimated by the following steps according to MLE:

Step 1: Suppose D contains n independent samples, $x_1, x_2, \ldots, x_n$; and let $p(x_k|\theta)$ denote the probability of sample x_k given the distribution with parameter vector $\theta=(\theta_1, \theta_2, \ldots, \theta_m)$. Build the likelihood function of θ, $L(D|\theta)$. Equation 7.1 is an example.

$$LL\ L(D|\theta) = \prod_{k=1}^{n} p(x_k|\theta) \tag{7.1}$$

Step 2: Transform the likelihood function into the log-likelihood function, $\ln L(D|\theta)$, for computational convenience.

Step 3: Solve the following differential equation, known as the likelihood equation:

$$\frac{\partial \ln L(D|\theta)}{\partial \theta_i} = 0 \tag{7.2}$$

Then $\widehat{\theta}$, the value of θ that best agrees with the actually observed data set, is obtained. Thus we obtain the estimated parameters for the distribution of interest.

If it is not known which distribution fits the data best, 1-sample non-parametric test methods are needed. At present, the commonly used methods include the chi-square test, the K-S test, the binomial test, the Wilcoxon signed ranks test, the sign test, the run test, and so on. However, the binomial test, the Wilcoxon signed ranks test, the sign test, and the run test cannot be applied within the analysis here. The binomial test works well only when the data is dichotomous; the sign test is used to test the hypothesis that there is "no difference" between two continuous distributions, which requires a known distribution; the Wilcoxon signed ranks test works on the assumption that the population probability distribution is symmetric; and the run test is developed to determine the randomness of the data. We choose the chi-square test and the K-S test because they can be applied to test the goodness-of-fit of normal, exponential, gamma, and Weibull distributions, and provide comparable results which lead to an identical evaluation criterion.

The1-sample K-S test is designed to test the null hypothesis in favor of the alternative hypothesis. It uses a statistic known as D-stat in order to test the hypothesis. The K-S test's appeal is its straightforward computation of the test statistic and the distribution-free characteristic. Similarly, the chi-square test can be used to test the significant difference between the sample data and the presumed distribution.

The K-S test and the chi-square test are used to determine the goodness-of-fit of the four distributions mentioned above. These two tests can provide results in two aspects: first, whether the null hypothesis that a certain distribution fits the sample data is rejected at a significance level of 5%; and second, the probability (referred to as the p-value), under assumption of the null hypothesis, of observing the given statistic. The result will be analyzed comprehensively to select a distribution to be used for reliability modeling with the characteristics of the distributions taken into account.

Additionally, because the exponential distribution is a special case of the Weibull distribution when the slope parameter $\beta = 1$, a goodness-of-fit test is only performed on normal, gamma, and Weibull distributions.

Among these distributions the Weibull distribution is the most widely utilized in reliability modeling of machinery facilities. The distribution is characterized by two parameters, a scale (η) and a slope (β). The scale parameter (η) is defined as the life of the product at which 63.2% of all facilities will fail, while the slope parameter (β) is defined as the mode of failure. Referring to the well-known bathtub curve, $\beta < 1$ indicates an early mortality, $\beta = 1$ a random failure, and $\beta > 1$ a wear-out failure [17]. If t represents the lifetime, the reliability of the facility can be calculated by

$$R(t) = \exp\left[-\left(\frac{t}{\eta}\right)^{\beta}\right] \tag{7.3}$$

7.3.2 Modeling the Improvement of Reliability after Maintenance

After the first life of a facility, it can only be reused if its reliability is still above a threshold below which remanufacturing or overhauling should be performed in order to restore the facility to a usable state. Therefore, it is crucial to maintain the facility before its reliability reaches the threshold.

According to Lie and Chun [18] maintenance can be divided into two major categories, corrective or preventive. Corrective maintenance (CM) is any maintenance that occurs when the system has failed. PM is any maintenance that occurs when the system is operating.

CM can be divided into two categories:

Minimal repair restores the system to the reliability it had when it failed. This is often called *bad as old*.

Corrective replacement restores the system time to zero; the reliability curve is that of a new system. This is often called *good as new*.

PM can also be divided into two categories:

Simple PM improves the reliability of a facility to a higher level, but not all the way to *good as new*.

Preventive replacement, like corrective replacement, restores the reliability to as new.

Herein, only simple PM is taken into consideration on the assumption that the maintenance is always implemented before any failure happens. This assumption is reasonable because prognosis serves the purpose of failure prevention. Additionally, the facility is intended to be reused and hence no preventive replacement will be carried out.

To better describe the reality that repaired systems are neither in "as good as new" nor "as bad as old" conditions, many imperfect maintenance models have been developed in the past decades to characterize mathematically the maintenance quality from various points of view.

Some assumptions are given below before presenting the repair models [19]:

1. PM is executed at time $t_1^{\mathrm{p}}, (t_1^{\mathrm{p}} + t_2^{\mathrm{p}}), \ldots, (t_1^{\mathrm{p}} +, \ldots, t_{k-1}^{\mathrm{p}} + t_k^{\mathrm{p}}), \ldots$ where t_k^{p} is the time interval between the $(k-1)$th and the kth PM.
2. PM is treated as imperfect maintenance. CM is carried out once the system fails between adjacent PMs, and it is regarded as minimal repair action.
3. $\lambda_k(t)$ denotes the failure intensity function in the kth preventive repair cycle, and t is reset to zero at the beginning of the next preventive repair cycle. $\lambda_1(t)$ represents the initial failure intensity function of a new system.
4. The time spent on maintenance is negligible.

There are four imperfect maintenance models that are widely used [20, 21].

Model I

The general idea is that the system's health condition is related to the virtual age (also called effective age), but not the actual working time. In the Kijima type I model, the virtual age of the system is formulated as:

$$V_k = V_{k-1} + a_k t_k^{\mathrm{p}} \tag{7.4}$$

where V_k is the virtual age of the system immediately after the kth preventive repair; a_k indicates the effect of the kth preventive repair action on the virtual age of the system. The corresponding failure intensity function of the kth preventive repair cycle is written as:

$$\lambda_k(t; a_1, \ldots, a_{k-1}) = \lambda_1(t + V_{k-1}) = \lambda_k \left(t + \sum_{i=1}^{k-1} a_i t_k^{\mathrm{p}} \right) \tag{7.5}$$

where t is the working time in every preventive repair cycle. The preventive repair action only reduces a partial virtual age of the system since the last one.

Model II

The Kijima type II model assumes that preventive repair actions will reduce all the virtual age of the system just before the repair. The virtual age of the system after the kth preventive repair is defined as:

$$V_k = a_k V_{k-1} \tag{7.6}$$

The failure intensity function of the kth preventive repair cycle is written as:

$$\lambda_k(t; a_1, \ldots, a_{k-1}) = \lambda_1(t + V_{k-1}) = \lambda_k\left(t + \sum_{i=1}^{k-1}(t_k^{\mathrm{p}}\prod_{j=i}^{k-1}a_i)\right) \tag{7.7}$$

Model III

This model assumes that after the preventive repair, the age of the system can be first brought to zero, but the failure intensity function will have a faster increasing trend than that of the previous repair cycle [22]. According to the classification in Wu and Zuo [23], it can be called the linear PM model, since the repair activities change the failure intensity function linearly. The failure intensity function of the system in the kth preventive repair cycle is given by:

$$\lambda_k(t; a_1, \ldots, a_{k-1}) = \lambda_1(t)\prod_{i=1}^{k-1}a_i, (a_i \geq 1) \tag{7.8}$$

Besides the three models mentioned above, another kind of approach could be applied for imperfect maintenance model selection which is categorized as data driven based methodology.

Model IV

To estimate the parameters of the imperfect repair model, the MLE can be used. Suppose the data are collected from N identical repairable systems. For the lth system, $n_{l,k}$ failures happen during the kth PM cycle, and the corresponding failure time in this PM cycle is denoted as $t^{\mathrm{f}}_{l,(k,1)}, t^{\mathrm{f}}_{l,(k,2)}, \ldots, t^{\mathrm{f}}_{l,(k,n_{l,k})}$, where $0 < t^{\mathrm{f}}_{l,(k,1)}, t^{\mathrm{f}}_{l,(k,2)}, \ldots, t^{\mathrm{f}}_{l,(k,n_{l,k})} \leq t_k^{\mathrm{p}}$. Assume that the system will be discarded or replaced by an identical new one at the end of the Hth PM action. If the data are failure truncated, that is, $t^{\mathrm{f}}_{l,(k,n_{l,k})} = t_k^{\mathrm{p}}$, the corresponding likelihood function relative to the failure time is written as:

$$L(\text{failure time}|\theta, a) = \prod_{l=1}^{N}\prod_{k=1}^{H}\prod_{i=1}^{n_{l,k}}\left(\lambda_k\left(t^{\mathrm{f}}_{l,(k,i)}\right)\exp\left(-\int_{t^{\mathrm{f}}_{l,(k,i-1)}}^{t^{\mathrm{f}}_{l,(k,i)}}\lambda_k(x)\mathrm{d}x\right)\right) \tag{7.9}$$

and if the data is time truncated, that is, $t^{\mathrm{f}}_{l,(k,n_{l,k})} \neq t_k^{\mathrm{p}}$, the likelihood function can be expressed as:

$$L(\text{failure time}|\theta, a) = \prod_{l=1}^{N}\prod_{k=1}^{H}\left(\prod_{i=1}^{n_{l,k}}\left(\lambda_k\left(t^{\mathrm{f}}_{l,(k,i)}\right)\exp\left(-\int_{t^{\mathrm{f}}_{l,(k,i-1)}}^{t^{\mathrm{f}}_{l,(k,i)}}\lambda_k(x)\mathrm{d}x\right)\right)\right.$$
$$\left.\exp\left(-\int_{t^{\mathrm{f}}_{l,(k,n_l,k)}}^{t_k^{\mathrm{p}}}\lambda_k(x)\mathrm{d}x\right)\right) \tag{7.10}$$

where the vector θ represents a set of parameters in the initial failure intensity function, and it is assumed to be known in our research; the vector a corresponds to the unknown parameters of the imperfect repair model, for example, $a_1, a_2, \ldots$, to be estimated. The estimators of the unknown parameters, denoted as a, can be computed by maximizing the logarithm of the equations mentioned above. With the estimates of the unknown parameters, the conditional survival distribution of the lth system after the $(i-1)$th failure of the kth PM cycle can be given by:

$$r_{l,(k,i)}(\mathrm{t}) = \exp\left(-\int_{t^{\mathrm{f}}_{l,(k,i-1)}}^{t-t^{\mathrm{f}}_{l,(k,i)}} \lambda_k(t; a)\mathrm{d}t\right) \tag{7.11}$$

To model the reliability improvement after PM, Malik's proportional age reduction (PAR) model is employed. According to Malik's model [24], the kth effective maintenance is presumed to reduce the last operation time $(t_k - t_{k-1})$ to $(1 - I_k)(t_k - t_{k-1})$.

In this model, the improvement factor I_k denotes the effect of the kth maintenance and is set between 0 and 1. If I_k goes to 0, the state of the maintained facility is as *bad as old*.

For example, if the simple PM is carried out at t_1 when reliability decreases to 0.8, the theoretical operation time that has elapsed is reduced to $(1 - I_1)t_1$ which is a portion of the actual operation time t_1 Therefore, the reliability of the facility is elevated to the level at time $(1 - I_1)t_1$. If the second simple PM is carried out at t_2 when reliability decreases to 0.7, the theoretical operation time that has elapsed between t_1 and t_2 is reduced to $(1 - I_2)(t_2 - t_1)$, as is shown in Figure 7.2, where $I_1 = 0.5$ and $I_2 = 0.2$.

It is also assumed that the improvement by the kth maintenance has no effect on that by the $(k-1)$th maintenance. If the reliability is modeled using Weibull distribution, after the kth maintenance is carried out, the reliability of a facility between t_k and t_{k+1}

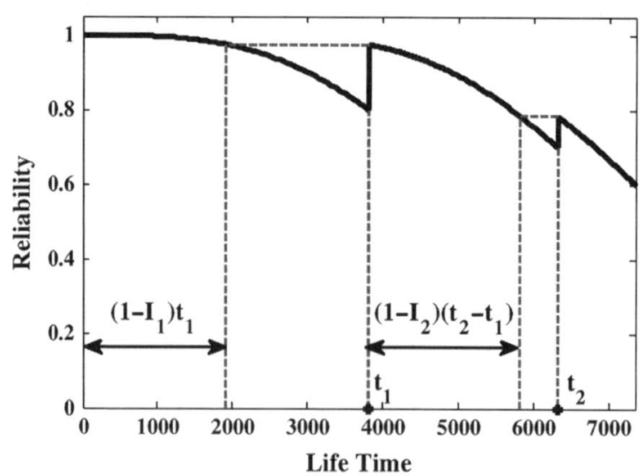

Figure 7.2 Illustration of proportional age reduction model

can be calculated by Equation 7.12

$$R_k(t) = \exp\left[-\left(\frac{t + T_k}{\eta}\right)^{\beta}\right] \tag{7.12}$$

where

$$T_k = -t_k + (1 - I_1) \cdot t_1 + \sum_{i=2}^{k}(1 - I_i) \cdot (t_i - t_{i-1}) \tag{7.13}$$

The improvement factor I_k could be estimated either by statistical methods [25] or by analyzing all the possible simple PM activities and their improvement effect on a facility [26]. For the latter, the simple PM activities are categorized into six types: lubricating, cleaning, calibrating, tightening, simple repairing, and consumed material resupplying. The improvement effect of these activities on the reliability of a facility is measured by improvement effect E_i, and the probability of a certain type of activity being taken is measured by P_i. Both parameters have their values limited between 0 and 1. The improvement factor can be calculated by Equation 7.14

$$I = \frac{1}{\sum_{i=1}^{6} P_i} \cdot \sum_{i=1}^{6} P_i E_i \tag{7.14}$$

It is assumed that the improvement factor is estimated by the maintainer who is experienced and, without any written calculation, able to give a relatively correct estimation of the improvement effect of maintenance work he/she carries out. Additionally, it is reasonable to assume that the value of the improvement factor decreases as the number of maintenances increases.

Even if the maintenance can be carried out when the reliability of the facility reaches a threshold below which the reliability is not acceptable for reuse, the facility cannot be maintained indefinitely and hence the facility cannot be reused indefinitely. The fact is that after several maintenances, the reliability of the facility cannot be improved to a relatively high level and the reuse of the facility is less profitable than purchasing a new one. Therefore, when this situation occurs, it is recommended that maintenance should no longer be carried out. In other words, the reuse of the facility should cease and remanufacturing or recycling should be implemented.

7.4 Modeling of Optimization Objective – Maintenance Cost

The main idea of prognosis-incorporating maintenance policies is to optimize the maintenance actions according to certain criteria, such as risk, cost, reliability, and availability.

Risk is defined as the combination of probability and consequence. There are some cases, for example, critical equipment at plant level, for which the risk cannot be estimated by cost. Under such circumstances, the reliability criterion would be appropriate. However, the risk criterion is usually equivalent to the cost criterion since the consequence is measured by cost in most cases. Hence cost-based optimization is appropriate in most situations.

The optimization objectives of maintenance actions studied mainly include minimal maintenance cost per unit time, that is, optimal maintenance cost rate or optimal system availability in a fixed time period. In this chapter, minimal maintenance cost rate, which is composed of direct maintenance cost and indirect production loss resulting from system shutdown for each unit time, is set as the cost-based optimization objective of maintenance.

In addition, the maintenance cost in a single maintenance activity is set as the short-term optimization objective. Maintenance activity, which includes a number of maintenance actions such as minor maintenance and replacement, is composed of set-up of maintenance, implementation of maintenance actions, and production recovery.

The maintenance cost of the kth maintenance activity consists of the direct maintenance cost C_{m}^{k} and the indirect production loss L_{p}^{k}. The direct maintenance cost, which includes the cost of maintenance actions for maintenance units C_{u}^{k} and set-up cost C_{s}^{k}, can be calculated by:

$$C_{\mathrm{m}}^{k} = C_{\mathrm{u}}^{k} + C_{\mathrm{s}}^{k} \tag{7.15}$$

$$C_{\mathrm{u}}^{k} = \sum_{i=1}^{M} (C_{\mathrm{p}}^{k,i} + C_{\mathrm{t}}^{k,i} + C_{\mathrm{h}}^{k,i} + C_{\mathrm{c}}^{k,i}) \tag{7.16}$$

where $C_{\mathrm{p}}^{k,i}$, $C_{\mathrm{t}}^{k,i}$, $C_{\mathrm{h}}^{k,i}$, and $C_{\mathrm{c}}^{k,i}$ are the cost of spare parts (or brand new facilities if replacement is carried out), maintenance tools, maintainers, and consumables for maintenance unit i. The cost of consumables, maintenance tools, and maintainers is time related.

The maintenance cost rate R_{C} in a time period T_{S} can be calculated by

$$R_{\mathrm{C}} = \frac{\sum_{k=1}^{N_{\mathrm{M}}} (C_{\mathrm{m}}^{k} + L_{\mathrm{p}}^{k})}{T_{\mathrm{S}}} \tag{7.17}$$

where, N_{M} is the total number of maintenance activities occurring in T_{S}.

It is assumed that maintenance tools and maintainers are assigned to a maintenance group according to the maximum numbers needed to maintain any one facility in this group. Therefore, the cost of maintenance tools and maintainers should be calculated by

$$C_{\mathrm{t}}^{k,i} = \sum_{j=1}^{N_{\mathrm{u}}^{i}} P_{\mathrm{t}} \times N_{\mathrm{t}}^{k,i} \times T_{\mathrm{m}}^{k,i} \tag{7.18}$$

$$C_{\mathrm{h}}^{k,i} = \sum_{j=1}^{N_{\mathrm{u}}^{i}} P_{\mathrm{h}} \times N_{\mathrm{h}}^{k,i} \times T_{\mathrm{m}}^{k,i} \tag{7.19}$$

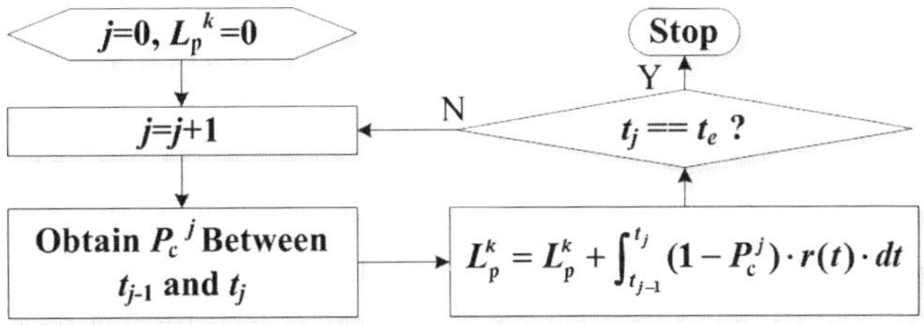

Figure 7.3 Flow chart for production loss calculation

where, N_{u}^{i} is the number of facilities in maintenance unit i; P_{t} and P_{h} are the unit price of using maintenance tools and maintainers; $N_{\mathrm{t}}^{k,i}$ and $N_{\mathrm{h}}^{k,i}$ are the numbers of maintenance tools and maintainers needed for maintenance unit i; $T_{\mathrm{m}}^{k,i}$ is the time needed to carry out all the maintenance actions in maintenance units i.

Additionally, production loss should be calculated from the perspective of the entire system. Hence the production recovery situation should be checked after maintenance of a unit is finished. Note that maintenance of different units may be finished at the same time, the time when the maintenances of one or more units are finished is set as t_j and t_0 is set as zero. The portion of production recovery at time t_j is denoted as P_{c}^{j}. Thus the production loss L_{p}^{k} can be calculated following the flow chart in Figure 7.3. In Figure 7.3, $r(t)$ stands for loss rate, that is, production loss per unit time with the entire system shut down, and can be calculated by

$$r(t) = r_0 \cdot 1.1^{\lfloor t/0.5 \rfloor} \tag{7.20}$$

The loss rate increases, from its initial value r_0, with maintenance time since the longer the production stays partly or entirely shut down, the bigger the opportunity cost.

7.5 Prognosis-Oriented Maintenance Decision-Making

In this section, we will present case studies to demonstrate the procedure of implementation of maintenance decision-making, which primarily includes prognosis for facility and maintenance scheduling.

7.5.1 Reliability Estimation and Prediction

To realize sustainable maintenance, first it is crucial to implement prognosis for facilities, which presents the assessment of reliability of the product and facility, facilitating the prediction of the end point of life.

Traditional approaches of reliability estimation are based on the distribution of historical time-to-failure data which, however, only reflects the statistical quality of a facility. Considering this disadvantage, it is recommended that condition monitoring data should also be used to reflect the quality and severity of degradation of a particular facility so that the reusability of used facilities can be estimated more specifically.

Therefore, the methodology we present is an efficient ANN-based prognosis combined with reliability methods, which predicts the RUL of a facility through mining the online condition monitoring data by utilizing back propagation ANNs and supports the decision-making for maintenance by referring to the reliability of the facility that is calculated through fitting a suitable life distribution versus the in-house time-to-failure data. Two thresholds are defined for both the RUL and the reliability of the facility to obtain the time of maintenance and guarantee sufficient reusability. The reliability improvement of the used facility after maintenance is modeled by adopting Malik's PAR model for imperfect maintenance. The credibility of the prediction results obtained by ANN is defined and calculated through analyzing their fluctuation, which reduces the impact of the fluctuation and makes the result more reliable. Utilizing the proposed methodology of prognosis, the performance of a facility can be evaluated dynamically based on both historical and online monitoring information and maintenance can be carried out at the right time so that the reuse of the facility can be guaranteed.

7.5.2 Case Study

Now the case study of reliability assessment and prediction for blade material specimens is presented to show the effectiveness of the ANN-based methodology, which is carried out using the following procedures: data acquisition, modeling and training, data test, and result analysis.

7.5.2.1 Data Acquisition

The material fatigue experiments of steam turbine blade specimens were conducted on a material testing system (MTS810) at the Harbin Turbine Company, under a cyclic strain of range ±0.45%. For every test cycle, the strain goes from −0.45 to +0.45% and then back to +0.45% again. Referring to GB/T 15248−1994, the fatigue failure occurs when the amplitude of stress is less than or equal to 20% of the amplitude at the first test cycle. There were 13 blade material specimens experiencing the run-to-failure test, cracks caused by fatigue were found on the material surface when the specimens were unloaded from the testing system. Thirteen sets of data are obtained in the test. Eight of them are used for life distribution fitting and network training as historical data and the remaining five sets are used as online condition monitoring data.

7.5.2.2 Reliability Modeling and Estimation

With MATLAB, we fit the in-house test data to normal, gamma, and Weibull distributions using the MLE method and apply the K-S test to determine their goodness of fit.

Table 7.1 Result of K-S test

	Normal	Gamma	Weibull
Null hypothesis	Rejected	Rejected	Rejected
P-value	0.7599	0.7472	0.7113

Table 7.2 Result of chi-square test

	Normal	Gamma	Weibull
Null hypothesis	Rejected	Rejected	Rejected
P-value	0.6089	0.5794	0.5239

The result is shown in Table 7.1. With the same method, the chi-square test is carried out. The result is shown in Table 7.2.

As shown in Tables 7.1 and 7.2, the K–S test and the chi-square test provide similar results. Normal distribution has the best goodness of fit, followed by gamma with Weibull last. However, the results show no remarkable difference between the distributions.

First, the difference between normal and Weibull distribution is merely 0.0486 through the K-S test and 0.0850 through the chi-square test.

Second, the P-P chart, shown in Figure 7.4, also demonstrates the difference between the distributions to be very slight.

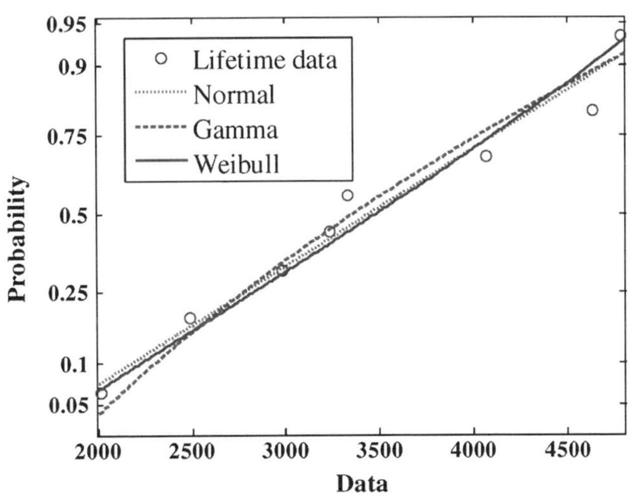

Figure 7.4 P-P chart of lifetime data

Now that there is no remarkable difference of goodness of fits between distributions, we choose Weibull to carry out the reliability modeling considering some of its advantages:

1. Weibull can well approximate normal when its slope parameter ranges from 3.25 to 3.61, especially when the slope parameter equals 3.60232, the percentiles of the two distributions are very close to each other.
2. Compared with gamma and normal, Weibull is easier to use. Moreover, Weibull has a simple, useful, and informative graphical plot of failure data, which is extremely important to engineering.
3. Weibull is more widely applied in reliability engineering of machinery equipment. As the data used in this case come from the torsion test of the blade material, Weibull is more suitable.
4. The data form a relative small sample. Weibull analysis can offer reasonably accurate failure analysis and failure forecasts with extremely small samples [27].

With all the considerations mentioned, Weibull is used for the reliability modeling. To estimate the reliability of the specimens, the time-to-failure data, that is, the maximum test cycles, of 8 out of the 13 material specimens are used to carry out the Weibull fitting. The parameters are calculated and the result is $\eta = 3798.5$ and $\beta = 4.2$.

The architecture of ANN-based prognosis is composed of network training and real-time prognosis, as shown in Figure 7.5. Network training involves sample data preprocessing, feature extraction, performance-evaluation network training, and remaining-life-prediction network training, after which a performance-evaluation neural network N_{PE} and a remaining-life-prediction network N_{RLP} are obtained, as

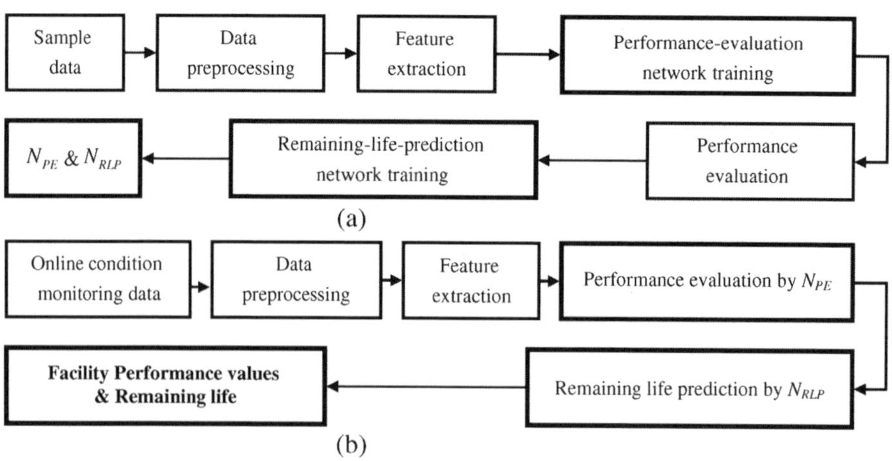

Figure 7.5 Architecture of the artificial neural network-based prognosis: (a) network training, (b) real-time prognosis

shown in Figure 7.5a. Real-time prognosis involves online condition monitoring data collection, data preprocessing, feature extraction, performance evaluation, and dynamic remaining life prediction, as shown in Figure 7.5b.

7.5.2.3 Data Test and Result Analysis

Historical data collected from the in-house test were used. Historical data are composed of feature data, the same type of data as online monitoring data, and actual remaining life. Feature data from one of the five earlier mentioned material specimens are used as input. As the material specimen underwent no maintenance during the in-house test, the final validation result is obtained by reorganizing the actual value and predicted value of the specimen's remaining life.

The result is shown in Figure 7.6 where the four dots represent four maintenance activities. In Figure 7.6a, the horizontal line represents the threshold of reliability, T_r, which is 0.8. The material specimen is maintained three times and hence reused three times. The improvement factor of the first maintenance is 0.7; the second, 0.6; and the third, 0.35. At the end of the fourth life (i.e., at the end of the third reusing life) period, the reliability of the specimen cannot be improved to an acceptable level, so it is considered more suitable to be remanufactured or recycled. In Figure 7.6b, the dashed line represents the actual remaining life, which is obtained by joining four pieces of actual remaining life data of the specimen according to the improvement of its reliability after maintenance activities, and the polyline with asterisks represents the predicted

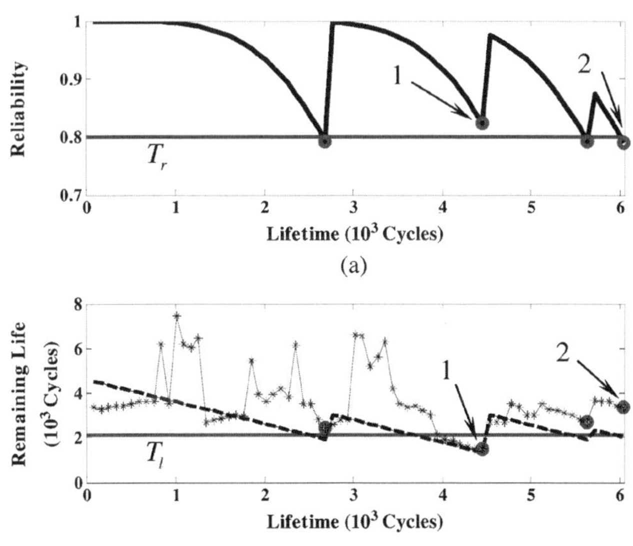

Figure 7.6 Validation result: (a) reliability evaluation, (b) remaining life prediction

value of the remaining life, which is obtained by joining the corresponding pieces of remaining life that are predicted utilizing four different remaining-life-prediction networks trained on the same training sample set.

The unit of lifetime and remaining life here is converted from the data collection interval into a test cycle so that the unit of lifetime here conforms to the unit in the reliability estimation. The horizontal line represents the threshold of the actual value of remaining life, T_l , which stands for 2129 test cycles. The cause of the second shutdown is that the value of the remaining life is predicted to be lower than T_l. The cause of the other shutdowns is that the reliability of the material specimen is very close to T_r even if the value of the remaining life is not predicted to be lower than T_l.

The accuracy of remaining life prediction is analyzed utilizing mean absolute deviation (MAD) and mean forecast error (MFE). MAD reflects the accuracy of prediction, whereas MFE reflects the unbiasedness of prediction. MAD, denoted as $\bar{E}$, and MFE, denoted as $\bar{e}$, can be calculated from Equations 7.21 and 7.22.

$$\overline{E} = \frac{\sum_{i=1}^{n} |\hat{y}_i - y_i|}{n} \tag{7.21}$$

$$\overline{e} = \frac{\sum_{i=1}^{n} (\hat{y}_i - y_i)}{n} \tag{7.22}$$

where $\widetilde{y}_i$ and y_i are the predicted value and the actual value of the ith remaining life prediction and n is the total number of life predictions performed from the beginning to the end of a facility's life. Additionally, the prediction accuracy of the remaining-life-prediction network has to be calculated in units of data collection intervals instead of test cycles because it was trained and used with the data collected in a certain interval.

According to the validation result, the overall MAD and MFE of the prediction are 14 and −10.6806, respectively. Also, the MAD and MFE of the prediction are 16.2653 and −12.0204, respectively, for the earlier 50 predictions, and 8.6087 and −7.8261, respectively, for the later 22 predictions. Therefore, it can be concluded that the prediction methods perform better in the later fatigue stage than in the initial stage. In fact it is just because of the low accuracy in the early prediction that ANN is combined with reliability methods to carry out the remaining life prediction.

The result shows that this methodology can guarantee the reusability of a facility efficiently. If the reliability method and T_r are solely used to make the maintenance decision, the chances are that the degradation of the facility cannot be detected and maintenance cannot be carried out in time. As point 1 in Figure 7.7 shows, the reliability is still far higher than T_r while the actual remaining life of the material specimen is lower than T_l. The facility may not be maintained until its remaining life is far

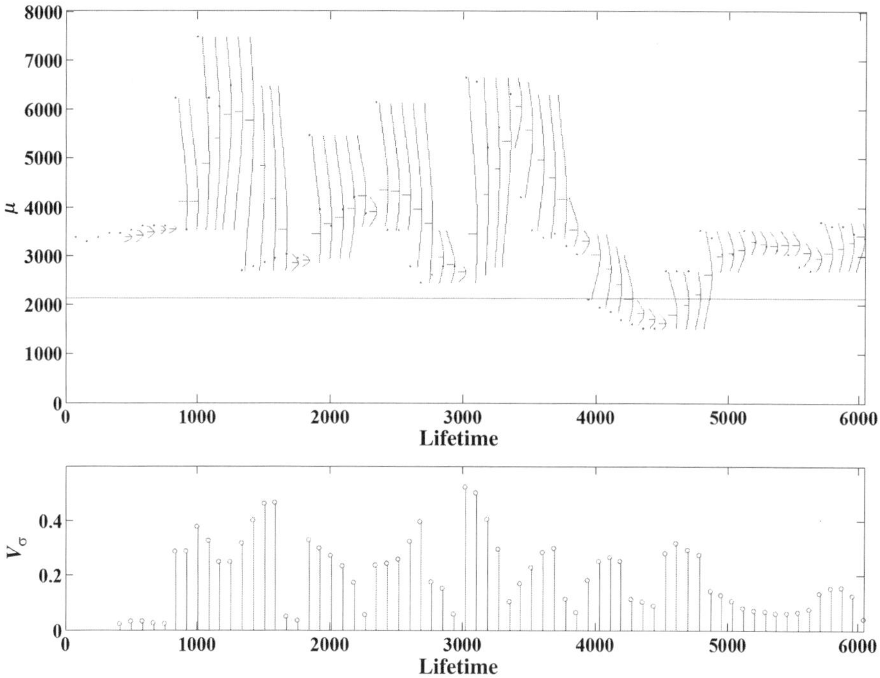

Figure 7.7 Analysis for credibility level

lower than T_l by referring to reliability only, which means the reusability cannot be guaranteed.

If the prognosis method and T_l are solely used, the reliability information is totally ignored. As point 2 in Figure 7.7 shows, the actual value of remaining life is very close to T_l, while the predicted value is still far higher than T_l. If the reliability information is ignored, the maintenance would not be carried out until the actual remaining life is far lower than T_l, which means the performance would degrade to an unacceptable level and the facility would not be reusable.

According to the presented methodology, thresholds for reliability and RUL, and credibility level (C_l) of the predicted value of remaining life are defined to make use of the results from the distribution estimation and the prognostics algorithm. In order to prove that the credibility level (C_l) is academically justifiable, we set every five prediction values in succession in Figure 7.6 as a data sample, and calculate its average value μ and coefficient of variation V_σ. The coefficient of variation, which assesses the representativeness of the average value μ, can be calculated by

$$V_\sigma = \frac{\sigma}{\mu} \tag{7.23}$$

where σ is the mean square deviation of the sample. A small value of V_σ means high representativeness.

We fit normal distribution to the samples and present their probability density function plots with average value μ (presented as short horizontal lines) in Figure 7.7. Also in this figure is the corresponding V_σ of each sample. As is shown in this figure, when the second maintenance is carried out, the average value of the predicted remaining life is below the threshold. The corresponding V_σ is very small, which means this prediction is very credible. On the contrary, when the predicted value fluctuates dramatically, the corresponding V_σ is very large, which means the prediction is not credible enough to be accepted. This conforms to the result obtained by referring to the credibility level (C_l). Thus this analysis shows that our method is academically justifiable.

Overall, the application results demonstrate that the proposed methodology provides sufficient condition information for reuse decision-making from both historical and online perspectives; a facility can be reused many times during its lifetime until its reuse is no longer economic, which can assist in the achievement of the goal of manufacturing with fewer resources and assets.

7.5.3 Maintenance Scheduling Based on Reliability Estimation and Prediction by Prognostic Methodology

The maintenance scheduling could be carried out after implementation of the prognosis method for reliability assessment. The maintenance scheduling method we introduce here uses the intelligent algorithm to find optimal solutions that aim at improving the reuse of facilities as well as saving maintenance cost and production loss. The main procedure of maintenance scheduling includes production system modeling and implementation of an intelligent algorithm.

We employ a genetic algorithm (GA) to find the optimal solution of maintenance scheduling. A flow chart for the hybrid genetic algorithm (HGA), which combines a simple GA with simulation annealing (SA), is shown in Figure 7.8. The initial population is created after initialization of the parameters. Then the fitness of the population

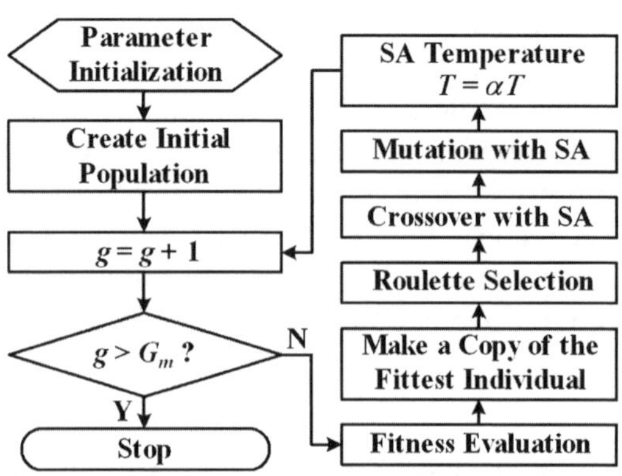

Figure 7.8 Flow chart of HGA

is evaluated, after which the optimal individual, that is, the optimal solution, of this generation is recorded. Subsequently, selection, crossover, and mutation operations are carried out. The optimization process by HGA is stopped when the population has evolved for G_m generations.

7.5.3.1 Solution Encoding

In this case, either a single facility that does not belong to any groups or a maintenance group is considered as a maintenance unit and assigned with an integer unit number. Hence integer encoding is utilized. In addition, the string that contains an individual's encoding is referred to as a chromosome, and each integer is referred to as a gene. If there are M units in one maintenance activity, feasible chromosomes are obtained by putting integers from 1 to M in random order. Examples of chromosomes will be presented to illustrate the operators.

7.5.3.2 Objective Function

The maintenance cost of the kth maintenance activity consists of direct maintenance cost C_{m}^{k} and indirect production loss L_{p}^{k}. The direct maintenance cost, which includes the cost of maintenance actions for maintenance units C_{u}^{k} and set-up cost C_{s}^{k}, can be calculated by Equations 7.15 and 7.16.

The maintenance cost rate R_{C} in a time period T_{S} can be calculated by Equation 7.17.

As for constraints of maintenance scheduling, it is assumed that maintenance tools and maintainers are assigned to a maintenance group according to the maximum numbers needed to maintain any one facility in this group. Therefore, especially, the cost of maintenance tools and maintainers should be calculated by Equations 7.18 and 7.19.

The loss rate increases from its initial value r_0 with maintenance time since the longer the production stays shut down, partly or entirely, the bigger the opportunity cost.

7.5.3.3 Fitness Function of Hybrid Genetic Algorithm

The fitness function of the HGA is mainly used to evaluate the individual fitness value. Usually, it only provides relative fitness values of the individuals to increase selective pressure. In this chapter, the fitness of each individual is not only used in the selection operation, but also used in the SA – Crossover operation and Simulate Annealing – Mutation Operation to compare the offspring individuals with parent individuals. Here an example is given to introduce the fitness function where the population consists of H individuals.

1. Calculate the corresponding direct maintenance cost C_{M}^{h} and indirect production loss L_{p}^{h} of each individual.

2. Calculate the pseudo-fitness value $\bar{f}_h$ (where $h=1, 2, \ldots, H$) of each individual according to Equation 7.24

$$\bar{f}_h = \left(\frac{C_{\mathrm{m}}^h + L_{\mathrm{p}}^h}{\sum_{r=1}^{H} \left(C_{\mathrm{m}}^r + L_{\mathrm{p}}^r \right)} \right)^{-1} \tag{7.24}$$

3. Carry out linear scaling on the pseudo-fitness value to amplify the disparity of different individuals' pseudo-fitness values and get the final fitness f_h (where $h=1, 2, \ldots, H$). Linear scaling can be realized by Equations 7.25–7.27.

$$f_h = \lambda \cdot \bar{f}_h + \xi + \delta \tag{7.25}$$

$$\lambda = \frac{\bar{f}_{avg}}{\bar{f}_{avg} - \bar{f}_{\min}} \tag{7.26}$$

$$\xi = \frac{-\bar{f}_{avg} \cdot \bar{f}_{\min}}{\bar{f}_{avg} - \bar{f}_{\min}} \tag{7.27}$$

where δ is a very small number, for example, 0.1, to avoid a zero fitness value; $\bar{f}_{avg}$ and $\bar{f}_{\min}$ denote, respectively, the average and minimal fitness values within the population. The function of linear scaling is to amplify the disparity of different individuals' fitness values and thus keep high population diversity, which is shown in Figure 7.9. In Equation 7.26, obviously, λ is a value greater than 1 in Figure 7.9, embodied as the slope greater than 1. It can also be seen that the disparity of individual fitness values is amplified after the linear scaling.

Note that if all the pseudo-fitness values of all individuals are the same, the linear scaling cannot be carried out, the pseudo-fitness of individuals is then the final fitness in this case.

7.5.3.4 Crossover and Mutation Operations

Moreover, the idea of SA is integrated into the crossover and mutation operations by accepting or discarding the degenerate chromosomes according to SA methods. The crossover and mutation operations with SA are presented in Figures 7.10 and 7.11, respectively. The population has $N=2L$ individuals.

The population has N individuals. Additionally, order crossover (two-point crossover) and inverse mutation are used. The procedure of order crossover is described as follows with the illustration of Figure 7.12.

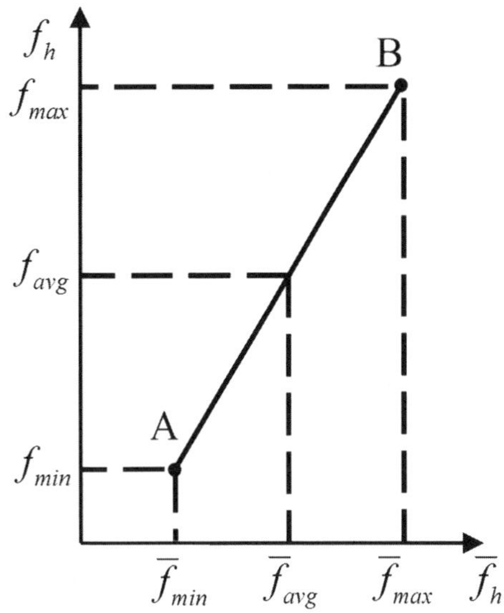

Figure 7.9 The linear scale modification of fitness

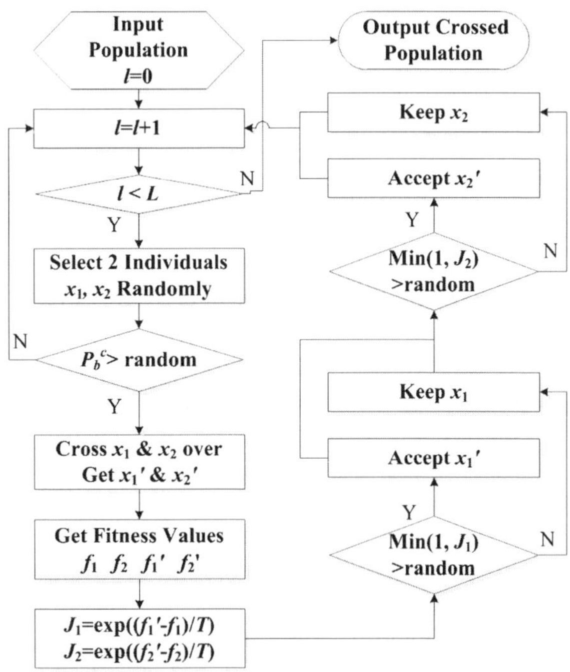

Figure 7.10 Flowchart of crossover operation with SA

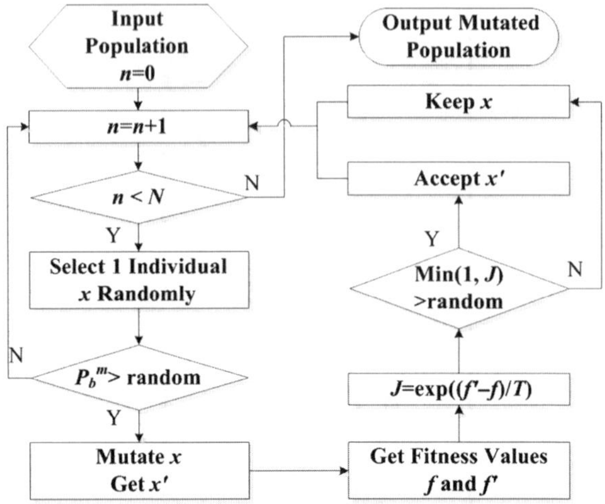

Figure 7.11 Flowchart of mutation operation with SA

Step 1	*Parent* 1	3	4	6	5	1	2
	Parent 2	5	6	1	3	2	4
Step 2	*Proto-child* 1		4	6	5		
	Proto-child 2		6	1	3		
Step 3	*Remain* 1	X	4	X	5	X	2
	Remain 2	X	X	1	3	2	X
			end point		*start point*		
Step 4	*Child* 1	1	4	6	5	2	3
	Child 2	4	6	1	3	2	5

Figure 7.12 The illustration of order crossover

Step 1: Select a substring from each of the parents at random. As shown in Figure 7.12, the second to fourth genes of each parent are chosen as a substring.

Step 2: Produce two proto-children by copying the substrings into the corresponding positions as in the parents.

Step 3: Delete all the genes contained in proto-child 1/2 from parent 2/1 to obtain remain 2/1.

Step 4: Place the genes of remain 2/1 into the unfilled positions of the proto-child 1/2, from the start point to the end point according to the inverse order of the genes in remain 2/1 in order to produce child 1/2 as shown in Figure 7.12.

Inverse mutation starts by randomly selecting two points in a chromosome. Genes located between the two points are then placed in reverse order.

7.5.4 Case Description

In this section, a case study on maintenance scheduling of a bearing production workshop is presented. The production system has 45 facilities, as shown in Figure 7.13. Facilities 0, 46, and 17 are input, output, and heat treatment, respectively, and it is assumed that their performances do not degrade with time. The arrows on the left connect the production lines for the outer race and those on the right connect those for the inner race. The bottom arrows connect the assembly line of the bearings. In Figure 7.13 the different types of facilities and the layout of the workshop are also presented. Facilities 1–16 carry out lathing processes, 18–35 grinding, 36 and

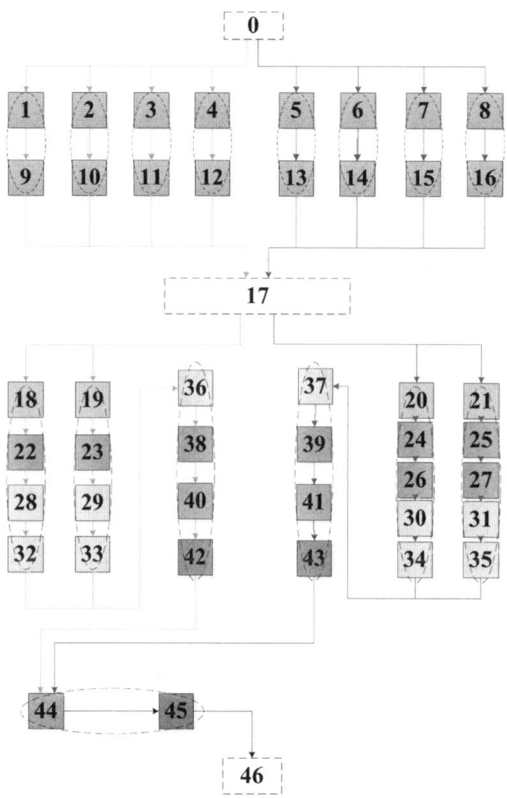

Figure 7.13 Production system for bearings

37 lapping, 38 and 39 demagnetizing, 40 and 41 cleaning, 42 and 43 sizing, 44 assembling, and 45 riveting. Based on the method of building structure dependence of a production system, the structure dependence of this bearing production system can be built. According to the rule-based group maintenance policy, 15 static groups can be formed, which are marked with dashed ellipses in Figure 7.13.

7.5.4.1 Parameter Settings

For each facility, the two parameters for reliability modeling, η and β, are derived from randomly generated simulation data; this is done for the facility's price and the resources and time needed for its minor maintenance, medium maintenance, overhaul, and replacement.

In this case study, the three thresholds, T_h^1, T_h^2, and T_h^3, are set as 0.9, 0.75, and 0.6, respectively; and L_R is set as 0.2; improvement factors for minor maintenance, medium maintenance, and overhaul are set as 0.2, 0.6, and 0.7; the compensation factor for medium maintenance, F_d, is calculated by Equation 7.28.

$$\begin{cases} F_d = 0.2^{\left(\frac{1}{2K_d}\right)}, & \text{if } K_m \le 3 \\ F_d = 0.1^{\left(\frac{1}{2K_d}\right)}, & \text{if } K_m > 3 \end{cases} \tag{7.28}$$

where K_m and K_d are the numbers of minor and medium maintenances for a single facility. Similarly, the compensation factor for overhaul F_o is calculated by Equation 7.29.

$$\begin{cases} F_o = 0.2^{\left(\frac{1}{K_o}\right)}, & \text{if } K_m \le 3 \\ F_o = 0.1^{\left(\frac{1}{K_o}\right)}, & \text{if } K_m > 3 \end{cases} \tag{7.29}$$

From Equations 7.28 and 7.29, it can be concluded that the two compensation factors increase with increasing numbers of medium maintenances and overhauls, which makes the compensation effect decrease at the same time. This is to simulate the practical situation that the maintenance effect will decrease as the number of maintenances increase. In addition, the compensation factor for overhaul tends to be smaller than that of medium maintenance, which means the maintenance effect of overhaul tends to be magnified more significantly. This is consistent with the practical situation that the maintenance effect of overhaul is more significant than the effect of medium maintenance.

The set-up cost C_s of each maintenance activity is set as 1000; the unit prices for four types of maintenance resources, that is, spare parts, tools, maintainers, and consumables, are set as 100, 50, 50, and 10, respectively; the initial value of the production loss rate r_0 is set as 1000.

For the HGA, population size N is set as $(M-1)M/2$, where M is the number of maintenance units in a maintenance activity; maximum evolution generation G_m is set as 100; crossover probability P_b^c and mutation probability P_b^m are set as 0.7 and 0.05, respectively; the initial value of the simulated annealing temperature T is set as 10^4, and the cool-down factor α is set as 0.9.

7.5.4.2 Simulation Result

A simulation is carried out to present how the proposed method can be used and to verify the advantage of a group maintenance policy. In the simulation, the maintenance scheduling is carried out for a time period of 1000 working days. A maintenance activity will be triggered once a facility needs overhaul or replacement. Simulation will be carried out in two scenarios. In the first scenario, only an opportunistic maintenance policy is followed, which means when a maintenance activity is triggered, all the facilities that need minor maintenance, medium maintenance, overhaul, and replacement will be maintained separately. In the second scenario, an opportunistic maintenance policy and a rule-based group maintenance policy are followed.

The Gantt charts and optimization process of the second maintenance activity in the two scenarios are presented as follows. According to the reliability of facilities and the three prescribed thresholds, there are 29 facilities that need maintenance. Facilities 1, 2, 5, 6, 13, 16, 20, 21, 23, 25, 28, 29, 32, 33, 35, 36, 37, 38, 40, 41, 42, and 43 need minor maintenance; facilities 22, 26, 27, 30, 31, and 39 need medium maintenance; facility 30 needs overhaul; and no facility needs replacement.

The Gantt chart for the optimal maintenance schedule under an opportunistic maintenance policy is presented in Figure 7.14. The maintenance tasks are scheduled separately and 3 hours are needed for the whole maintenance activity, as shown in the figure.

The Gantt chart for the optimal maintenance schedule under an opportunistic maintenance policy and a rule-based group maintenance policy is presented in Figure 7.15.

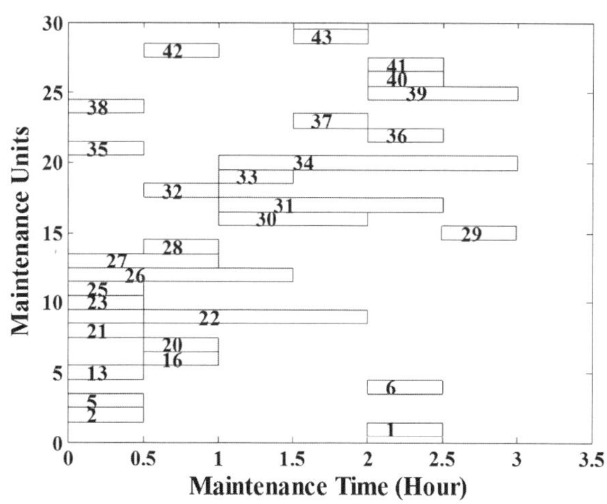

Figure 7.14 Gantt chart for the optimal schedule under opportunistic maintenance policy

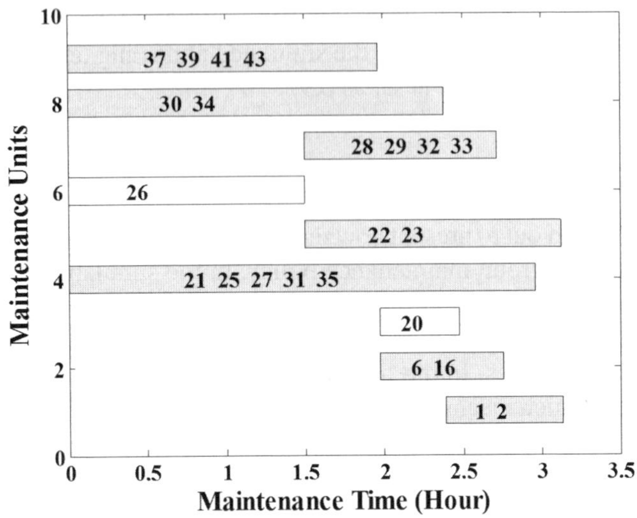

Figure 7.15 Gantt chart for the optimal schedule under opportunistic maintenance policy and rule-based group maintenance policy

Facilities 5 and 13 both need minor maintenance, and are included in one static group, thus they are left out from this maintenance activity according to the rule-based group maintenance policy. The same applies to facilities 36, 38, 40, and 42. The remaining facilities are either separated into different maintenance groups or left as a single facility to form maintenance units. The facilities 20 and 26 are left single to form units 3 and 6. Some units are formed into a static maintenance group, that is, units 4 and 9; and some units, such as units 1 and 2, are formed into dynamic maintenance groups. More than 3 hours are needed for the whole maintenance activity, as shown in the figure.

In Table 7.3, the optimal maintenance costs for the second maintenance activity under the two different maintenance policies are listed. It can be seen that the opportunistic maintenance combined with rule-based group maintenance policy is effective in reducing maintenance cost. The same conclusion can be reached from Table 7.4 where the optimal maintenance cost rates for the whole operation period of 1000 days under the two different maintenance polices are listed.

In this chapter, we first reviewed the development of maintenance. The changing role and new perspective of maintenance facilitate the implementation of new techniques

Table 7.3 Optimal maintenance cost under different maintenance policies

Maintenance policy	OM	OM&RGM
Optimal maintenance cost	11111	11005

Table 7.4 Optimal maintenance cost rate under different maintenance policies

Maintenance policy	OM	OM&RGM
Optimal maintenance cost rate	103.3	100.9

in maintenance decision-making. As a result, we have attempted to present recent research in prognosis-incorporating maintenance decision-making, which is good for sustainable manufacturing since it enhances facility reuse – one important part in the 6R of a sustainable manufacturing system.

With the rapid development of micro-electro-mechanical systems technology, implementation of such a method will be a future trend. The fast and robust on-line signal processing algorithms are crucial to the design of an intelligent device, which has the capability of continuously monitoring its own health using on-line data acquisition, on-line signal processing and on-line prognostic tools. This will no doubt stimulate increasing research interest in this area.

7.6 Maintenance Decision-Making Considering Energy Consumption

With high energy consumption, industry is crucial to the development of the economy. From the perspective of sustainable development, lowering the energy consumption is essential and extremely urgent. Since equipment is the main source of energy consumption within industrial processes and degradation of equipment performance leads to increasing energy consumption, then it is necessary to maintain equipment performance through an appropriate maintenance strategy. Maintenance scheduling taking account of energy consumption will contribute to energy conservation. In this section, a method for multi-objective maintenance time decision-making with energy consumption considered is illustrated. It includes building the energy consumption model for a single machine then establishing the model of systematic energy consumption and objective function, and finally introducing a sliding bearing production system as a case study. The MOCLPSO-based method, introduced in Section 6.3, is used in the case study.

7.6.1 Energy Consumption Modeling

7.6.1.1 Energy Consumption Modeling for One Facility

Equipment wear is inescapable during a continuous operation process and the outward manifestation of that is abrasion. We divide the process of wear into three stages based on the normal working conditions: running-in period, normal wear stage, severe wear stage. The relationship between wear and operating time is shown in Figure 7.16.

Wear of equipment components is closely related to the equipment energy consumption.

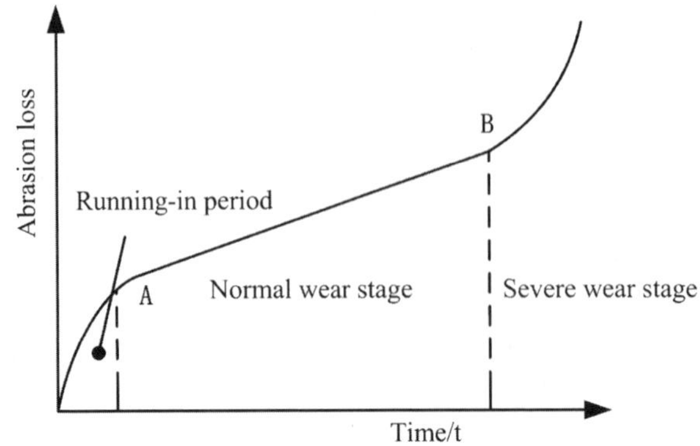

Figure 7.16 Schematic of empirical relationship between wear and time

First, wear is a process which can lead to energy loss through heat dissipation, elastic deformation, and plastic deformation [28].

Secondly, wear contributes to the change in clearance and properties of the contact surface, intensifying vibration. As a result, energy consumption in the form of mechanical energy increases and the impact of vibration will also accelerate the wear of equipment [29].

Referring to the literature [30], the relationship between wear and energy consumption can be described as:

$$e = aW^b \tag{7.30}$$

where e is energy consumption per unit of wear, W is weight loss due to wear, and a, b are constants.

Since

$$e = \frac{E}{W} \tag{7.31}$$

where, E is total energy consumption.

Equation 7.30 can be written as:

$$E = aW^\beta \tag{7.32}$$

where, $\beta = b + 1$.

According to the literature [31], the vibration severity of the time domain signal can characterize the vibration energy, as described in Equation 7.33.

$$\text{VCRS} = \sum_{t=t_1}^{t_n} \log(\sigma_{(\text{rms})t} / \min(\sigma_{(\text{rms})t})) \tag{7.33}$$

where, VCRS is the vibration cumulative relative scale, σ_{rms} is the root mean square value of the vibration velocity.

Wear of the gear box can be determined by measuring the mass fraction of elements in the oil, as described in Equation 7.34.

$$\mathrm{WCRS} = \lambda \sum_{t=t_1}^{t_n} \log(G_{it}/\min(G_{it})) \tag{7.34}$$

where, WCRS is the wear cumulative relative scale, G_{it} is the mass fraction of the element i at time t, and λ is a proportionality coefficient.

As the experimental result shows, wear and vibration are highly correlated, and there is an approximate linear relationship between time and both VCRS and WCRS.

Suppose the relationship between VCRS and time t is described as:

$$\mathrm{VCRS} = kt + c \tag{7.35}$$

where, k and c are constants.

Since the vibration signal in the literature [30] is a discrete signal, the serialized result of Equation 7.33 is shown as Equation 7.36

$$\mathrm{VCRS} = \int_{t_1}^{t_n} \lg(\sigma_{(\mathrm{rms})t}/\min(\sigma_{(\mathrm{rms})t}))\mathrm{d}t \tag{7.36}$$

Accordingly, the serialized result of Equation 7.34 is shown as Equation 7.37

$$\mathrm{WCRS} = \lambda \int_{t_1}^{t_n} \log(G_{it}/\min(G_{it}))\mathrm{d}t \tag{7.37}$$

Suppose the relationship between VCRS and WCRS is described by Equation 7.38:

$$\mathrm{VCRS} = \eta \mathrm{WCRS} + \varsigma \tag{7.38}$$

where, η and ς are constants.

The substitution result of Equations 7.36–7.38 is Equation 7.39

$$\int_{t_1}^{t_n} \log(\sigma_{(\mathrm{rms})t}/\min(\sigma_{(\mathrm{rms})t}))\mathrm{d}t = \eta\lambda \int_{t_1}^{t_n} \log(G_{it}/\min(G_{it}))\mathrm{d}t + \varsigma \tag{7.39}$$

Take the derivative of Equation 7.39, then take the exponential transformation result as shown in Equation 7.40

$$\sigma_{(\mathrm{rms})t}/\min(\sigma_{(\mathrm{rms})t}) = (G_{it}/\min(G_{it}))^{\lambda\eta} \tag{7.40}$$

Replace the $\sigma_{(\mathrm{rms})t}$ and G_{it} in Equation 7.40 with E and W, the result is shown in Equation 7.41

$$E = \alpha W^{\beta} \tag{7.41}$$

where, α and β are constants.

Equation 7.41 coincides with the result in the literature [30], so Equation 7.42 can represent the functional relationship between energy consumption and wear.

Considering the normal work energy consumption of the equipment, the relationship between the total energy consumption of the equipment and wear can be described by Equation 7.42

$$E = E_0(t) + \alpha W^{\varphi} \tag{7.42}$$

where, $E_0(t)$ is the normal work energy consumption of the equipment, which can be calculated by

$$E_0(t) = P_0(t) \cdot t \tag{7.43}$$

where, $P_0(t)$ is the normal output power of the equipment which, in this section, we suppose to be a constant recorded as P_0.

For the purpose of simulating the wear of mechanical equipment, Equation 7.44 is introduced,

$$W(t) = kt + c + \lambda e^{\omega t} \tag{7.44}$$

where, k, c, and λ are constants.

Equation 7.44 is composed of two parts: a linear function and an exponential function. The linear function is used to simulate the wear during the normal wear stage, while the exponential function is applied to simulate the wear during the severe wear stage. As discussed above, since equipment will undergo debugging and grinding-in before leaving the factory, the users just need to focus on the normal and severe wear stages.

The calculation of equipment energy consumption $E(t)$ can be summarized from Equations 7.42 and 7.44:

$$E(t) = E_0(t) + \alpha[kt + c + \lambda e^{\omega t}]^{\varphi} \tag{7.45}$$

Equation 7.45 is the model of "energy consumption–time," the derivative result is the "energy consumption of unit time–time" model. One group of simulation results is shown in Figure 7.17. The constants above can be determined by statistical analysis of historical data in practical application.

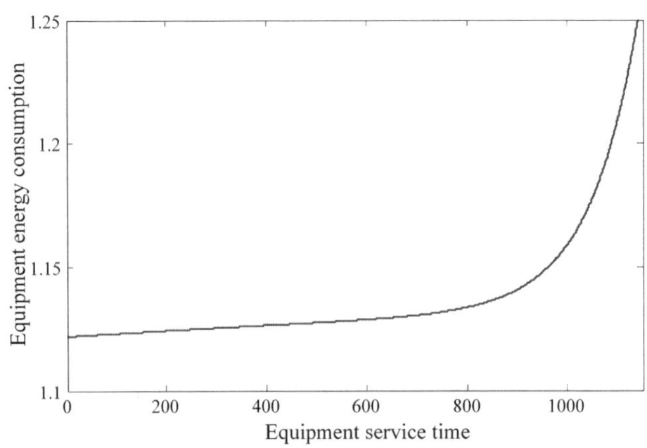

Figure 7.17 Example of relationship between energy consumption and time

As shown in Figure 7.17, in the early stages, the equipment energy consumption per unit of time is relatively stable. However, when the running period reaches a certain time, taking 800 days as an example, the equipment energy consumption per unit of time goes up obviously, as a consequence of accelerated wear. The simulation result is in agreement with the pattern seen in actual use.

7.6.1.2 System Energy Consumption Model

Since the system reliability and cost models have been established in earlier chapters, only the energy consumption model is established in this section.

The total energy consumption of a production system in a period of time is the combination of each device's energy consumption in the system. It can be calculated by:

$$E_S = \sum_{j=1}^{m} E^j \tag{7.46}$$

where, E_S is the total energy consumption of the system during the simulation time.

E^j is the total energy consumption of equipment j during the simulation time, it can be calculated by:

$$E^j = \int_0^{T_{\text{total}}} e_j(t) \cdot \mathrm{d}t \tag{7.47}$$

where, $e_j(t)$ is the power of equipment j at time t.

7.6.2 Implementation

7.6.2.1 Sliding Bearing Production System

This section is a case study of a sliding bearing production system producing mainly radial sliding bearings As is shown in Figure 7.18, the bearing assembly includes a bearing bush, set screw, bearing cover, bearing seat, oil cup, bolt, and so on. The bearing bush is produced from a tin-base bearing alloy, the bush back from carbon steel bar, and the bearing cover and bearing seat are castiron. The structural parameters are shown in Table 7.5, while the codes of the components and some other information are provided in Table 7.6.

According to Table 7.6, this production system mainly produces three components: bearing covers, bearing seats, and bearing bushes, while other components are obtained through outsourcing. As a consequence, this system consists of four production lines: bearing cover, bearing seat, and bearing bush production lines; and the assembly line. The manufacturing process and required equipment are shown in Tables 7.7–7.10.

According to Tables 7.7 and 7.8, with a productivity of 24 units per hour under normal conditions, all the equipment is put into production. The production system consists of 44 facilities, as shown in Figure 7.19. With the production lines being designed

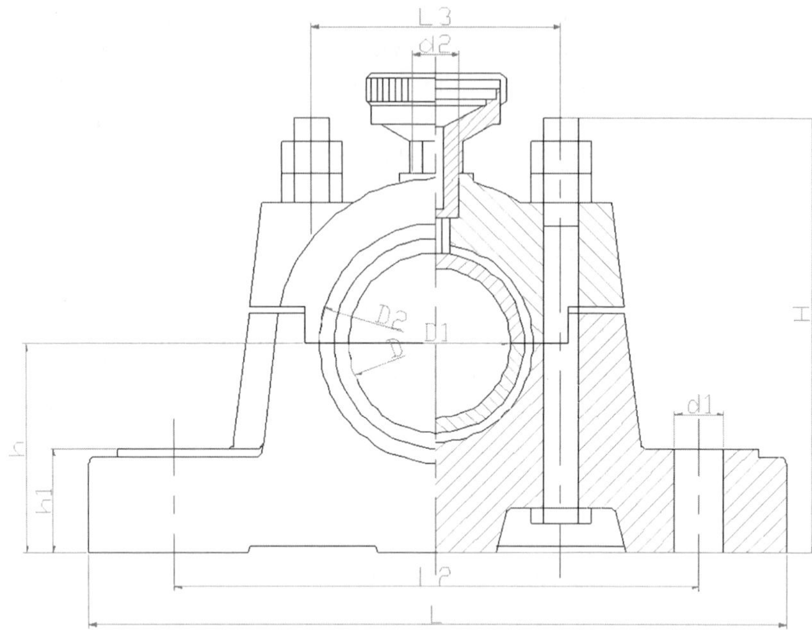

Figure 7.18 Schematic of radial sliding bearing

Table 7.5 Parameters of the product

Code	D	D1	D2	H≈	h	h1	d1	d2	L	L2	L3
HD2060	60	50	80	130	60	25	24	M14	240	190	100

Table 7.6 Information on raw material and product components

Code	Name	Material	Material specification	Remarks
D	Upper bearing bush	ZSnSb11Cu6 + HT200	Ø70 barstock	
E	Lower bearing bush	ZSnSb11Cu6 + HT200	Ø70 barstock	
F	Set-screw			Outsourcing
G	Top bearing cover	HT200		
H	Bearing seat	HT200		
I	Oil cup			Outsourcing
J	Bolt			Outsourcing
K	Spring washer			Outsourcing
L	Nut			Outsourcing

Table 7.7 Facilities in bearing seat production line

Number	Process	Details of process	Facility model	Amount	Productivity
1	Milling	Rough mill Ø60 end face	Horizontal milling machine X6025	2	20
2	Milling	Fine mill seat	Horizontal milling machine X6025	3	10
3	Milling	Fine mill two Ø60 end face	Horizontal milling machine X6025	2	15
4	Drilling	Drill Ø60 hole, chamfer 2.5 × 45°	Vertical drilling machine Z5163	4	7.5
5	Drilling	Drill 2 × Ø11 holes	Radial drilling machine Z025 × 1/10	2	15
6	Drilling	Drill 2 × Ø24 holes	Radial drilling machine Z025 × 1/10	1	30
7	Assembly	Assemble bearing seat cover and seat	Vice bench	1	30
8	Boring	Fine bore Ø60	Horizontal boring machine T617A	2	12
9	Test			2	20

Table 7.8 Facilities in bearing cover production line

Number	Process	Details of process	Facility model	Amount	Productivity
1	Milling	Rough mill Ø60 end face	Horizontal milling machine X6025	2	15
2	Milling	Fine mill upper end face and two Ø60 end face	Horizontal milling machine X6025	4	7.5
3	Drilling	Drill 2 × Ø11 and Ø11.9 holes	Radial drilling machine Z025 × 1/10	2	12
4	Drilling	Drill Ø60 hole, chamfer 2.5 × 45°	Vertical drilling machine Z5163	4	7.5
5	Benchwork	Tapping M14 × 1.5	Vertical drilling machine Z5163	2	20
6	Test			2	20

as a U-shape, the buffer caches of raw materials and products in the process set are arranged on both sides of the main thoroughfare. The position coordinate of each facility is shown in Figure 7.19 and the overall arrangement of this production system is given in Figure 7.20. In Figure 7.20, each box with a number represents a single machine. For instance, facility No. 0 represents system input, while facility No. 45 represents system output. Information on the other equipment is shown in Table 7.11.

Table 7.9 Facilities in bearing bush production line

Number	Process	Details of process	Facility model	Amount	Productivity
1	Fine lathing	Fine lathe surface of bearing bush	Horizontal lathe CA6140	3	10
2	Milling	Mill bearing bush	Horizontal milling machine X6025	2	12
3	Fine machining	Mill split surface and oil groove, locate half slot, chamfering, and nick	Vertical lift platform mill machine X5012	4	6
4	Test			2	15

Table 7.10 Facilities in assembly line

Number	Process	Details of process	Facility model	Amount	productivity
1	Bearing seat assembly	Assemble the bearing cover and seat, install oil cup and bolt	Vice bench	2	20
2	Bearing bush assembly	Assemble the bearing bush, fix the bearing bush with set screw, lubricate bearings	Vice bench	3	10
3	Test			2	20

7.6.2.2 Method of Setting Simulation Parameters of the Production System

1. *Parameters of equipment reliability*

   The two parameters of the Weibull distribution, which is used as the equipment reliability function, are determined according to the literature [32]. The scale parameter of the equipment, η, is set between 100 and 1000 according to the durability of the equipment; the shape parameter, β, is set between 1 and 3 according to the aging rate of the equipment.
2. *Parameters of maintenance cost*

   The price of the equipment is set according to the current market price. The maintenance cost for one piece of equipment contains the cost of a replacement part, consumables, and so on, and is set as follows: minor maintenance cost about 1% of the price of the equipment, medium maintenance cost about 10%, and major maintenance cost about 60%. The price of maintenance personnel and maintenance tools are 150 and 50 yuan/h. The pure profit of each product is 15 yuan.
3. *Parameters of equipment energy consumption*

   We assume parameters of equipment wear are set as follows: $k=1.2$, $c=500$, $\omega=0.01$, the equipment will pass into the severe wear stage when its reliability

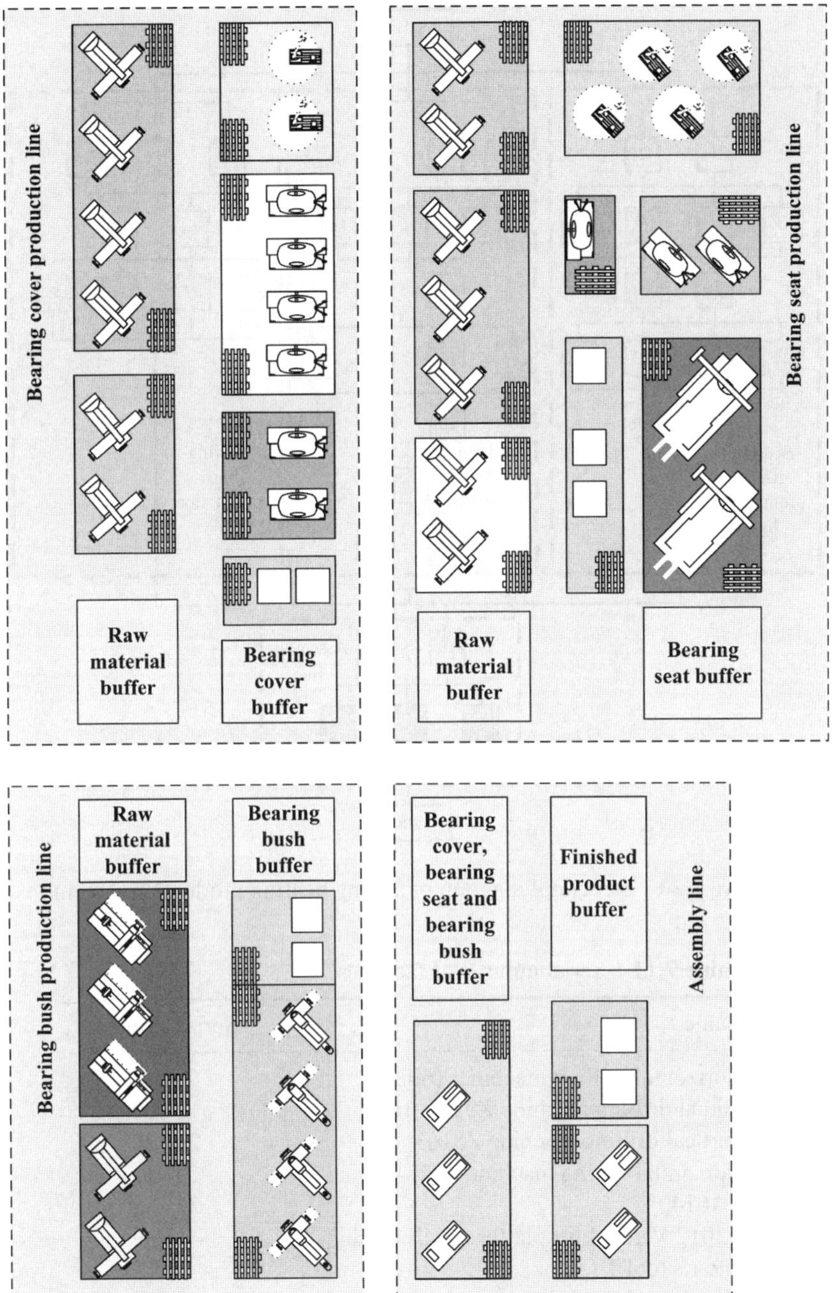

Figure 7.19 Schematic of production system layout

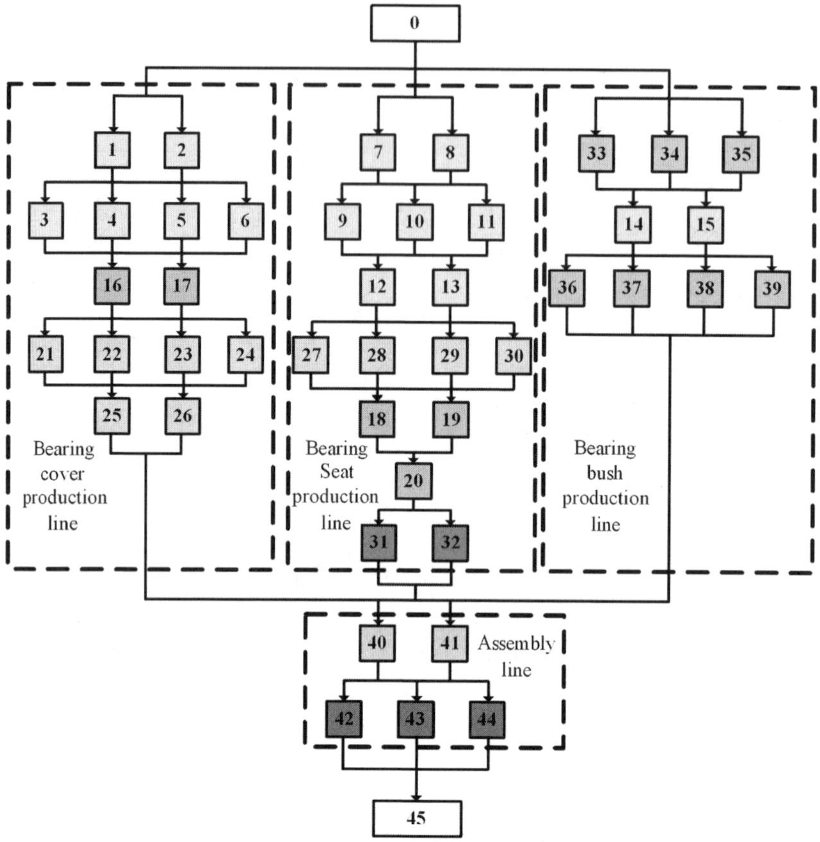

Figure 7.20 Structural diagram of sliding bearing production system

Table 7.11 Serial number of facilities

Name	Serial number
Horizontal milling machine X6025	1–15
Radial drilling machine Z025 × 1/10	16–20
Vertical drilling machine Z5163	21–30
Horizontal boring machine T617A	31, 32
CA6140	33–35
X5012 Vertical lift platform mill machine	36–39
Fitter's tool 1	41, 42
Fitter's tool 2	43–45

falls to 0.5. The time before the equipment reaches the severe wear stage can be calculated by

$$t_{\text{turn}} = \eta \cdot (-\ln 0.5)^{1/\beta} \tag{7.48}$$

Assume the equipment starts to wear severely when the slope of the equipment wear curve reaches $2k$, λ can be calculated by

$$\lambda = \frac{k}{\omega \cdot \exp(\omega \cdot t_{\text{turn}})} \tag{7.49}$$

The normal equipment energy consumption is set according to the equipment's rated power, while the other two parameters are $\alpha = 0.2$, $\varphi = 1.3$.

4. *Other parameters*
   The capacity of the buffer caches between the production and assembly lines are 50. The numbers of maintenance personnel and maintenance tools are determined according to the total maintenance resources needed by each maintenance unit in every maintenance activity, in this case, the ratio r_{MR} is set between 10 and 40%.
5. *Objective function*
   In general, a multi-objective optimization problem is composed of n decision variables, M objective functions, and K constraint conditions, in this case the objective of optimization is:

$$\min y = f(x) = [f_1(x), f_2(x), f_3(x)] \tag{7.50}$$

where the decision vector $x = (x_1, x_2, \cdots, x_{45}) \in X$, the target vector $y = (y_1, y_2, y_3) \in Y$, y_1 represents the reliability index, y_2 represents the maintenance cost, y_3 represents the energy consumption, X is the decision space, and Y is the target space.

In a multi-objective optimization problem, there are always conflicts among the objectives, optimization of one objective might cause degradation of another. Therefore balance among these objectives is the optimization target.

7.6.3 Verification and Conclusions

The first problems in maintenance scheduling are when to start the maintenance activity, which equipment needs maintenance and what kind of maintenance is needed.

In this section, the optimization result of the Pareto-space-based MOCLPSO method is analyzed.

The parameters of the algorithm are set as shown in Table 7.12

The result of the program is shown in Figures 7.21–7.23. Figure 7.21 shows the variation in the number of particles in the Pareto front with the increase in iterations in the outfile. In general, the number of particles increases gradually with increasing iterations then the rate of increase of particles gradually slows with further increase in iterations. However, there are frequent fluctuations in the rate of increase of particles.

Table 7.12 Parameters of Pareto-space-based MOCLPSO

Parameter	Value
Simulation time (day)	1000
Population quantity	200
Number of outfile	100
Number of iterations	200
w_{max}	0.9
w_{min}	0.5
c_{1i}	2.5
c_{1f}	0.5
c_{2i}	0.5
c_{2f}	2.5

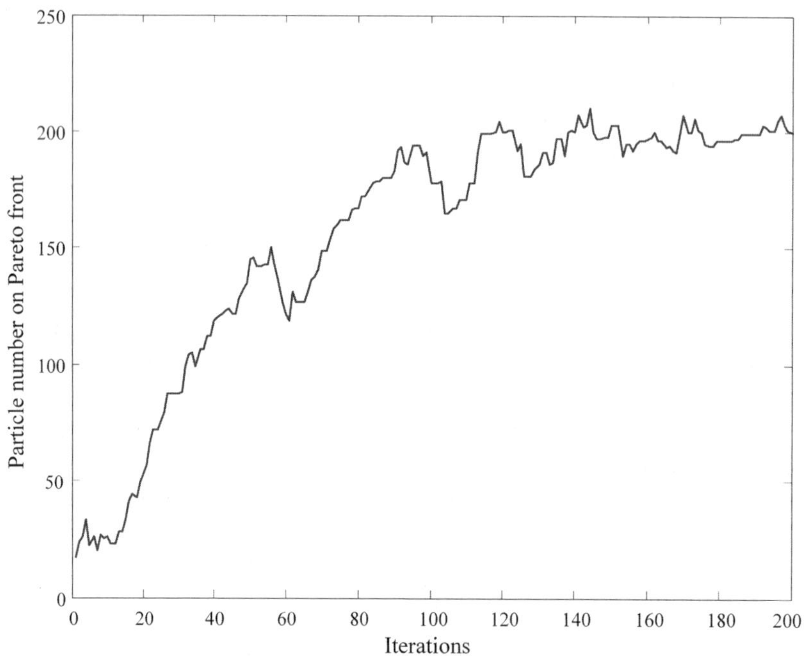

Figure 7.21 Number of particles in the Pareto front versus number of iterations

At the initial stage of iteration, due to the randomness of the initial population and outfile, the calculated particles in the Pareto front are few in number and of poor quality, thus being easily replaced by particles of a new population. In Figure 7.21, it is obvious that the number of particles in the Pareto front did not increase rapidly during the 1st to 15th iterations. This means at the initial stage of iteration, there is much elimination in the process of updating the outfile. After the 15th iteration, new particles are gained in the Pareto front and they are difficult to be replaced due to their good quality. Therefore the number of particles in the Pareto front rises stably while the weeding-out process decreases.

In the process of iteration, there is a possibility for particles to rush out of the current Pareto front, due to the existence of an inertia factor and the mechanism of self-variation.

Figure 7.22 shows the mean value of simulation results for the particles in the Pareto front for each iteration, for (a) the system average daily maintenance cost, (b) the mean value of the system reliability, and (c) the system average daily energy consumption. The mean value of the simulation results for particles in the Pareto front shows the overall trend of the movement of particles in the Pareto front.

1. The variation diagram of mean maintenance cost corresponds to the particles in the Pareto front.
2. The variation diagram of the mean reliability value corresponds to the particles in the Pareto front.
3. The variation diagram of mean energy consumption corresponds to the particles in the Pareto front.

In general, the three objectives changed to a different degree after the iterations. At the initial stage of iteration, the three objectives show an obvious trend of optimization due to the constant appearance of particles in the Pareto front: the system average daily maintenance cost decreased, the mean value of the system reliability increased, the system average daily energy consumption decreased. In the middle and later stages of iteration, the optimization rates of the three objectives slow down since the central particles in the Pareto front are found gradually.

It can be concluded from Figure 7.22 that as the iteration time increases, the three objectives are optimized to a different degree: the system average daily maintenance cost and system average daily energy consumption decreased, while the mean value of the system reliability increased, which means the proposed methodology for multi-objective maintenance time decision-making with energy consumption considered is valid.

One of the Pareto optimal solutions obtained using the above Pareto space comparison method will be discussed as an example to deepen the understanding of the optimization results.

The corresponding maintenance scheduling to the Pareto optimal solution is shown in Table 7.13, since there are 45 facilities, we listed the maintenance scheduling result of 4 facilities as an example.

Figure 7.23 shows the changing trend of the corresponding system reliability. Figure 7.24 shows the changing trend of the system daily energy consumption. From Figures 7.23 and 7.24, it can be concluded that the proposed methodology for

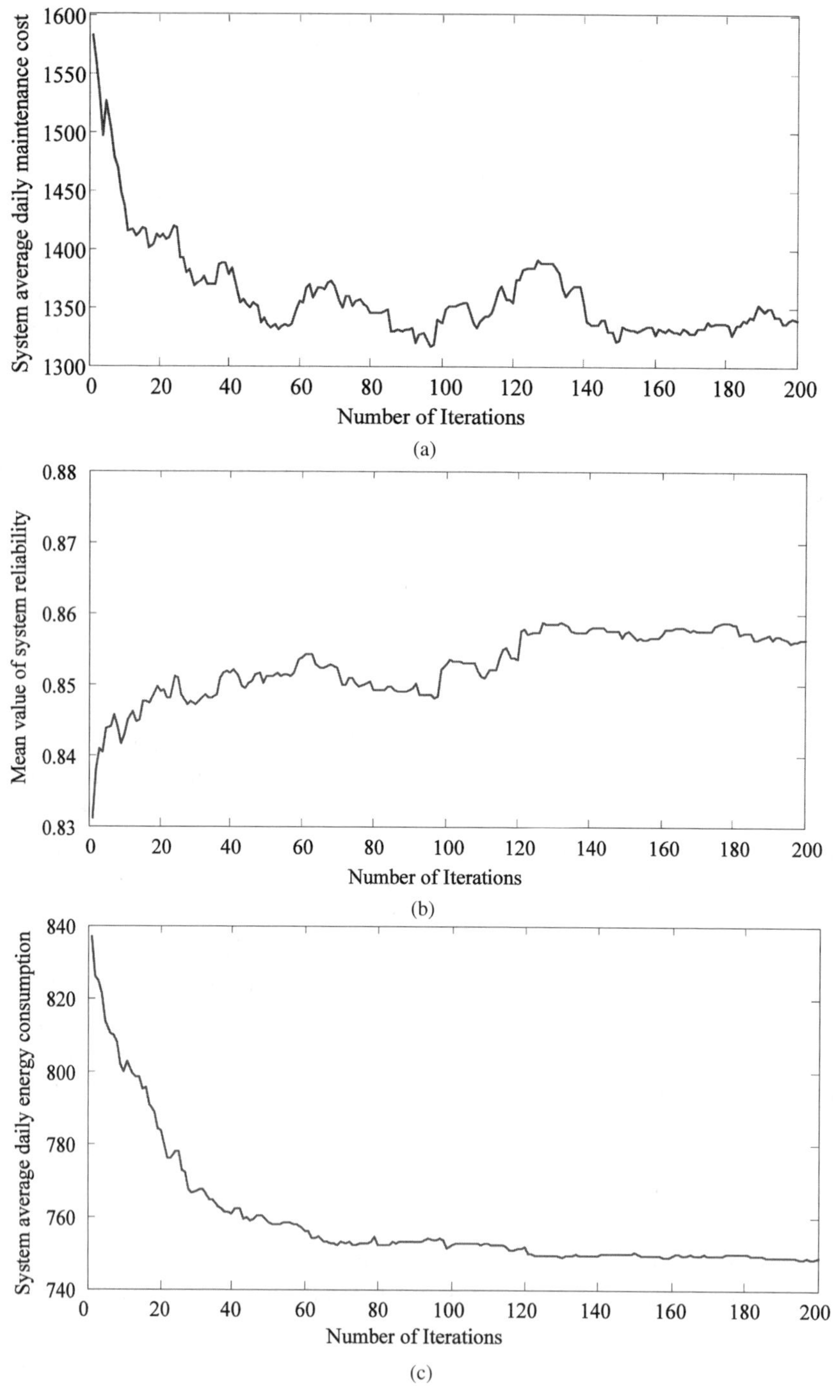

Figure 7.22 Variation diagrams of objectives' mean value corresponding to the particles in the Pareto front in an iterative process. (a) System average daily maintenance cost, (b) mean value of system reliability, (c) system average daily energy consumption

Table 7.13 Maintenance scheduling result

Maintenance time	Facility1	Facility 2	Facility 3	Facility 4
295	Maintenance free	Maintenance free	Maintenance free	Maintenance free
337	Maintenance free	Medium maintenance	Medium maintenance	Medium maintenance
421	Medium maintenance	Minor maintenance	Minor maintenance	Medium maintenance
491	Medium maintenance	Medium maintenance	Maintenance free	Medium maintenance
533	Maintenance free	Medium maintenance	Maintenance free	Minor maintenance
631	Medium maintenance	Maintenance free	Replacement	Medium maintenance
687	Medium maintenance	Major maintenance	Minor maintenance	Medium maintenance
743	Medium maintenance	Maintenance free	Minor maintenance	Medium maintenance
757	Maintenance free	Minor maintenance	Maintenance free	Maintenance free
827	Medium maintenance	Minor maintenance	Minor maintenance	Medium maintenance
869	Maintenance free	Maintenance free	Minor maintenance	Medium maintenance
897	Medium maintenance	Minor maintenance	Minor maintenance	Medium maintenance

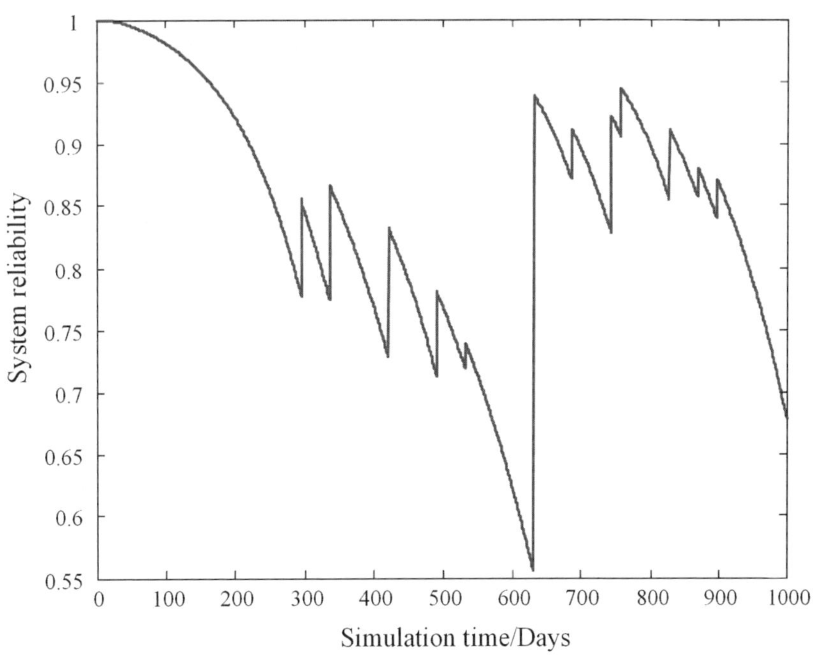

Figure 7.23 System reliability versus simulation time

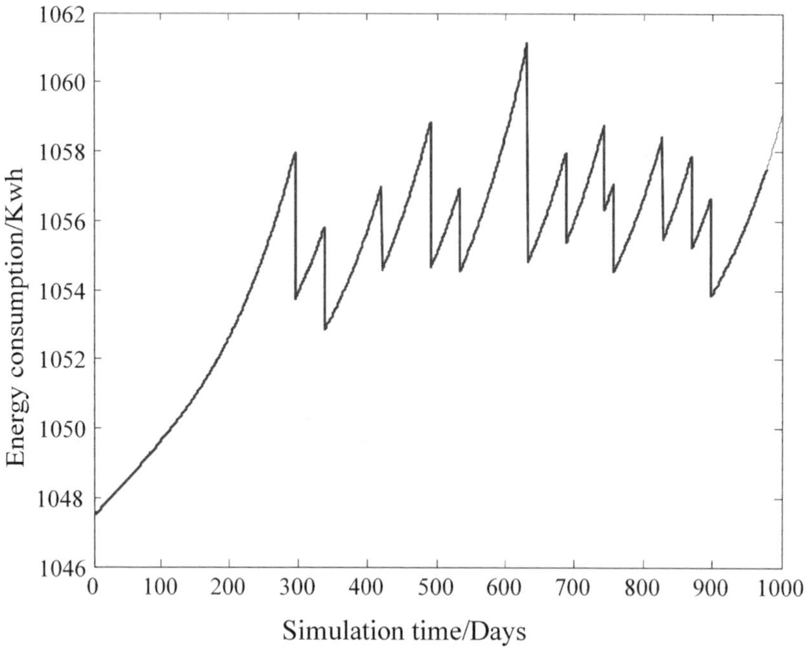

Figure 7.24 System energy consumption versus simulation time

multi-objective maintenance time decision-making with energy consumption considered can balance system reliability, system energy consumption, and maintenance cost, so that the system is kept working under relatively low energy consumption and with relatively high reliability, while the maintenance cost is relatively inexpensive.

References

1. Arai, T. and Shimomura, Y. (2004) Proposal of service CAD system-a tool for service engineering. *CIRP Annals-Manufacturing Technology*, **53** (1), 397–400.
2. Seliger, G., Buchholz, A., and Grudzien, W. (2002) Multiple usage phases by component adaptation. Proceedings of the 9th CIRP International Seminar on Life Cycle Engineering, Erlangen, Germany, pp. 47–54.
3. Kaebernick, H., Kara, S. and Sun, M. (2003) Sustainable product development and manufacturing by considering environmental requirements. *Robotics and Computer-Integrated Manufacturing*, **19** (6), 461–468.
4. Mangun, D. and Thurston, D.L. (2002) Incorporating component reuse, remanufacture, and recycle into product portfolio design. *IEEE Transactions on Engineering Management*, **49** (4), 479–490.
5. Murayama, T. and Shu, L.H. (2001) Treatment of reliability for reuse and remanufacture. Proceedings EcoDesign 2001: Second International Symposium on Environmentally Conscious Design and Inverse Manufacturing, IEEE, 2001, pp. 287–292.

6. Anityasari, M. and Kaebernick, H. (2008) A concept of reliability evaluation for reuse and remanufacturing. *International Journal of Sustainable Manufacturing*, **1** (1), 3–17.
7. Murayama, T., Yamamoto, S., and Oba, F. (2004) Mathematical model of reusability. 2004 IEEE International Symposium on Electronics and the Environment, May, 2004. Conference Record, pp. 183–188.
8. Meeker, W.Q. and Escobar, L.A. (1998) *Statistical Methods for Reliability Data*, John Wiley & Sons, Inc., New York.
9. Ohta, S. and Sato, T. (2005) Reliability prediction of re-used electronics circuit boards. Fourth International Symposium on Environmentally Conscious Design and Inverse Manufacturing, 2005. Eco Design 2005, IEEE, pp. 620–621.
10. Takata, S., Kirnura, F., Van Houten, F.J.A.M. *et al.* (2004) Maintenance: changing role in life cycle management. *CIRP Annals-Manufacturing Technology*, **53** (2), 643–655.
11. Jardine, A.K., Lin, D. and Banjevic, D. (2006) A review on machinery diagnostics and prognostics implementing condition-based maintenance. *Mechanical Systems and Signal Processing*, **20** (7), 1483–1510.
12. Heng, A., Zhang, S., Tan, A.C. *et al.* (2009) Rotating machinery prognostics: state of the art, challenges and opportunities. *Mechanical Systems and Signal Processing*, **23** (3), 724–739.
13. Lee, J., Ni, J., Djurdjanovic, D. *et al.* (2006) Intelligent prognostics tools and e-maintenance. *Computers in Industry*, **57** (6), 476–489.
14. Yan, J. and Wang, P. (2007) *Blade Material Fatigue Assessment Using Elman Neural Networks*, ASME.
15. Satish, B. and Sarma, N.D.R. (2005) A fuzzy BP approach for diagnosis and prognosis of bearing faults in induction motors. Power Engineering Society General Meeting, 2005. IEEE, June, 2005, pp. 2291–2294).
16. Myung, I.J. (2003) Tutorial on maximum likelihood estimation. *Journal of Mathematical Psychology*, **47** (1), 90–100.
17. Anityasari, M., Bao, H., and Kaebernick, H. (2005) Evaluation of product reusability based on a technical and economic model: a case study of televisions. Proceedings of the 2005 IEEE International Symposium on Electronics and the Environment, IEEE, May, 2005, pp. 199–204.
18. Lie, C.H. and Chun, Y.H. (1986) An algorithm for preventive maintenance policy. *IEEE Transactions on Reliability*, **35** (1), 71–75.
19. Liu, Y., Huang, H.Z. and Zhang, X. (2012) Data-driven approach for imperfect maintenance model selection. *Reliability*, **61** (1), 101–112.
20. Kijima, M. (1989) Some results for repairable systems withgeneral repair. *Journal of Applied Probability*, **26** (1), 89–102.
21. Gasmi, S., Love, C.E. and Kahle, W. (2003) A general repair, proportional-hazards, framework to model complex repairable systems. *IEEE Transactions on Reliability*, **52** (1), 26–32.
22. Nakagawa, T. (1988) Sequential imperfect preventive maintenance policies. *IEEE Transactions on Reliability*, **37** (3), 295–298.
23. Wu, S. and Zuo, M.J. (2010) Linear and nonlinear preventive maintenance models. *IEEE Transactions on Reliability*, **59** (1), 242–249.
24. Malik, M.A.K. (1979) Reliable preventive maintenance scheduling. *AIIE Transactions*, **11** (3), 221–228.
25. Shin, I., Lim, T.J. and Lie, C.H. (1996) Estimating parameters of intensity function and maintenance effect for repairable unit. *Reliability Engineering & System Safety*, **54** (1), 1–10.
26. Tsai, Y.T., Wang, K.S. and Teng, H.Y. (2001) Optimizing preventive maintenance for mechanical components using genetic algorithms. *Reliability Engineering & System Safety*, **74** (1), 89–97.
27. Abernethy, R.B. (2000) *The New Weibull Handbook*, 4th edn, Published by the author, November 2000. ISBN 09653062-1-6.

28. Qi Kesi, H. (1984) in *Tribology-Analysis of Friction, Lubrication, Abrasion Science and Technology* (translated Z. Liu, X. Wang, and S. Chen *et al.*), China Machine Press, Beijing, pp. 250–266.
29. Zhang, B., Wang, A., Den, X. *et al.* (2012) Research on MTBF prediction and test of wear-out failure of main spindle in numerical control machine tool. *Machine Tool and Hydraulics*, **40** (11), 149–151.
30. Zhao, G., Zhao, Y. and Wang, Y. (1996) Measurement of wear energy consumption and establishment of the analytical model. *Experimental Technology and Management*, **13** (4), 43–46.
31. Feng, W., Xie, X. and Liu, C. (2010) Energy loss based relevance modeling of gear abrasion and vibration. *Vibration, Test and Diagnosis*, **30** (4), 458–461.
32. Bloch, H.P. and Fred, K.G. (1994) *Practical Machinery Management for Process Plants*, Machinery Failure Analysis and Troubleshooting, 2nd edn, vol. **2**, Gulf Publishing Company, Houston, TX.

8

Case Studies

8.1 Improved Hilbert–Huang Transform Based Weak Signal Detection Methodology and Its Application to Incipient Fault Diagnosis and ECG Signal Analysis

Weak signals themselves are not clear-cut and consist of information of an imperfect quality. Generally, two aspects can be considered: (i) the weak signal is premature with small amplitude and generated from the early stage of irregular operating and (ii) the signals are obfuscated by confounding factors and with a high level of background noise although they have significant amplitudes. Corresponding to the above two points, we validate the performance of the proposed Hilbert–Huang transform (HHT) method using two kinds of signals: (i) a vibration signal with small amplitude recorded from an incipient rotor imbalance fault; and (ii) a noisy physiological signal with low signal-to-noise ratio (SNR) caused by noise from instrument amplifiers, ambient electromagnetic signals from cables, and power-line interferences.

8.1.1 *Incipient Fault Diagnosis Using Improved HHT*

Aiming at identifying fault features from the early stage of a rotor degradation process, experiments were conducted on a Bently rotor test rig, shown in Figure 8.1. The testbed consisted of two acceleration transducers (left), two eddy current sensors (center), a three-phase induction motor (right), and control electronics. The length of the shaft is 430 mm and the diameter of the shaft is 10 mm. There are 16 screw holes uniformly distributed on the face of the mass wheel in order to add standard weights. Imbalance faults of the test rig were simulated by gradually increasing the number of standard weights, and the rotor ran from a norm state to a drastically imbalanced state. The vibration signals were probed by acceleration transducers mounted on the bearing support and eddy current sensors fixed on a bracket near the mass wheel.

The rotor imbalance faults were simulated by adding 0.4, 3.6, and 5.4 g standard weights to the screw hole of the mass wheel, and the 0.4 g imbalance operation was

Machinery Prognostics and Prognosis Oriented Maintenance Management, First Edition. Jihong Yan.

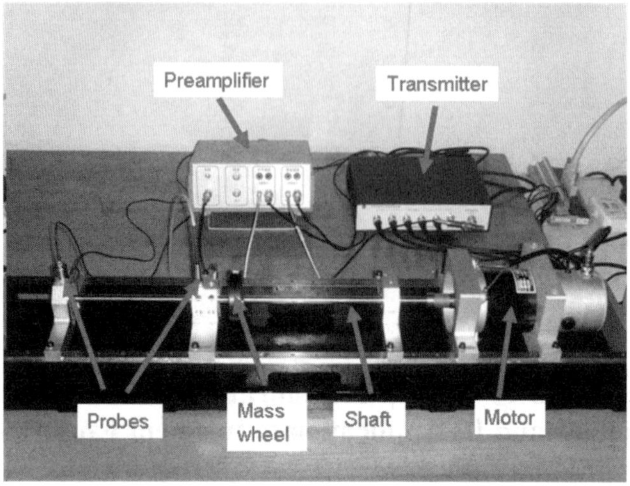

Figure 8.1 Bently rotor testbed

regarded as the early rotor failure. The speed of rotation was 2400 rpm and each imbalance state included approximately 50 samples. The vibration data collection system consisted of a high bandwidth preamplifier, a transmitter, and a data recorder with a sampling frequency of 1 kHz per channel.

The comparison of the normal state and incipient rotor imbalance fault is shown in Figure 8.2. The normal state has slight vibration with amplitude of approximately

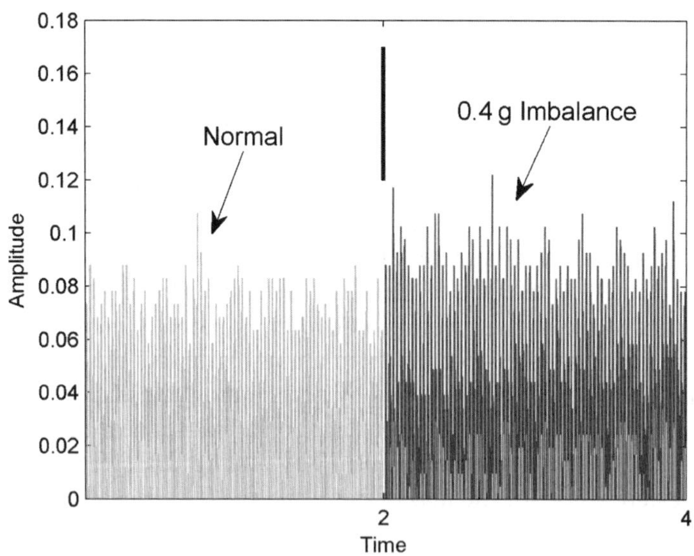

Figure 8.2 Vibration signal of the normal state and the early stage of a rotor imbalance fault

0.07 V, and the minimal initial imbalance of the testbed has an amplitude of approximately 0.09 V, that is, there is little difference between the norm state and the initial imbalance state. The method discussed in Section 3.3.7 was applied to detect weak features from the incipient rotor failure. Comparative studies of Huang's stopping criterion and the proposed correlation analysis based stopping criterion were performed to analyze the simulated rotor faults. The signal analysis based on Huang's stopping criterion, shown in Figure 8.3 and Table 8.1, had 10 sub-modes and the Hilbert spectrum had great distortions on the time location at 0.2, 0.4 and 0.9 s. Nevertheless, as shown in Figure 8.4 and Table 8.1 the proposed improved empirical mode decomposition (EMD) method decomposed the vibration signal into three IMFs (intrinsic mode functions), and clearly identified the main feature of the incipient rotor failure, which had a slight fluctuation around 40 Hz.

The computational efficiency of the improved HHT method and Huang's routine was also discussed. All the mentioned routines for identifying the incipient rotor fault

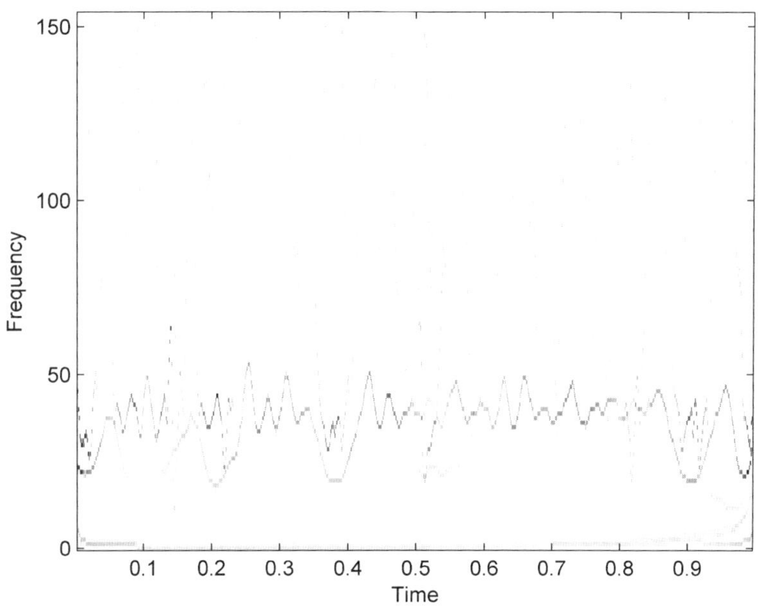

Figure 8.3 Signal decomposition based on Huang's stopping criterion

Table 8.1 Comparative study of two stopping criteria on analysis of the incipient rotor imbalance fault

Algorithm	Numbers of IMFs	Time consumed(s)
Huang's stopping criterion	10	0.1231 ± 0.0020
The proposed stopping criterion	3	0.0420 ± 0.0016

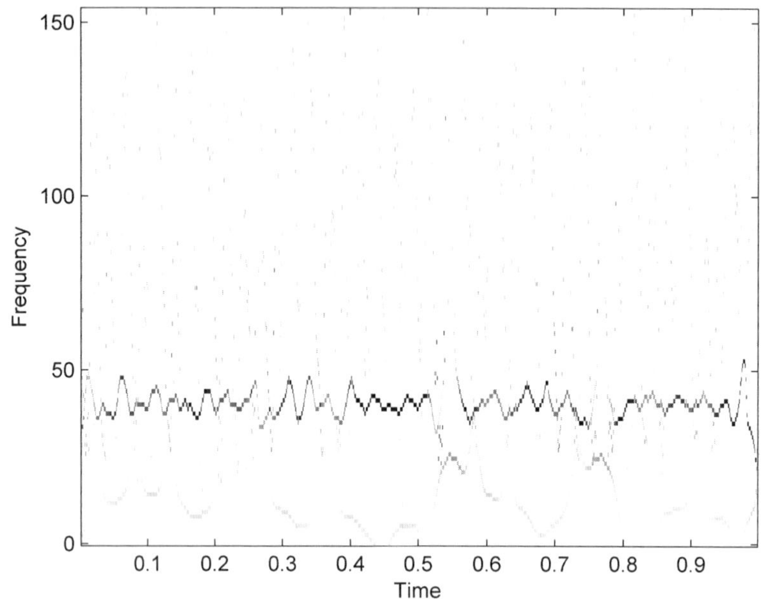

Figure 8.4 Signal decomposition based on the proposed stopping criterion

features were performed under the same operating environment. The performance tests were made in a machine with 2.88 GB of memory and Pentium(R) G620 CPU, running 32 bit Windows 7 operating system, and the MATLAB version was 7.10.0. The weak mechanical signal was analyzed 100 times, and statistical scores are shown in Table 8.1. It can be seen from the table that the analysis of the degradation process based on Huang's stopping criterion took 0.1231 s with standard deviation 0.002 s, while the analysis of the degradation process based on the proposed stopping criterion took only 0.0420 s with standard deviation 0.0016 s.

8.1.2 HHT in Low SNR Scenario

The performance was tested against a set of arbitrarily chosen ECG samples from the MIT-BIH Arrhythmia Database and ECG signals with high levels of background noise [1]. The database contains 48 half-hour excerpts of two-channel ambulatory ECG recordings, obtained from 47 subjects studied by the BIH Arrhythmia Laboratory. The 48 recordings were digitized at 360 samples per second per channel with 11-bit resolution over a 10 mV range.

In most reports in the literature, clean ECG signals were taken and some artificially generated Gaussian noises or shock signals were added to the original signal, then mixed noisy signals were used to validate the performance of the developed methods. However, a real ECG signal may contain complex components and the noise may be different in nature to the artificial noise. Therefore, to simulate real-world situations as well as to validate the performance of the proposed method for detecting weak features from a noisy signal with a high level of background noise, the investigated signals (Equation 8.1) are considered as clean signals corrupted by the extracted noise from the MIT-BIH Arrhythmia database.

$$x_{\text{signal}}(t) = x_{\text{ECG}}(t) + k * A_{\text{noise}}(t) \tag{8.1}$$

where, $x_{\text{signal}}(t)$ is the noisy signal, $x_{\text{ECG}}(t)$ is the clean ECG signal, $A_{\text{noise}}(t)$ is the extracted noise, and k is the multiplying factor to modulate the level of the noise, here k was set as 20.

As shown in Figure 8.5a, the clean ECG signal numbered 112 was taken for investigation, and the interval between the two R-wave peak values of the investigated ECG signal was 0.725 s, which corresponds to the principal frequency (1.367 Hz). However, by adding noise (Figure 8.5b) extracted from the database to the clean ECG signal, the investigated noisy ECG signal (Figure 8.5c) has a high noise level with SNR = 15 dB and key features of the noisy ECG signal were nearly submerged by the background noise. Comparative studies of Huang's stopping criterion and the proposed method for analysis of the weak features of the investigated noisy ECG signal were performed. The Hilbert–Huang spectrum (Figure 8.6) clearly represented the frequency information corresponding to the peak values of the ECG signal. The approach based on Huang's stopping criterion decomposed the investigated signal into 10 sub-modes. However, it distorted the main frequency of 1.367 Hz at both ends of the ECG signal and frequency aliasing appeared around 5 Hz. As shown in Figure 8.7, the proposed method employing a wavelet analysis embedded sifting process and a

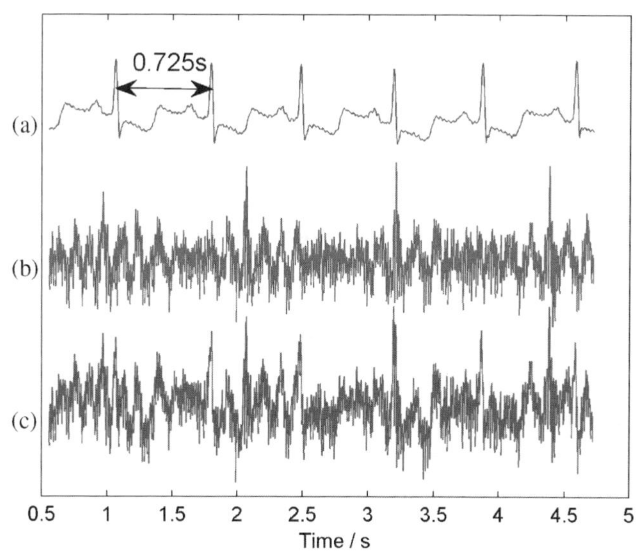

Figure 8.5 (a) Clean ECG, (b) noise, and (c) noisy signal

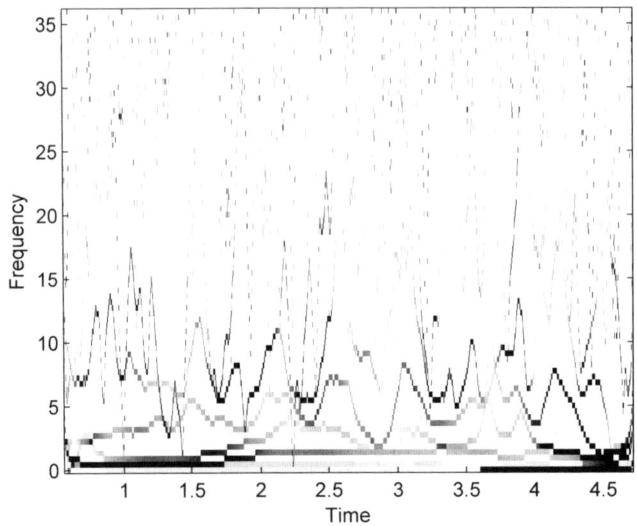

Figure 8.6 ECG signal decomposition based on Huang's stopping criterion

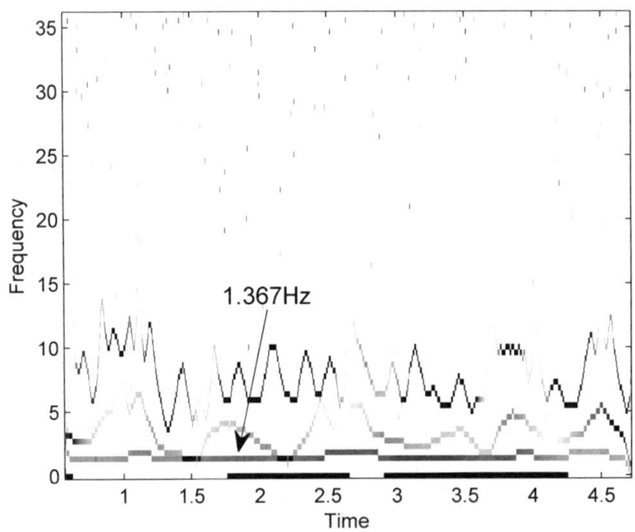

Figure 8.7 ECG signal decomposition based on the proposed stopping criterion

correlation analysis based stopping criterion decomposed the signal into five IMFs, and the main frequency with 1.367 Hz was effectively detected from the ECG signal. It also matched well with the impulse features.

Similarly, comparative studies of the computational efficiencies of the three methods for analysis of the ECG signal were discussed. All the mentioned routines for identifying the incipient rotor fault features were performed under the same operating

Table 8.2 Comparative study of two stopping criteria on analysis of an ECG signal

Algorithm	Numbers of IMFs	Time consumed(s)
Huang's stopping criterion	10	0.1542 ± 0.0017
The proposed stopping criterion	5	0.0547 ± 0.0010

environment discussed in the previous section. Table 8.2 clearly shows the analysis of the investigated ECG signal based on Huang's stopping criterion took 0.1542 s with standard deviation 0.0017 s, while the identification of weak features based on the proposed stopping criterion took only 0.0547 s with standard deviation 0.0010 s.

8.1.3 Summary

This research proposed a wavelet analysis embedded sifting process and a correlation analysis based stopping criterion aiming to overcome the end effects and remove redundant IMFs of the classical HHT. Comparative studies showed that the proposed method is superior to signal extension based improved EMD methods in dealing with the end effects problem, and more efficient than the widely used standard deviation based stopping criterion in removing redundant IMFs. The results of analysis of incipient mechanical failure and weak ECG signal confirmed that the proposed improved HHT is a promising tool for detecting weak signals with low SNR, and the high computing efficiency makes the tool an alternative way for on-line condition monitoring. Future work will focus on developing a systematic method for threshold selection in the terminating function, and improving the stability and performance of HHT from other aspects of the EMD method, such as theoretical foundation and optimized interpolation approaches.

8.2 Ant Colony Clustering Analysis Based Intelligent Fault Diagnosis Method and Its Application to Rotating Machinery

The ant colony clustering based fault diagnosis method proposed in Chapter 4 was applied to vibration signals acquired from a Bently rotor test bed to validate its functionality of fault diagnosis.

8.2.1 Description of Experiment and Data

A mass wheel is fixed in the middle of the rotor. There are 16 screw holes uniformly distributed on the face of the rotor mass wheel in order to add imbalance mass. Vibration signals were probed by eddy current sensors fixed on the mass wheel, which is shown in Figure 8.8. In the experiment, the rotor speed was 2700 rpm, and the sampling frequency1000 Hz. Each group of experiment data sets collected had three

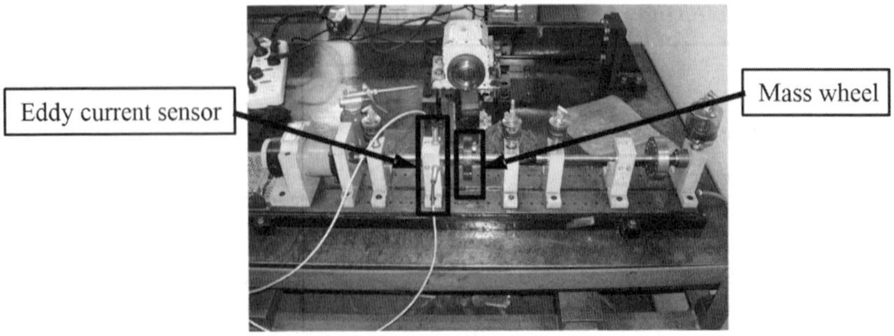

Figure 8.8 Bently rotor test bed

conditions – no mass, 0.6 g mass, and 1.2 g mass. Fifteen groups of data sets were obtained from the experimental system.

Nine groups of experimental data were used to train the fault diagnosis model and the remaining six groups of data were used for testing.

8.2.2 Model Training for Fault Diagnosis

After a large amount of data has been collected from experiment, it cannot be directly input into the classifier because too many features can cause dimensionality, furthermore, irrelevant and redundant features degrade the performance of the classifier.

8.2.2.1 Feature Extraction Using WPT

In this case, a wavelet packet transform (WPT) is employed to extract features from the vibration signals. The vibration signals can be decomposed into 2^i frequency sub-bands, with the bandwidth in Hz for each sub-band defined by

$$\Delta f = f_s/(2 \times 2^i) \tag{8.2}$$

where f_s is the sampling frequency and i represents the decomposition level of WPT.

As a result, the frequency intervals of each sub-band can be computed by

$$((n-1)2^{-i-1}f_s,\ n2^{-i-1}f_s]\ ,\ n = 1, 2, \cdots, 2^i \tag{8.3}$$

The base band is 45 Hz because the rotor speed is 2700 rpm, and integer harmonics $2f_r, 3f_r \cdots$ are also determined. Through adjusting i, the base band f_r and integer harmonics $2f_r, 3f_r \cdots$ are decomposed into different sub-bands. Therefore, vibration signals are decomposed into four levels, in which Daubechies wavelet packet is employed as the mother wavelet. The energy spectrum in different sub-bands is obtained, as shown in Figure 8.9, where the second sub-band (31.25–62.5 Hz) has a high energy representing a working frequency (45 Hz) reflecting the operation condition of the rotor. It is not clear whether sub-bands after sub-band number 5, such as the sub-bands

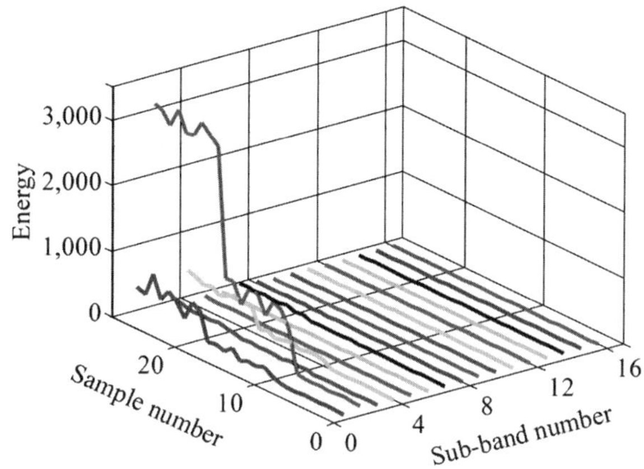

Figure 8.9 Energy spectrum in all sub-bands

6–8, belong to integer harmonics of the base band containing a small amount of energy, and whether sub-bands 9–16 belong to high-frequency noise containing a small amount of energy. Three-dimensional graphics shows the overall trend of rotor conditions in the time and frequency domains, however, the relevance of the energy spectrum in various sub-bands cannot be analyzed from the graph. As for the signals acquired from practical applications, syntonic and linear relationships are apparent because of the emergence of resonance, which reflects hidden characteristics of the system. Therefore, the energy spectrum must be transformed in order to contribute to extracting features further.

Various sub-bands cannot be compared owing to a larger gap between the energy values of these sub-bands. The influence of some sub-bands may be neglected, causing incorrect results in the analysis. Therefore, the energy value of the total sub-bands is normalized. A comparison of the preprocessed data, two different sub-bands of vibration signal: 31.25–62.5 Hz, 93.75–125 Hz, is shown in Figure 8.10.

Figure 8.10 illustrates that the energy in different sub-bands follows a similar trend, which shows that there are resonant relations in different sub-bands, and extracting these interrelated sub-bands is conductive to reducing redundant information. Useful information should be provided as far as possible to increase the accuracy and comprehensibility for back-band research.

8.2.2.2 Feature Selection Using IACCA

In this study, major features were extracted by the improved ant colony clustering algorithm (IACCA) in the frequency domain. As described in Section 4.4.5, on the basis of data analysis and expert experiences, the parameters of the ant colony algorithm were set as: $\alpha = 0.23$, ant number $= 10$, size of the grid 10*10, size of the neighbor 3*3. The maximal comparison probability was set as $P_{\max} = 0.9$ and the

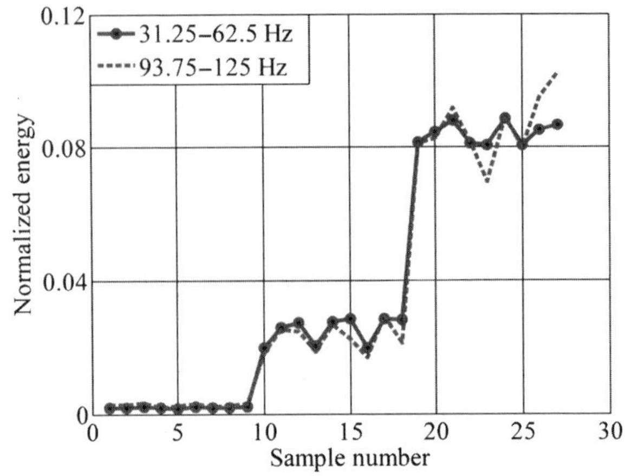

Figure 8.10 Similarity comparison in different sub-bands

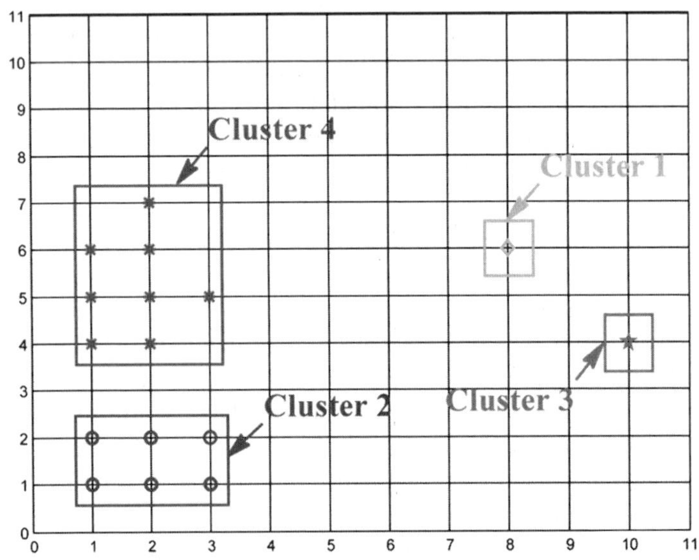

Figure 8.11 Clustering results obtained by IACCA

maximum iteration $I_{max} = 400$. The clustering results are shown in Figure 8.11. One row and column is enlarged at the edge of the grid for a clear display.

Correspondingly, the clustering results with specific sub-band number are shown in Table 8.3.

Table 8.3 indicates that the cluster categories of the first eight sub-bands are different. Therefore, the clustering results of the three algorithms need to be analyzed further. Additionally, compared with ACCA, iterations of the IACCA are reduced to 400 times, and convergence of the IACCA is strengthened.

Table 8.3 Clustering results of FCM, ACCA, and IACCA in the frequency-domain

	FCM				ACCA			IACCA			
Iterations	/				1000			400			
Cluster number	1	2	3	4	1	2	3	1	2	3	4
Sub-band number	1,5	2,3, 4,7	6,8	9,10,11, 12,13,14, 15,16	1,2,3,4, 6,7,8	5	9,10,11, 12,13,14, 15,16	1	2,3,4, 6,7,8	5	9,10,11, 12,13,14, 15,16

According to the specific sub-band number of the IACCA in Table 8.3, feature patterns for each cluster are illustrated in Figure 8.12.

Figure 8.12 shows that similar sub-bands are clustered by the improved ant colony algorithm. These identified interrelated sub-bands are conducive to reducing redundant information. The first cluster (0–31.25 Hz), as shown in Figure 8.12a, is

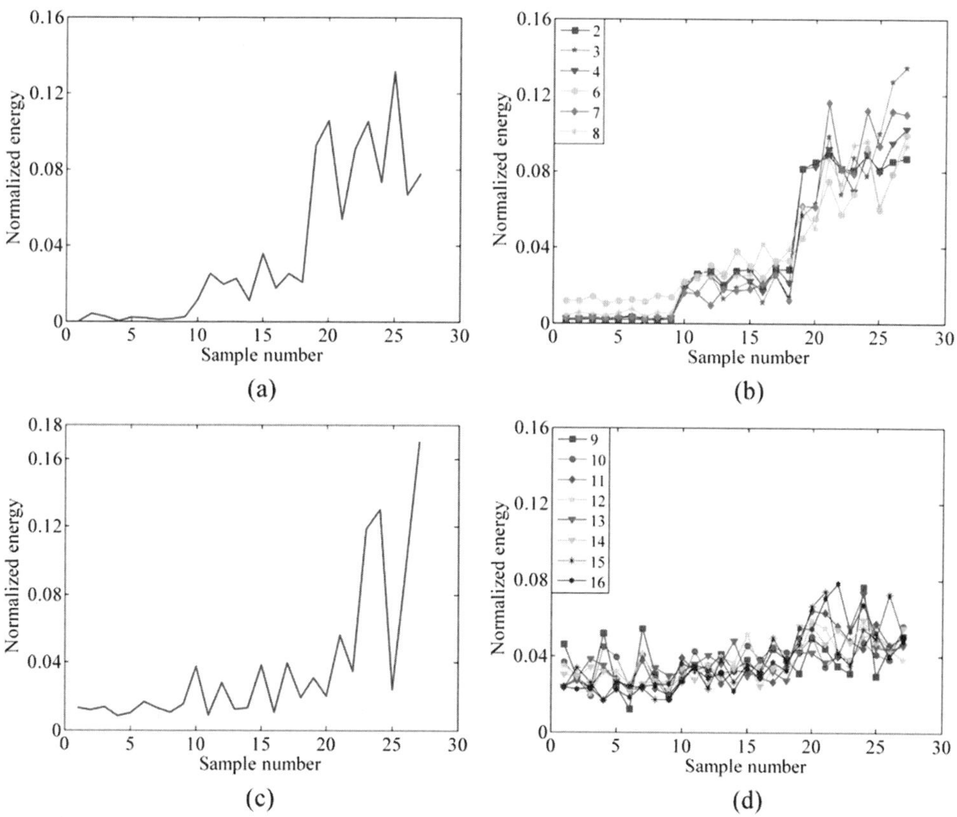

Figure 8.12 Patterns of four clusters obtained: (a) Pattern of the first cluster, (b) patterns of the second cluster, (c) pattern of the third cluster, and (d) patterns of the fourth cluster

the initial part of the low-frequency. Although there is an increasing trend, it belongs to an interference sub-band, which is not a feature of the rotor imbalance condition. For the second cluster (see Figure 8.12b), the base band and harmonic component correspond with the results of clustering from the frequency domain (31.25–125 Hz, 156.25–250 Hz) perspective; according to the energy spectrum, energy values contained in this cluster account for 87.53% of the total; moreover, the energy values of the cluster sub-bands are gradually increasing from the feature pattern perspective, reflecting gradual degradation of rotor performance and indicating the imbalance conditions of the rotor gradually increasing. For the third cluster (125–156.25 Hz) (see Figure 8.12c), although a three-harmonic is in the cluster, it belongs to an interference sub-band because of overlapped frequency characterization of the wavelet packet decomposition. In addition, the cluster sub-band does not reflect a three-harmonic component. For the fourth cluster (250–500 Hz) (see Figure 8.12d), the trend of the energy spectrum is similar in the cluster, as well as changing gently, and therefore it belongs to high-frequency noise. Based on the above analysis, the clustering results of IACCA are correct. Therefore, the second cluster sub-bands represent crucial features reflecting the operating conditions of the rotor.

8.2.2.3 Fault Model Establishment

After feature selection using IACCA, the crucial information containing the second, the third, the fourth, the sixth, the seventh, and the eighth sub-bands is extracted to contribute to improving the performance of fault classification. In this study, each group of experiment data sets collected had three conditions – no mass, 0.6 g mass, and 1.2 g mass, respectively. Three types of operating conditions of the rotor can be reflected by the six sub-bands extracted. According to the three given conditions, the fault diagnosis model was trained based on nine groups of experimental data. Eventually, the fault model is established by combining the extracted major sub-bands with given fault prototypes, as shown in Figure 8.13, where each solid line represents one category of operating condition of the rotor, and each node represents one sub-band.

8.2.3 Fault Recognition

Vibration signals acquired from the rotor are decomposed by WPT, after which sub-bands of signals are clustered by the improved ant colony algorithm, and sub-bands of each cluster are analyzed from a pattern perspective for extracting major features reflecting imbalance conditions of the rotor. Finally, the imbalance conditions of the rotor are recognized using the Euclidean nearness degree based on the established fault model. As described in step 4 in Section 4.4.6, the values of the Euclidean nearness degree are calculated for each testing data, and 18 testing data are

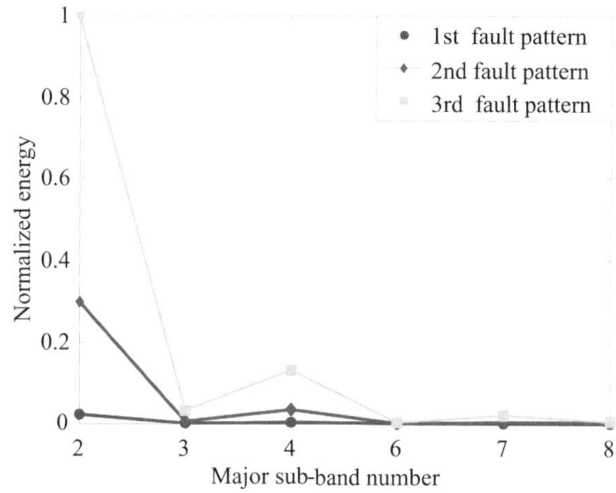

Figure 8.13 Fault diagnosis model

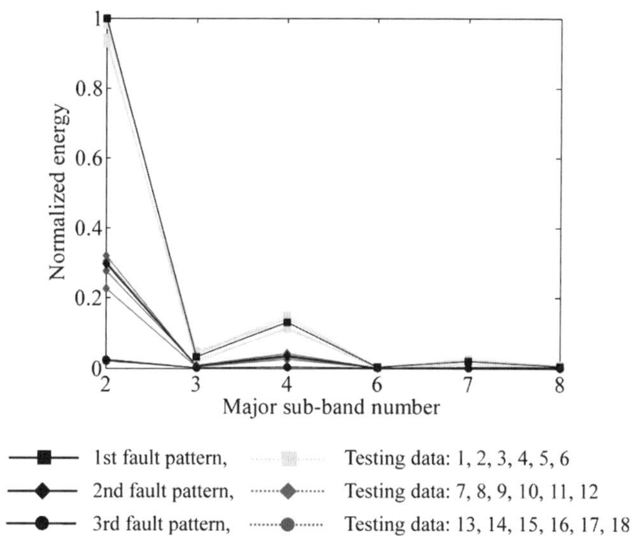

Figure 8.14 Fault recognition result

divided into 3 fault categories. The fault recognition results are shown in Figure 8.14, where each solid line represents one category imbalance condition of the rotor, each node represents one sub-band, and each dashed line represents one testing data. The x-axis represents the major sub-band number reflecting imbalance conditions of the rotor and the y-axis represents the normalized energy of each major sub-band.

Correspondingly, the fault recognition results with specific fault categories of testing data are shown in Table 8.4.

Table 8.4 Fault recognition results of testing data

Fault category	First	Second	Third
Testing data	1,2,3,4,5,6	7,8,9,10,11,12	13,14,15,16,17,18
Accuracy (%)	100	100	100

The testing data of the first fault category represent the normal operating condition of the rotor, the second represent a moderate imbalance condition (0.6 g mass), and the third represent a severe imbalance condition (1.2 g mass) in Table 8.4. From Table 8.4 we can see that the testing data are classified into three fault categories according to the fault diagnosis model established, and the accuracy of the fault recognition results is 100%.

8.2.4 Summary

This study proposes a novel intelligent fault diagnosis method based on ant colony clustering analysis. The novelty of this methodology lies in using WPT and ant colony clustering analysis to mine major features reflecting the operating conditions of equipment from the pattern of the frequency bands and establishing the fault model on the basis of the extracted features from the pattern. The application illustrates that the established model is of good accuracy which is meaningful and practical for fault recognition. Furthermore, an IACCA is proposed to adjust the comparison probability dynamically and detect outliers. Compared with other clustering algorithms, the algorithm has higher convergence speed to meet the requirements of real-time analysis as well as further improvement of accuracy, and the simulation validates the IACCA. The effectiveness and feasibility of the proposed method have been verified by vibration signals acquired from a rotor test bed.

In this study, three fault conditions (none mass, 0.6 g, and 1.2 g mass) are considered, more rotor unbalance conditions, such as 0.1 g, … ,0.5 g, 0.7 g, … , 1.1 g, and so on, will be explored in the next step. Moreover, we plan to apply similar methods to different application objects, such as bearings, turbine rotors, and so on, to validate the proposed method in the fault diagnosis field.

8.3 BP Neural Networks Based Prognostic Methodology and Its Application

To illustrate the effectiveness of the back propagation neural network (BPNN) based intelligent prognostic method, we applied the networks to real material fatigue data collected from a bunch of stress–strain experiments. The experiments were conducted to simulate the material fatigue process of the last stage blade of a steam turbine, at room temperature for reference.

Table 8.5 Chemical components of 0Cr17Ni4Cu4Nb

C	Si	Mn	Cr	Ni	Cu	Nb	S	P
≤0.07	≤1.0	≤1.0	15.5–17.5	3.0–5.0	3.0–5.0	0.15–0.45	≤0.03	≤0.035

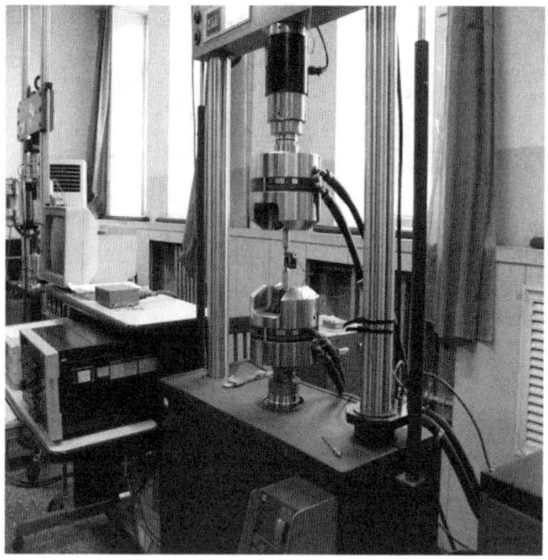

Figure 8.15 Material testing system 810

8.3.1 Experimental Test Conditions

The experiment was completed at the Harbin Turbine Company, the experimental material was 0Cr17Ni4Cu4Nb and its chemical components are shown in Table 8.5.

The material fatigue test was carried out using a MTS 810 servo-hydraulic testing machine, shown in Figure 8.15, whose control and data acquisition were performed by a computer. Material fatigue tests were carried out under strain control, the load on the material was increased continuously until the corresponding strain measurements reached the pre-set level. The material pieces used in this experiment are shown in Figure 8.16.

A low cycle fatigue test was completed, based on the national standard GB/T 15248–1994. Figure 8.17 illustrates the relationship between strain and stress with the pre-set strain range at ±0.45%. The solid curve corresponds to the behavior of a brand new material (the first testing cycle), the stress values are 530 and −550 MPa when the strain reaches upper and lower boundaries at ±0.45%. As for the last testing cycle, shown as the dashed curve, the strain reaches its margins at ±0.45% with stress at 220 and −420 MPa, respectively, which is much less than the first testing cycle's margin stress. Figure 8.17 reveals the influence on the strain–stress relationship caused by material fatigue. The material condition is defined as "fatigue" at the cycle

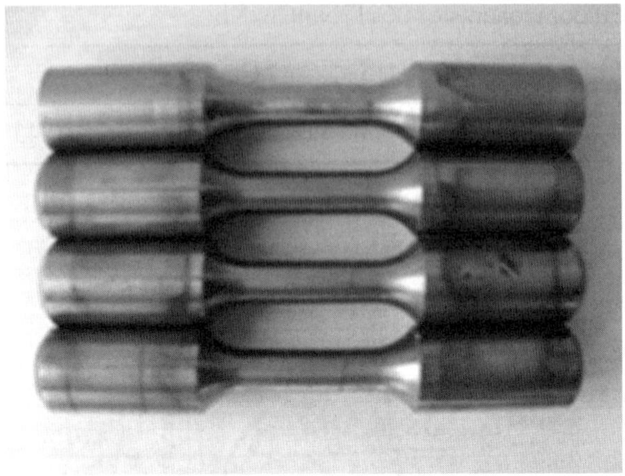

Figure 8.16 Alloy material pieces after fatigue testing

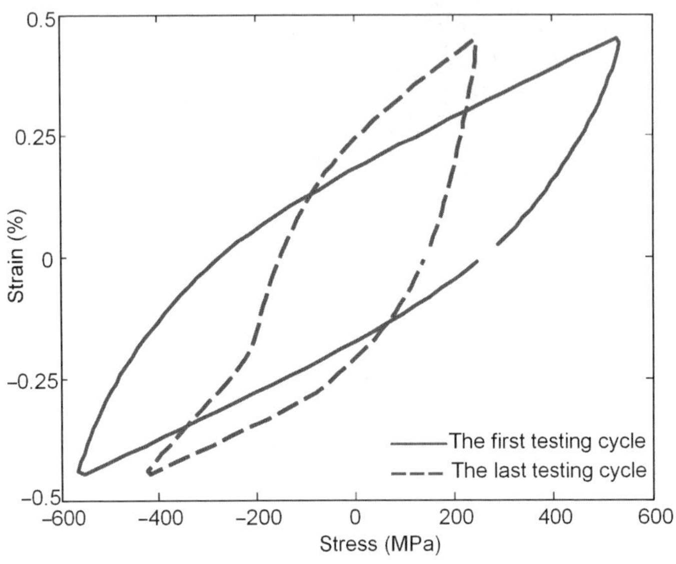

Figure 8.17 Strain–stress curves

where the maximum stress measurement is less than 50% of the reference stress (the twentieth cycle's maximum stress value).

8.3.2 BP Network Model Training

Fifty samples were obtained from the Harbin Turbine Company, 35 were used to model M_E and M_P, and a data set of 15 samples was used for validation. The specific procedures in the steam turbine's blade fatigue life prediction are as follows:

1. *Data pre-processing*: raw data filtering is performed.
2. *Feature extraction*: since the blade's fatigue data belong to a lower-varying signal, the maximum stress, minimum stress, and sum of the absolute stress were extracted and normalized as features for the blade's performance degradation process.
3. *Performance assessment*: according to submodule 3 in model training, first, compute the bounds of the hidden nodes: because the dimension of the input vector is 3×1, the output is the result of performance evaluation, between 0 and 1. According to equation 5.31, the bound of the hidden nodes is from 3 to 12. Secondly, build an $N_C = 10$ networks model for each hidden node to train, the average value of 10 models as the final result of the network, comparing with each model's MSE (mean square error) to extract the best network model M_E.

   According to the above steps, by programming and simulating in Matlab, the result of the MSE is as shown in Figure 8.18. The minimum error is 0.1027 with the number of hidden nodes being 11, so choose this model as the optimal BP performance assessment model. And then, through simulation, deliver the performance evaluation results of each material sample, which are used as the inputs of the life prediction model.
4. *Life prediction network model*: firstly, select the value N, the number of testing cycles for each blade experiment (average number of testing cycles of the 35 material samples is 57.3), therefore select $N = 6$ as the width of the window; secondly, calculate the hidden neural nodes, for example, when $N = 6$, select $N_I = 5$, $N_O = 1$, $N_H = 3 \sim 12$; thirdly, build a $N_C = 10$ model to train and calculate

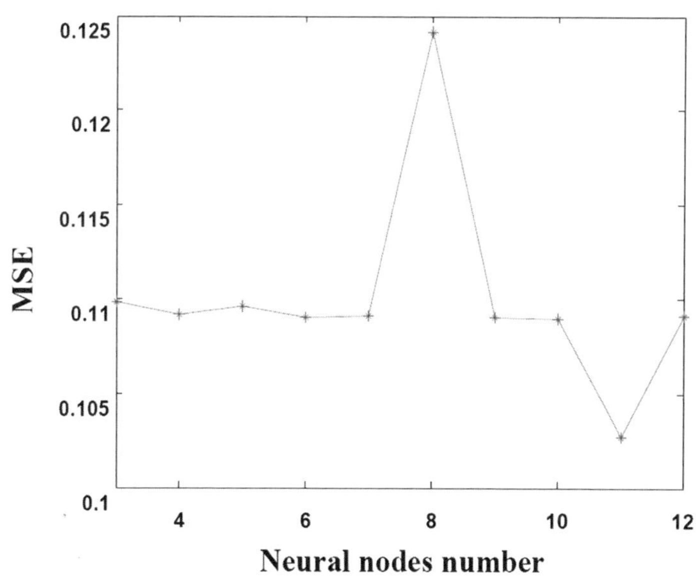

Figure 8.18 MSE of performance assessment model

the average remaining life and total average error based on the equation:

$$\overline{E}_{\text{avg}} = \frac{\sum_{j=1}^{S} \overline{E}_j}{S} \tag{8.4}$$

where $\overline{E}_j$ is the average error of each sample calculated by Equation 5.32, S is the total number of samples, $S = 35$. Finally, compare $\overline{E}_{\text{avg}}$ with different hidden neural nodes to choose the optimal model M_P.

According to the above step, realized through the program and simulated in Matlab, the result of $\overline{E}_{\text{avg}}$ is shown in Figure 8.19, when the number of hidden neural nodes equals 10, the total average error is a minimum, therefore the optimal BP life prediction model M_P is with $N_H = 10$.

8.3.3 BP Network Real-Time Prognostics

The remaining 15 samples were used to validate the established models M_E and M_P. Here, the results of 1 of the 15 material samples are given as an example to illustrate the real-time prognostics process. After acquiring real-time data, data pre-processing and feature extraction are performed, then performance assessment is conducted by normalizing the extracted features and feeding them into the model M_E, the performance evaluation result is shown in Figure 8.20.

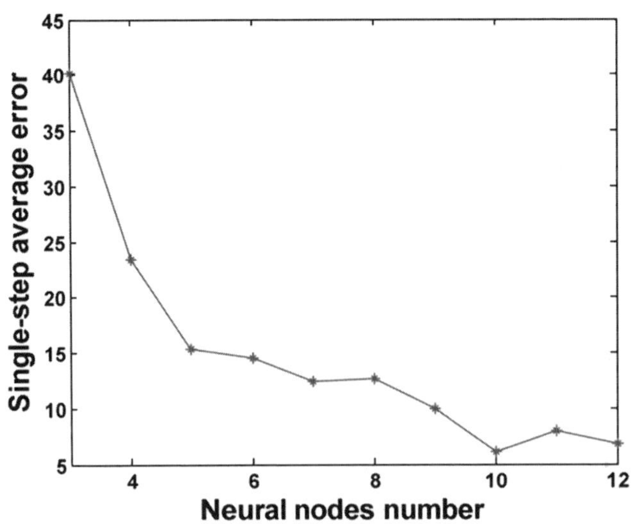

Figure 8.19 Single-step average error of life prediction model

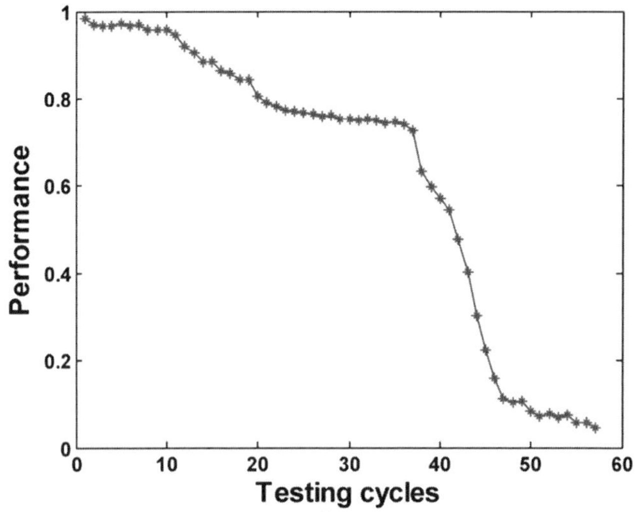

Figure 8.20 Performance of identified sample

Dynamic life prediction: select $K = 9$, the learning rate is 0.01, $N_C = 10$, and use the gradient algorithm to adjust the weights and biases of M_P. Use M_P' as introduced in Section 5.3.2.4 to carry out the prediction. The length of the input vector of M_P is 5, in this case, when the predictive time is smaller than 5, there is not enough data to adjust weights and biases, so use M_P to carry out the prediction instead of M_P', then use the average remaining life of the 35 samples at the first four steps as the corresponding remaining life. The life dynamic prediction result is shown in Figure 8.21, where the asterisk curve represents the predicted remaining life and the solid curve represents the actual remaining life. Obviously, early stage prediction error is larger as less information is available, however, with prediction time elapsed, more useful information becomes available, and the prediction accuracy is getting better.

8.3.4 Error Analysis for Prediction

According to Equations 5.33 and 5.34, obtain $\mu = -0.8393$, $r^2 = 0.6829$ in this case.

8.3.5 PDF Curve for Life Prediction

Actually, after each predictive time point, there is a probability of failure, as introduced in Section 5.2, three probability density function (PDF) curves are given for illustration at prediction times $t = 12$, $t = 24$, $t = 36$, respectively.

As shown in Figure 8.22, the PDF curves are getting narrower and narrower with time elapsing, which indicates that the life prediction results from the BP-based prediction model are converging, furthermore, the remaining life distribution also

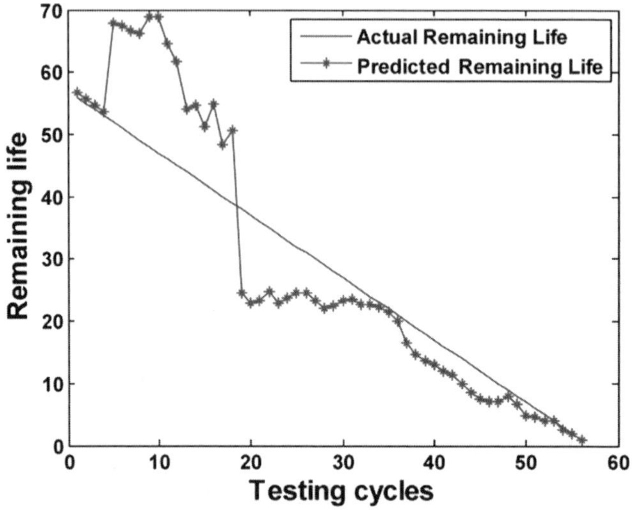

Figure 8.21 Remaining life of identified sample

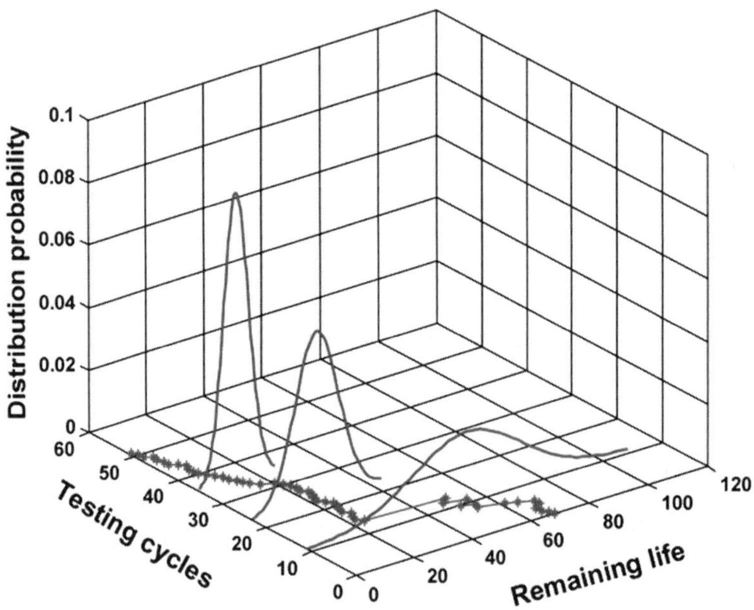

Figure 8.22 PDF curve of remaining life

provides a decision-making time for predictive maintenance and spare parts ordering and even inventory management.

The prediction errors of the other 14 material samples are shown in Table 8.6, given by the single step prediction error $\overline{E}$, the average error μ, and the certainty factor r^2 for predictive time $t = 1–30$, $t = 31$ to the last point, respectively.

Table 8.6 Prediction error of the other 14 samples

Samples		1	2	3	4	5	6	7	8	9	10	11	12	13	14
1–30	$\overline{E}$	10.2	10.1	10.1	9.7	10.1	10.3	10.0	9.9	10.2	9.9	11.3	11.0	10.8	11.2
	μ	−6.2	−5.4	−4.7	−4.8	−4.4	−6.2	−6.1	−5.7	−5.2	−6.0	−6.4	−7.6	−6.5	−6.4
	r^2	−0.3	−0.4	−0.5	−0.5	−0.51	−0.4	−0.3	−0.4	−0.3	−0.3	−0.2	−0.2	−0.2	−0.2
31–last	$\overline{E}$	2.8	2.9	2.2	2.3	2.4	2.6	1.8	2.5	2.4	2.0	3.2	3.3	2.4	2.8
	μ	−3.1	−2.0	−0.7	−1.2	−0.8	−2.7	−2.8	−2.2	−2.2	−2.4	−1.5	−2.7	−2.2	−1.6
	r^2	0.77	0.87	0.96	0.93	0.95	0.82	0.81	0.87	0.84	0.85	0.90	0.80	0.86	0.89

Table 8.6 shows that when the prediction time is between 1 and 30, the single-step prediction average error $\overline{E}$ and the average error μ are large and the certainty factor r^2 is small, however, when the prediction time is between 31 and the last testing cycle, $\overline{E}$ and μ are small and r^2 is close to 1. The results show the accuracy is improving gradually as more useful information is available, furthermore, the effectiveness of the proposed BPNN-based intelligent prognostic method is validated.

8.3.6 Summary

The proposed intelligent prognostic framework and BPNN-based methodology are generic, applicable for equipment/components performance assessment and residual life prediction. The result of the blade's performance assessment and life prediction demonstrated the effectiveness of the methodology. It should be noted that the proposed dynamic life prediction method enhanced the generalization ability. As for the inherent defects of the BP algorithm, such as ease of falling into a local minimum, slow convergence speed, and so on, an improved BP algorithm is being produced to overcome these. In addition, an intelligent prognostic method for insufficient/incomplete data is also an important research direction.

8.4 A Dynamic Multi-Scale Markov Model Based Methodology for Remaining Life Prediction

8.4.1 Introduction

Equipment degradation and unexpected failures impact the three key elements of competitiveness – quality, cost, and productivity [2]. Maintenance has been introduced to help to reduce downtime and rework and to increase consistency and overall business efficiency. However, traditional maintenance costs constitute a large portion of the operating and overhead expenses in many industries [3]. More efficient maintenance strategies, such as condition-based maintenance (CBM) are being implemented to handle the situation. It is said that CBM can reduce the maintenance costs by approximately 25% [4]. In order to achieve this efficient maintenance strategy, prognostics is employed, which is built upon diagnostics and is the process of estimating remaining useful life (RUL) of a machine by predicting the progression of a diagnosed anomaly. Since, generally, machines go through degradation before failure occurs, monitoring the trend of machine degradation and assessing performance allow the degraded behavior or faults to be corrected before they cause failure and machine breakdowns. Therefore, advanced prognostics focuses on performance degradation monitoring and RUL prediction so that the failures can be predicted and prevented [5].

8.4.2 Methods of Signal Processing and Performance Assessment

The first two steps for prognostics are feature extraction and selection, as well as performance assessment. Capturing degradation information via vibration signals acquired by condition monitoring techniques is widely used in prognostics. The methods for these steps based on vibration signals are introduced as follows. Feature extraction using short-time Fourier transform (STFT) has been introduced in Section 4.3.2.3.

8.4.2.1 Feature Selection Using a Competitive Neural Network Model

The purpose of feature selection is to select the typical frequency bands as inputs of a performance assessment model. In recent years, unsupervised competitive neural networks (CNNs) have been recognized as a powerful tool for pattern analysis and clustering [6, 7]. These networks are mainly based on the winner-take-all (WTA) mechanism, where competitive signals, acting among all the elements of the network, are required.

To obtain competitive behavior, for each input pattern, a global search is required to locate it among all the units of the network. In this research, we use a CNN model to classify frequency bands into several categories. The CNN has two layers of nodes, the input layer and the competitive layer. Each node in the competitive layer has a weight vector with m weight values, corresponding to the m values of an input pattern denoted as $x = (x_1, x_2, \ldots, x_m)$. The training process consists of repeatedly feeding the input data to the network through the nodes in the input layer. The one competitive neuron with a minimum distance from the pattern is considered as the winner of the competition; the activation value of the winning neuron is set to one, while the activation values for all other neurons are set to zero. Competitive learning begins with all network weights initialized to some small, random value. Training proceeds by repeatedly exposing the network to the entire set of input vectors.

Herein, the Euclidean distance between a node in the competitive layer and an input pattern is chosen as a similarity measure. Frequency bands obtained by STFT [8] are regarded as inputs of the CNN. After competitive learning, these frequency bands with similar variation trend are clustered as one category. Finally, the frequency bands in the category with minimal dispersion degree are selected as typical features.

8.4.2.2 Performance Assessment Using a BP Neural Network

After features have been selected, neural networks are used to assess the performance. BPNN is the most widely used for its excellent calculating efficiency in artificial neural network (ANN) domains. A typical three-layer BPNN consisting of an input layer, a hidden layer, and an output layer, is powerful for multi-feature fusion. Previous papers [9, 10] have used BPNN to implement feature fusion. Each layer of the BPNN is composed of several neurons and the layers are interconnected by sets of correlation weights. The procedure of the BPNN is that the error at the output layer propagates backward to the input layer through a hidden layer in the network to obtain the final desired outputs. Traditionally, BPNN employs a gradient algorithm to adjust the weights according to gradient error, resulting in slow training speed and easy plunges into local minima. In order to accelerate training speed and avoid spurious local minima, a conjugate gradient algorithm was adopted in this research. Considering the fact that a three-layer BPNN can approximate any continuous function in a closed set, we choose the simplest BPNN structure with one hidden layer as performance assessment model. In this research, input variables of BPNN are the frequency band data and the output is the performance value between 0 (failure) and 1 (normal).

8.4.3 Markov-Based Model for Remaining Life Prediction

8.4.3.1 Markov Model and Weighted Markov Model

Consider a stochastic process $\{X_n, n = 1, 2, \ldots\}$ that takes on a finite or countable number of possible values. Unless otherwise mentioned, this set of possible values of the process will be denoted by the set of non-negative integers $\{1, 2, \ldots\}$. If $X_n = i$, then the process is said to be in state i at time n. Suppose that whenever the process is in state i, there is a fixed probability P_{ij} that it will next be in state j. That is

$$P\{X_{n+1} = j | X_n = i, X_{n-1} = i_{n-1}, \ldots, X_2 = i_2, \quad X_1 = i_1\}$$
$$= P\{X_{n+1} = j | X_n = i\} = P_{ij} \tag{8.5}$$

for all states $i_0, i_1, \ldots, i_{n-1}, i, j$ and all $n \geq 0$. Such a stochastic process is known as a Markov chain. Equation 8.5 can be interpreted as stating that, for a Markov chain, the conditional distribution of any state X_{n+1}, given the past states $X_1, X_2, \ldots, X_{n-1}$ and the present state X_n, is independent of the past states and depends only on the present state. This is called the Markovian property. The value P_{ij} represents the probability that the process will, when in state i, next make a transition into state j. Since probabilities are non-negative and since the process must make a transition into some state, we have that

$$P_{ij} \geq 0, \qquad i, j \geq 0; \qquad \sum_{j=1}^{\infty} P_{ij} = 1, \qquad i = 1, 2, \ldots$$

If the process has a finite number of states, which means the state space $S = \{1, 2, \ldots, i, j, \ldots, s\}$, then the Markov chain model can be defined by the matrix of one-step transition probabilities, denoted as

$$P = \begin{bmatrix} P_{11} & P_{12} & \ldots & P_{1s} \\ P_{21} & P_{22} & \ldots & P_{2s} \\ \vdots & \vdots & \ldots & \vdots \\ P_{s1} & P_{s2} & \ldots & P_{ss} \end{bmatrix}$$

The initial probability is computed by

$$P_{ij} = N_{ij}/N_i$$

where N_{ij} denotes the transition times from state i to state j and N_i denotes the number of the random variables $\{X_n, n = 1, 2, \ldots, m\}$ belonging to state i.

The Markov chain model adopts a state vector and state transition matrix to deal with the prediction issue. Suppose the state vector of moment $t - 1$ is P_{t-1}, the state vector of moment t is P_t and the state transition matrix is P, then the relationship is:

$$P_t = P_{t-1} \cdot P, \; t = 1, 2, \ldots, K \tag{8.6}$$

Update t from 1 to K, then

$$P_K = P_0 \cdot P^K \tag{8.7}$$

where P^K is the state vector at moment K.

Equation 8.6 is the basic Markov prediction model, if the initial state vector and the transition matrix are given, which allows calculation of any possible future state vector. Conventionally, the state with maximal probability is chosen as the next step state, known as the maximal probability rule.

The procedures of establishing the basic Markov model for prediction are as follows:

Step 1: Divide the states of the series and confirm the initial vector;
Step 2: Compute the transition matrix P;
Step 3: Solve the result of the Kth state transition vector according to $P_K = P_0 \cdot P^K$;
Step 4: Confirm the Kth state using the maximal probability rule.

Note that the maximal probability rule only takes into account the information of the state with maximal probability by ignoring other information. This approach results in inaccurate estimation of the stochastic process, especially when the probabilities of different states are close to each other. For instance, let the state transition vector P_K be (0.2 0.19 0.21 0.22 0.18). According to the maximal probability rule, the value of the series at a current instant should belong to the fourth state and the following calculation will only consider the information of state 4. It can be seen that the probabilities are so close that the influence caused by information of other states should not be ignored. The theory of grade characteristic value depicted as follows is an alternative method to take into account the influence of all the states in the state vector.

A function is characterized by two parameters, the state variable i ($i \in S = \{1, 2, \ldots, m\}$) representing the divided grade (herein it denotes the state of the Markov chain) and a membership value d_i representing the normalized probability of the value of the random variable X_n at a certain moment belonging to the ith state, which is shown as Equation 8.8. We called H the grade characteristic value. The membership value d_i can be calculated by $d_i = p_i^{\eta} / \sum_{k=1}^{m} p_k^{\eta}$, where p_i is the ith element of the state vector P and η is the influence coefficient of the maximal probability. In general, the value is $\eta = 2$ or $\eta = 4$. The larger the value, the stronger the influence that will be generated by the maximal probability. The essential of Equation 8.8 is that the states are weighted by the membership values so that all the states are considered.

$$H = \sum_{i=1}^{m} i \times d_i \tag{8.8}$$

When the grade characteristic value is obtained, the prediction value of the random variable is determined by

$$\begin{cases} T_i H / (i + 0.5) & H > i \\ B_i H / (i - 0.5) & H \le i \end{cases} \tag{8.9}$$

where i is the state number corresponding to the maximal probability of the state vector P; T_i and B_i are the upper and lower limits of the state interval corresponding to state i, respectively.

Additionally, considering the former moments' influence on the current moment, k-order autocorrelation coefficients are used to construct a weighted Markov model. The procedures of constructing a weighted Markov model for prediction are:

Step 1: Calculate the k-order autocorrelation coefficient of the input series, and normalize the results as the weighted coefficients of the Markov model according to Equations 8.10 and 8.11.

k -order autocorrelation coefficient:

$$r_k = \frac{\sum_{i=1}^{n-k} (x_i - \bar{x})(x_{i+k} - \bar{x})}{\sqrt{\sum_{i=1}^{n-k} (x_i - \bar{x})^2 \cdot \sum_{i=1}^{n-k} (x_{i+k} - \bar{x})^2}} \tag{8.10}$$

Weighted coefficient:

$$w_k = |r_k| / \sum_{k=1}^{m} |r_k| \tag{8.11}$$

Step 2: Divide the states of the series (how to perform state division is discussed in Section 8.4.3.2) and confirm the initial vector.

Step 3: Compute the Markov state transition matrices from the first to the kth step according to the state series.

Step 4: Calculate the ith state probability $p_i^{(k)}$ of the next moment using the state transition matrices from the first to the kth, respectively, where i indicates the ith state, k indicates the kth step.

Step 5: Compute the weighted sum as the final prediction state vector P of next moment, where $P_i = \sum_{k=1}^{m} w_k \cdot p_i^{(k)}$.

Step 6: Calculate the prediction value using the theory of grade characteristic value.

8.4.3.2 FCM Clustering Algorithm

State division is the process of determining the mapping from a random variable to state space. How to obtain state division is a crux for the Markov model. Traditionally, it is performed by a hard state division approach described as: let $X = \{x_1, x_2, \cdots, x_n\}$ be the random sequence; let $S = \{1, 2, \ldots, j, \ldots, m\}$ denote the state space; given $a_0 < a_1 < \ldots < a_m$, if a random variable $x_i \in [a_{j-1}, a_j]$, where $1 \leq i \leq n, 1 \leq j \leq m$, then the variable x_i belongs to state j. However, the division of $[a_{j-1}, a_j]$ depends on people's experience, which affects prediction accuracy. The fuzzy c-means (FCM) algorithm can cluster an unlabeled data set into a number of clusters such that similar subgroups are assigned to one cluster automatically according to the internal relations of the data [11, 12], which can be used to divide states of the Markov model. It is briefly depicted as follows:

Consider a set X formed by n feature vectors, that is, $X = \{x_1, x_2, \cdots, x_n\}$. FCM clustering is to divide X into c clusters $(2 \leq c \leq n)$. Let $V = \{v_1, v_2, \cdots, v_c\}$ be the set of c clusters. The certainty of the kth feature vector belonging to the ith cluster is measured by the membership function u_{ik}, $u_{ik} \in [0, 1]$, $\sum_{i=1}^{c} u_{ik} = 1$. $U = [u_{ik}]$ is the membership function matrix. The objective function of the FCM clustering algorithm is

$$J_m(U, V) = \sum_{k=1}^{n} \sum_{i=1}^{c} u_{ik}^m d_{ik}^2 \tag{8.12}$$

where $d_{ik} = ||x_k - v_i||$ is the Euclid space distance between element k and the cluster center i; m is the weighted exponent on u_{ik} to control the fuzziness or amount of cluster overlap. The target is to adjust (U, V) iteratively to gain the minimal objective function value.

8.4.3.3 Multi-Scale Markov Model for Remaining Life Prediction

In previous literature, the Markov model always utilizes a single sample for prediction, and forecasts the latter value by using the former data of a time series, which cannot get the overall trend of the series. Therefore, a prediction model based on a single sample is effective for short-term forecast but is inaccurate for long-term prediction. A multi-sample prediction method has the ability to obtain overall information of the series which provides the possibility for long-term prediction.

In this research, we combined the multi-sample prediction approach with the Markov model. Several historical samples are used to get historical state space which includes information reflecting the overall development trend of the series. However, if only historical data are used, model parameters are not affected by real-time data. In order to consider the influence of real-time data, we propose a dynamic prediction model which is composed of two models constructed, respectively, by historical samples and real-time data. These two models are combined by a weighted coefficient which determines the influence of historical samples and real-time data on the final prediction results.

However, the amount of data of historical samples is much larger than that of the real-time sample. Therefore, multi-scale theory is employed, which is successfully used in the signal processing field for such as wave analysis. As a useful tool to get the joint time–frequency distribution of vibration signals, wave analysis observes different frequencies with different scales so that it can get any changes in the high frequency area. Consulting the multi-scale theory, we divide the historical samples and real-time sample with different states numbers. The historical samples are of a large amount of data and wide span. Consequently, we divide them into fewer states of a large scale to locate the data in state space roughly and also to reduce the calculation work. As to the real-time sample, it is divided into more states of small scales to get the detailed information. Finally, taking advantage of the dynamic prediction model and multi-scale theory, we establish a dynamic multi-scale Markov model (DMMM) whose structure is shown in Figure 8.23.

The procedures of using DMMM for remaining life prediction are as follows:

Step 1: Input the real time performance series y and n historical samples; choose performance values of the current moment and its former k moments $y(t-k)$ to $y(t)$ as the input series of the DMMM for current moment t, where k is a positive integer ($k < t$).

Step 2: Calculate the prediction value of the next moment using the DMMM.

Step 3: Compare the prediction value with a preset failure threshold. If the prediction value exceeds the threshold, then stop and record the update number as the remaining life. Otherwise, update the input series by adding the new prediction value as the last input data and removing the first one, then return to step 2.

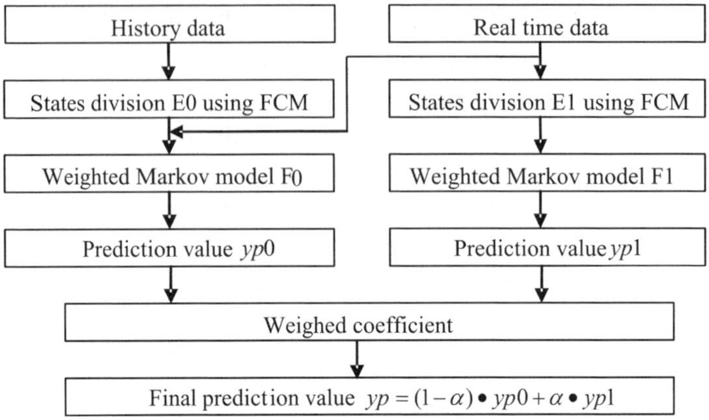

Figure 8.23 Configuration of DMMM

In the process of constructing the DMMM, the coefficient α is an important parameter reflecting the historical trend and the real-time performance of the model. We define it between 0 and 1. The bigger the coefficient, the stronger the historical trend. Otherwise, the real-time performance is stronger. Therefore, an appropriate coefficient is crucial for the model construction. In this research, we used the historical samples to train the DMMM obtaining the coefficient. First, the coefficients $\alpha_1 \sim \alpha_{11}$ are valued between 0 and 1 in steps of 0.1. For each value, calculate the remaining life errors between prediction and actual value of the historical samples at all moments. Find the coefficient α_i corresponding to the minimal mean error. Then value the coefficients $\alpha'_1 \sim \alpha'_{11}$ between α_{i-1} and α_{i+1} in steps of 0.01. Calculate the remaining life errors as above. Finally, we choose the coefficient α'_j corresponding to the minimal error mean as the weighted coefficient of the DMMM.

8.4.3.4 Prediction Error Analysis

The proposed model does not just predict the remaining life at a single moment. It predicts the remaining lives of multiple moments from the current moment t_0. Therefore, we take the mean absolute deviation (MAD) of the predicted remaining life as the criterion to evaluate the algorithm accuracy.

$$\mathrm{MAD} = \sum_{t=1}^{n} |\hat{y}_t - y_t|/n \tag{8.13}$$

where $\hat{y}_t$ indicates the prediction value of moment t; y_t represents the corresponding true value; and n is the total number of prediction moments of each sample.

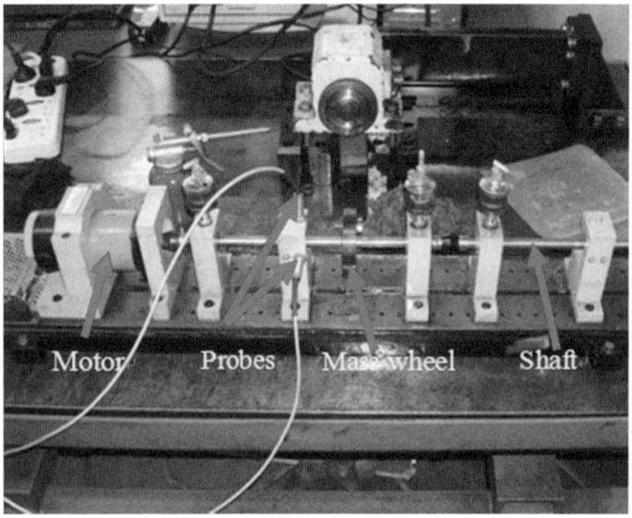

Figure 8.24 Bently-RK4 testbed

8.4.4 Experiment and Validation

8.4.4.1 Experimental Set-up

In order to validate the effectiveness of the DMMM methodology, a performance degradation experiment was designed based on a Bently-RK4 rotor imbalance testbed shown in Figure 8.24. The diameter of the shaft is 10 mm and the length of the shaft is 560 mm. The rotor mass wheel is 800 g and its diameter is 75 mm. There are 16 screw holes uniformly distributed on the face of the mass wheel in order to add imbalance mass. Performance degradation is simulated by increasing the number of the set-screws when the rotor moves from a balance state to an allowable imbalance state. The vibration signals are probed by eddy current sensors fixed on the mass wheel. In the experiment, the rotational speed was 2700 rpm and the sampling frequency 1 kHz. Vibration signals of five degradation processes are collected and each signal includes approximately 96 000 sampling points.

8.4.4.2 Signal Processing and Performance Assessment

In order to get the joint time–frequency distribution, STFT is applied as described in Section 4.3.2.3. A Hanning window is chosen as the window function $g(n)$. The window moving step N is valued as 1024 points, determining that the Fourier transform is performed for every 1024 points which we call a degradation cycle. Therefore, each signal for a degradation process (about 96 000 points) is divided into approximately

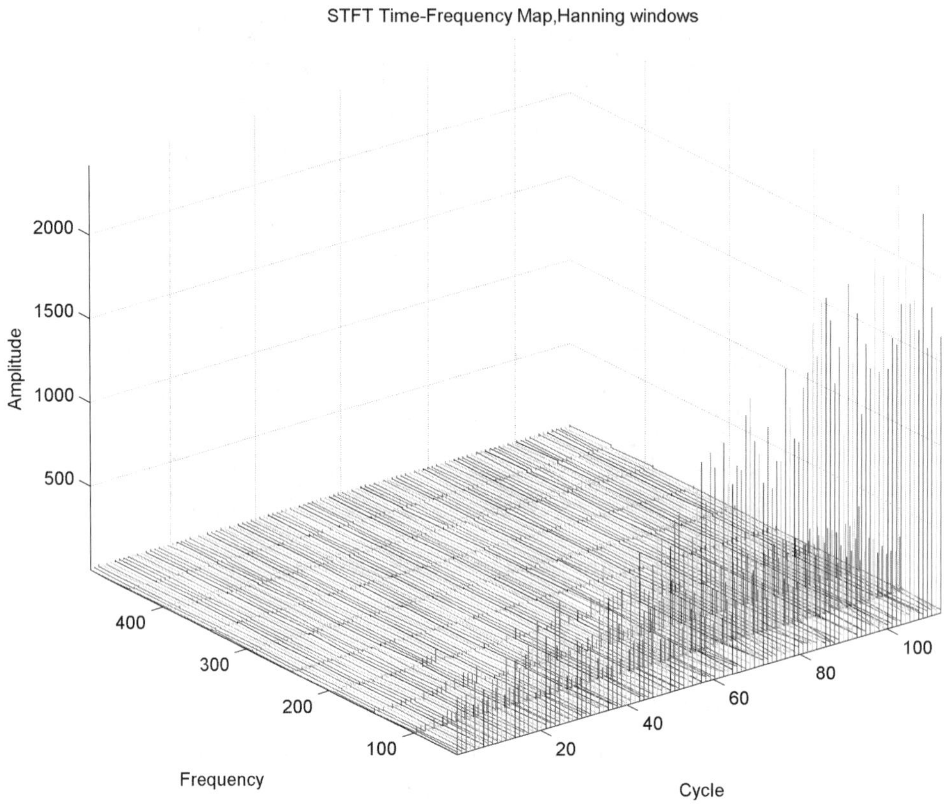

Figure 8.25 Joint time-frequency distribution of a degradation process

94 cycles. Since the sampling frequency is 1 kHz and the amplitude frequency is symmetrical in a cycle, we just implement STFT between 0 and 500 Hz. Considering the basic frequency to be 45 Hz, we divide the whole frequency into 16 frequency bands. The joint time–frequency distribution of a degradation process is shown in Figure 8.25.

The sum of the energy of each frequency band is calculated and chosen as the feature including the degradation information. For instance, the 16 frequency bands of the degradation process mentioned above are shown in Figure 8.26. For each figure of the frequency band, the horizontal axis represents a degradation cycle, the vertical axis represents energy.

Then, 16 frequency bands are classified into 4 categories using the CNN model. The clustering results of the 16 frequency bands and the dispersion degrees of these categories are listed in Table 8.7.

The table indicates that the second category corresponds to the minimal dispersion degree. Therefore, the second, third, and fifth frequency bands are selected as typical features.

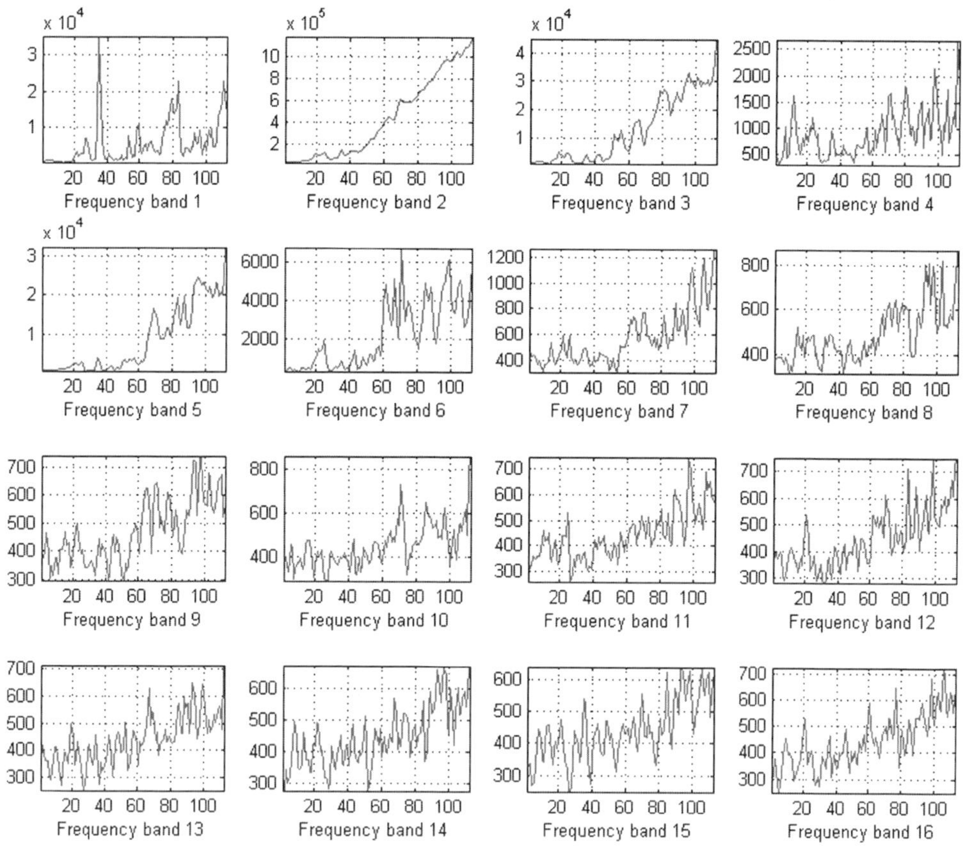

Figure 8.26 Time–energy figures for 16 frequency bands of a degradation process

Table 8.7 Clustering results and the dispersion degrees

	First category	Second category	Third category	Fourth category
Frequency band	1, 4	2, 3, 5	6	7–16
Dispersion degrees	0.0776	0.0571	0.0931	0.1050

After feature selection, the performance assessment model should be trained. The selected features of the degradation processes 2, 4, and 5 are chosen to train the performance assessment model, and those of degradation process 1 and 3 are used to test the trained model arbitrarily. A conjugate gradient algorithm is adopted to optimize the network parameters. The maximal training number is set as 5000. And the minimal training MSE is preset as 10^{-6}. Since the number of input nodes of the performance assessment model, equal to the number of typical features, is 3, and that of the output node is 1, according to Equation 5.31, the number of hidden nodes ranks from

Table 8.8 Training MSEs for different hidden nodes

Hidden node	3	4	5	6	7	8	9	10	11	12
Training MSE $\times 10^{-1}$	1.342	1.276	1.262	1.259	1.256	1.253	1.256	1.255	1.253	1.252

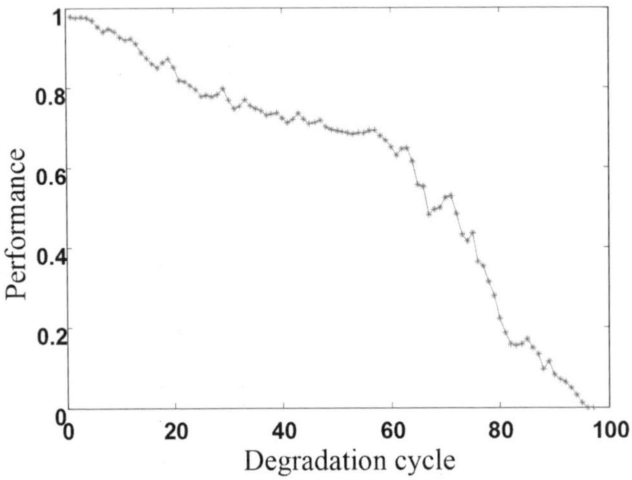

Figure 8.27 Assessment results of a degradation process

3 to 12. For each hidden node, 10 BPNN models are established. Training MSEs of performance assessment models for different hidden nodes are listed in Table 8.8.

Table 8.8 shows that the training MSE with 12 hidden nodes is minimal (Herein, we traverse the hidden nodes empirically calculated by Equation 5.31). Therefore, the structure of the performance assessment model is a three-layer BPNN with 12 hidden nodes. The assessment results of one degradation process using the trained performance assessment model are shown in Figure 8.27.

8.4.4.3 Remaining Life Prediction Using Markov Models

In this section, DMMM is validated using the results of performance assessment obtained in Section 8.4.4.2. We transform the performance value to increment as the input of DMMM for the performance curve is monotonically decreasing, inappropriate for state division. According to the description in Section 8.4.3.3, three degradation processes are used to construct the DMMM. In order to confirm the weighted coefficient α, first we utilize these three degradation processes to obtain the historical state space. Then each degradation process is considered as a real-time sample to implement the remaining life prediction. For each moment t, we choose the data consisting of the performance values at the current moment and its former 19 moments as the

Table 8.9 MADs of 0.1 step

α	0	0.1	0.2	0.3	0.4	0.5	0.6	0.7	0.8	0.9	1
MADs	9.63	9.40	9.01	8.17	7.76	7.51	7.00	6.70	7.712	9.25	20.97

Table 8.10 MADs of 0.01 step

α	0.6	0.61	0.62	0.63	0.64	0.65	0.66	0.67	0.68	0.69	0.70
MADs	7.00	7.15	6.74	6.49	6.28	6.61	6.31	6.33	6.58	6.78	6.63
α	0.71	0.72	0.73	0.74	0.75	0.76	0.77	0.78	0.79	0.80	
MADs	6.43	7.00	7.36	6.79	7.48	7.49	7.04	6.82	7.07	7.12	

input series of the DMMM for the current moment t. The state number of the input series is set as 8 and that of the historical state space is set as 4. Considering the performance curve declines sharply from approximately the 60th moment, we predict the remaining life beginning with the 58th moment for each sample. When the coefficient step is given as 0.1, the MADs of all the prediction moments are listed in Table 8.9.

The α corresponding to minimal mean error is 0.7. Therefore, the next searching range is from 0.6 to 0.8. The step reduces to 0.01. Then, list the results as in Table 8.10. This shows that when α' is valued as 0.64, the mean error is the smallest. Consequently, the final coefficient is chosen as 0.64.

After determining the coefficient, we use the remaining two samples as real-time data to test the prediction effect. According to the training process, we still choose 20 data as the inputs of DMMM at each prediction moment. The state number of real time data and historical samples is 8 and 4. The prediction results of a testing degradation process are shown in Figure 8.28. The line with asterisks represents the predicted remaining life and the solid line represents the actual remaining life. The errors between the predicted and true values are shown in Figure 8.29.

The MAD of the degradation process is 5.96. In order to have an insight into the deviations, we inspect the MAD values every 10 cycles. The segmented MADs are listed in Table 8.11.

This indicates that the prediction deviation is becoming smaller with time elapsing; in other words, the methodology is of good convergence.

For the purpose of validating the weighted coefficient influence on the prediction results, we set the coefficient α as 0 and 1, respectively. The MADs of the two testing degradation processes are calculated and listed in Table 8.12.

Table 8.12 shows that the MADs are minimal when the dynamic weighted coefficient is 0.64, determined by the training process. This means that the proposed DMMM considering both historical information and real-time information is better than the model considering only one aspect of these two. Therefore, the dynamic weighted method can improve the prediction effect.

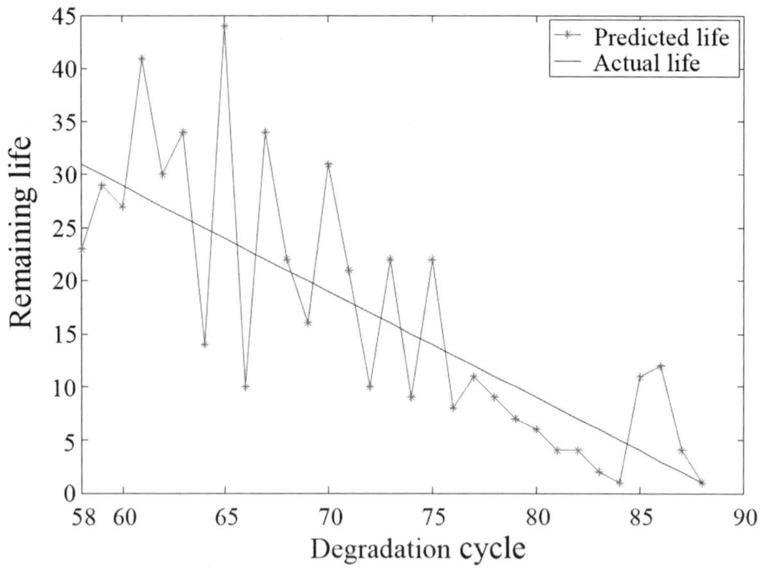

Figure 8.28 Prediction results of a testing degradation process

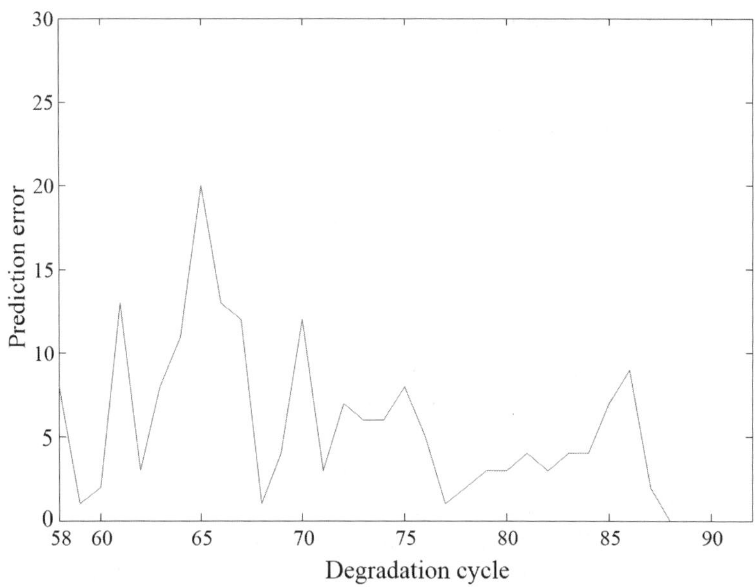

Figure 8.29 Prediction errors of a testing degradation process

Table 8.11 Segmented MADs of a testing degradation process

Degradation cycle	58–67	68–77	78–87	88
Segmented MADs	9.10	5.30	4.10	0

Table 8.12 MADs with different α

	$\alpha = 0$	$\alpha = 0.64$	$\alpha = 1$
MAD of sample 1	10.52	5.96	16.68
MAD of sample 2	10.91	7.60	13.83

Table 8.13 MADs with different state divisions

	(4, 4)	(4, 8)	(8, 8)
MAD of sample 1	11.81	5.96	17.13
MAD of sample 2	10.66	7.60	16.66

In order to investigate the influence of scales on prediction results, different state combinations (4, 4), (4, 8), (8, 8) are considered. In the parentheses, the first variable represents the state number of the historical data and the second variable represents the state number of the real-time data. The MADs are listed in Table 8.13.

It can be seen that the multi-scale division method has better prediction performance. Consequently, the proposed DMMM is valid. Additionally, the basic Markov model is used to predict the remaining life of the two testing degradation processes as a comparison. The input data are divided by the hard state division approach. When the states number is 4, the MADs of these two testing samples are 19.52 and 22.00. And when the states number is 8, the MADs are 29.32 and 36.41. Comparing the results with that of DMMM, which are 5.96 and 7.60, it can be easily concluded that the proposed DMMM is better than the basic Markov model.

8.4.5 Summary

This research proposed a systematic prognostics scheme based on neural networks combined DMMM. A performance degradation indicator is designed by the multi-feature fusion technique based on neural network models. Based on this indicator, the remaining life prediction is implemented by a DMMM. The novelty of this methodology lies in using a FCM algorithm to deal with state division and combining a dynamic prediction method and multi-scale theory with the Markov model. The proposed approach is validated by real-world vibration signals collected from a Bently rotor testbed. The results show that the proposed methodology is of high accuracy, which is effective for remaining life prediction. This research gives an example of combined approaches for remaining life prediction of a rotor machine, which can provide critical information for prognostics and health management systems and offer a great opportunity in terms of reducing the overall life-cycle cost.

Further work focuses on optimizing the weighted coefficient by an optimization algorithm and obtaining more vibration signal data in order to get the actual probability function (PDF) of remaining life. The methodology should be applied to different objects, such as bearings, turbine rotors, and so on, to validate also the actual prediction capability.

8.5 A Group Technology Based Methodology for Maintenance Scheduling for a Hybrid Shop

8.5.1 Introduction

Proper maintenance scheduling not only reduces maintenance cost, but also increases the availability, reliability, and life span of facilities. Current research on maintenance scheduling is mainly concerned with preventive maintenance (PM) scheduling [13], including periodic maintenance [14, 15], CBM [16, 17], and so on, due to its effectiveness to avoid or mitigate the consequences of failure of facilities.

Particularly, for multiunit systems, research on PM focuses on opportunistic maintenance (OM) [18, 19] and group maintenance (GM) [20–23]. Under OM, the failure of a subsystem results in a possible opportunity for other subsystems to undertake maintenance. And under GM, facilities are maintained in groups under certain conditions, so that more reasonable logistics of spare parts and a smaller scale scheduling problem can be achieved [23]. However, for either OM or GM, little research is conducted on complex systems, and methods for grouping facilities are scarcely studied.

In this section, we proposed a novel methodology for maintenance scheduling of a complex system based on GT, in which OM and clustering-based group maintenance (CGM) are combined. The structural dependence of facilities is studied and described with a structure model. Hierarchical clustering (HC) [23, 24] is employed to group facilities according to factors such as their similarities and interrelationships. A Tabu search (TS) is applied to optimize the weight allocation of the considered factors in clustering. A case study of a complex series–parallel production system is presented to verify the methodology.

8.5.2 Production System Modeling

The models of facility performance and maintenance effect for this case have been introduced in Section 6.2.3.2. The production system structure used in this case has been presented in Section 6.2.2. The maintenance cost model will be introduced in the following.

The maintenance cost of the kth maintenance activity consists of direct maintenance cost C_{m}^{k} and indirect production loss L_{p}^{k}. Direct maintenance cost, including the cost of maintenance actions for maintenance units C_{u}^{k} and set-up cost C_{s}^{k}, can be calculated by Equations 8.14 and 8.15.

$$C_{\mathrm{m}}^{k} = C_{\mathrm{u}}^{k} + C_{\mathrm{s}}^{k} \tag{8.14}$$

$$C_{\mathrm{u}}^{k} = \sum_{i=1}^{M} (C_{\mathrm{p}}^{k,i} + C_{\mathrm{t}}^{k,i} + C_{\mathrm{h}}^{k,i} + C_{\mathrm{c}}^{k,i}) \tag{8.15}$$

where $C_{\mathrm{p}}^{k,i}$, $C_{\mathrm{t}}^{k,i}$, $C_{\mathrm{h}}^{k,i}$, and $C_{\mathrm{c}}^{k,i}$ are the cost of spare parts, maintenance tools, maintainers, and consumables for maintenance unit i.

Commonly, the productivity of a production system $P(t)$ at time t depends on its bottleneck. In this research, it is assumed that there is no buffer between any two connected work stages, production of the system has been balanced, and facilities in the same work stage have the same productivity. Hence, the L_{p}^{k} can be calculated by Equation 8.16.

$$L_{\mathrm{P}}^{k} = P_0 \times (t_k - t_{k+1}) - \int_{t_k}^{t_{k+1}} P(t)\mathrm{d}t \tag{8.16}$$

where P_0 is the normal productivity of the system; t_k is the time when the kth maintenance activity starts; and t_{k+1} is when the maintenance activity ends. $P(t)$ equals the lowest productivity of all work stages at time t.

8.5.3 Clustering-Based Grouping Method

The description of this method is shown in Section 6.3.2.1. Facilities that need maintenance in one maintenance activity can be grouped according to their similarities under a certain level. However, for different production systems with different characteristics, fixed weight allocation of the considered factors in clustering may not achieve a reasonable grouping result. For example, in a series system, the consideration of the structural positions of facilities loses its importance. Furthermore, the quantity and types of facilities that need maintenance vary from one maintenance activity to another. Even a facility in a different maintenance activity may have different maintenance need. Hence, weight allocation should be considered in the clustering process.

In this research, weight allocation is optimized each time a maintenance activity is carried out via TS due to its property of fast convergence. In addition, a hybrid genetic algorithm [25] is employed for scheduling after grouping.

8.5.4 Application

8.5.4.1 Case Description and Parameter Settings

In this section, a case study on the maintenance scheduling of a sliding bearing production system with 24 facilities is presented and the maintenance cost is set as the objective of maintenance scheduling, which should be minimized. As shown in Figure 8.30

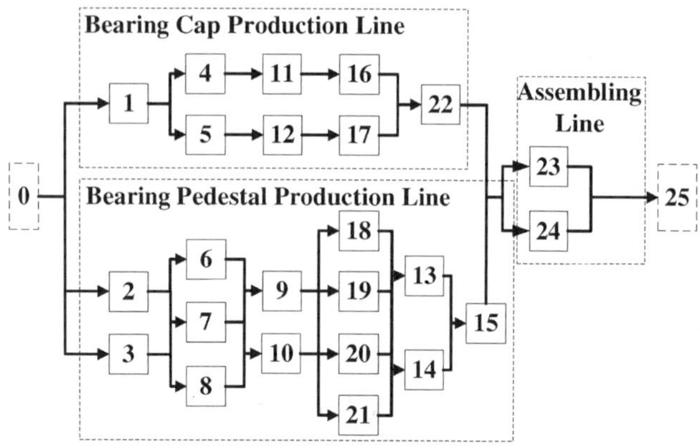

Figure 8.30 Sliding bearing production system

facilities 0 and 25 are input and output, respectively, which are assumed to have no maintenance need. Milling machines are labeled from 1 to 10, vertical drilling machines 11 to 15, radial drilling machines 16 to 22, and boring machines 23 and 24. The layout of the workshop is also presented in Figure 8.30. All the facilities form three production lines, that is, a bearing cap production line, a bearing pedestal production line, and an assembling line.

It is assumed that there are enough spare parts and consumables, while maintenance tools and maintainers are limited and are outsourced according to the maintenance need of the maintenance activity. Particularly in this research, the total number of maintainers or tools equals one-third of the total need if all maintenance actions are carried out simultaneously. In addition, tools and maintainers assigned to a maintenance group are according to the maximum need to maintain any one facility in this group.

For each facility of the same type, the two parameters for reliability modeling, η and β, are derived from randomly generated simulation data subject to the same distribution; and all facilities of one type have the same price and the resources and time needed for each kind of maintenance actions.

The three thresholds, T_{h}^{1}, T_{h}^{2}, and T_{h}^{3}, are set as 0.9, 0.75, and 0.6, respectively; and L_{R} is set as 0.2.

The set-up cost C_{s} of each maintenance activity is set as 1000; the unit prices for four types of maintenance resources, that is, spare parts, tools, maintainers, and consumables are set as 100, 50, 50, and 10, respectively; the normal production value v_0 is set as 1000/h.

8.5.4.2 Advantage Measurement of GM

With GT, several advantages can be gained when maintaining a group of facilities. Time can be saved by maintaining facilities within a close distance; similarities in structure and failure mode of a certain type of facility can be utilized to accelerate maintenance; similar maintenance processes of a certain maintenance type can be carried out on a group of facilities simultaneously so that the efficiency can be improved. In this research, a reduction factor is introduced to quantify the advantage, which is the weighted average of three subfactors, that is, reduction factors considering distance, facility type similarity, and maintenance need similarity among facilities in one group.

The reduction factor considering distance can be obtained by first averaging the distances between any pair of facilities in that group. Set N_g^k as the number of facilities in maintenance group *k;* the average distance can be calculated by Equation 8.17.

$$D_{\mathrm{avg}}^k = 2\sum_{i=1}^{N_g^k-1}\sum_{j=i+1}^{N_g^k} D_{\mathrm{dis}}^{i,j}/[N_{\mathrm{g}}^k \cdot (N_{\mathrm{g}}^k - 1)] \tag{8.17}$$

Suppose the possible maximal, mean, and minimal values of distance between any two facilities in the shop are $D_{\mathrm{avg}}^{\mathrm{max}}$, $D_{\mathrm{avg}}^{\mathrm{mean}}$, and $D_{\mathrm{avg}}^{\mathrm{min}}$. Assume that when the average distance in group *k* equals $D_{\mathrm{avg}}^{\mathrm{min}}$ or $D_{\mathrm{avg}}^{\mathrm{max}}$, the maintenance time of this group will be reduced by 30% or increased by 30%. Then the reduction factor considering distance in maintenance group *k* can be calculated by a function $f_1(\cdot)$ obtained by fitting a quadratic curve to two data sets, that is, $\{D_{\mathrm{avg}}^{\mathrm{min}}, D_{\mathrm{avg}}^{\mathrm{mean}}, D_{\mathrm{avg}}^{\mathrm{max}}\}$ and $\{0.7, 1, 1.3\}$. An example is shown in Figure 8.31.

Similarly, the average similarity in facility type and maintenance type in one group $S_{\mathrm{p,avg}}^k$ and $S_{\mathrm{n,avg}}^k$ can be calculated by Equation 8.18.

$$S_{x,\mathrm{avg}}^k = 2/[N_{\mathrm{g}}^k \cdot (N_{\mathrm{g}}^k - 1)]\sum_{i=1}^{N_g^k-1}\sum_{j=i+1}^{N_g^k} S_x^{i,j} \tag{8.18}$$

It is assumed that when the average similarity of group *k* in facility type or maintenance type equals 1, the time needed for maintenance actions in this group can be reduced by 40 or 30%, respectively. The reduction factor considering facility type and

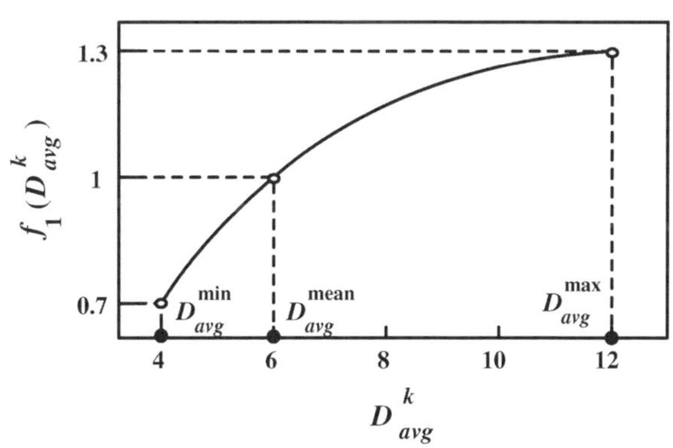

Figure 8.31 $f_1(\cdot)$ obtained by fitting to {4, 6, 12} and {0.7, 1, 1.3}

maintenance type in group k can be calculated by $f_2(S^k_{\text{p,avg}})$ and $f_3(S^k_{\text{n,avg}})$. Function $f_2(\cdot)$ is obtained by fitting a linear function to data sets $\{0, 1\}$ and $\{1, 0.6\}$, and function $f_3(\cdot)$ is obtained by fitting a linear function to data sets $\{0, 1\}$ and $\{1, 0.7\}$.

Finally, the reduction factor F_{dus} in group k can be calculated by Equation 8.19.

$$F^k_{\text{dus}} = W_1 \cdot f_1(D^k_{\text{avg}}) + W_2 \cdot f_2(S^k_{\text{p,avg}}) + W_3 \cdot f_3(S^k_{\text{n,avg}}) \tag{8.19}$$

where W_1, W_2, and W_3 are weights of the three sub-reduction factors, particularly in this case, set as 0.4, 0.4, and 0.2. The time needed for any maintenance actions in maintenance group k is reduced by $(1 - F^k_{\text{dus}})$.

8.5.4.3 Simulation and Result Analysis

The maintenance scheduling is carried out for a time period of 1000 working days in three scenarios, that is, only OM, OM and rule-based group maintenance (RGM) [26], and OM and CGM.

Four maintenance activities occur in the simulation. The total cost and cost of each maintenance activity under the three maintenance policies are shown in Table 8.14. GM costs less, not only because of the advantage of group technology that shortens the maintenance time, but also due to the smaller scale of the scheduling problem with which satisfactory results can be obtained more easily. Especially, CGM achieves the least cost.

Compared with RGM, CGM possesses more flexibility by adjusting its weight allocation on five factors in the clustering process. In the third maintenance activity, facilities 2, 8, 10–12, 15, 23, and 24 need minor maintenance; facilities 13, 14, 18–20, and 22 need overhaul; and no facility needs replacement. The grouping and scheduling results under OM & RGM and OM & CGM are shown in Figures 8.32 and 8.33, respectively. Among the facilities, the number of facilities that call for minor maintenance and medium maintenance are relatively balanced, which are 7 and 5 respectively, and facilities requiring maintenance are mainly vertical drilling machines and radial drilling machines, with 5 and 7 of each. By optimization, a weight allocation of (0.12, 0.2, 0.24, 0.06, 0.38) is obtained. Among the weights, those for maintenance

Table 8.14 Optimal maintenance cost in three scenarios

Maintenance activity	Maintenance policy		
	OM	OM & RGM	OM & CGM
1	22 443	24 892	21 052
2	17 508	18 265	16 510
3	27 081	25 455	23 481
4	42 863	39 203	37 529
Total	109 895	107 815	98 572

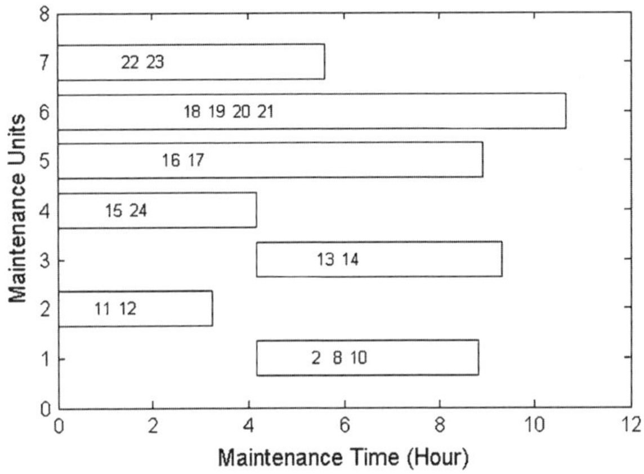

Figure 8.32 Gantt chart of the third maintenance activity under OM & RGM

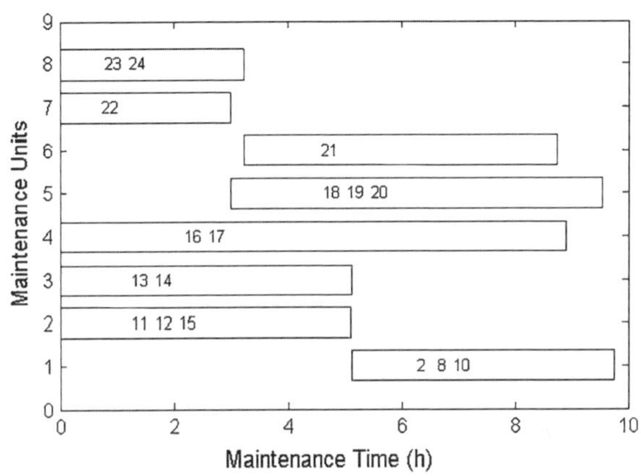

Figure 8.33 Gantt chart of the third maintenance activity under OM & CGM

type and facility type are relatively larger, so time can be reduced by grouping facilities with the same maintenance type need or facility type. To avoid too many facilities grouped together, a large weight for maintenance time is obtained. As shown in Figure 8.32, under OM and RGM, the group comprised of facilities 18–21 is unreasonable because of its long time consumed, while, as shown in Figure 8.33, under OM and CGM, facility 21 is singled out and no group's maintenance lasts more than 9 hours.

8.5.5 Summary

In this research, a novel maintenance methodology based on GT for complex systems is proposed.

A structure model of the system is established to describe the structural dependence between facilities, upon which the production loss during a maintenance activity can be calculated with higher consistency with practice.

In the methodology, comprehensive consideration of the clustering factors leads to more satisfactory grouping results. The flexibility derived from an optimized weight allocation of such factors enhances the methodology's adaptability to different systems and varying maintenance requirements. Furthermore, more factors could be included in clustering to expand the consideration in grouping, and the influence of such factors on maintenance could be analyzed. In this way, a system's characteristics could also be studied, upon which an optimized RGM could be obtained, which is often more easily implemented in practice.

In the future, similarity measurements in clustering will be investigated and refined, and the considered factors analyzed and selected. Moreover, the methodology to extract the characteristics of a system in terms of maintenance by analyzing the considered factors and their corresponding weight will be developed.

References

1. Goldberger, A.L., Amaral, L.A.N., Glass, L. *et al.* (2000) Components of a new research resource for complex physiologic signals. *Circulation*, **101** (23), 215–220.
2. Yan, J., Koc, M. and Lee, J. (2004) A prognostic algorithm for machine performance assessment and its application. *Production Planning & Control*, **15**, 796–801.
3. Gebraeel, N. and Lawley, M. (2004) Residual life predictions from vibration-based degradation signals: a neural network approach. *IEEE Transactions on Industrial Electronics*, **51**, 694–699.
4. Camci, F. (2005) Process monitoring, diagnostics and prognostics using support vector machines and hidden markov model. PhD thesis. Department of Industry Engineering, Wayne State University, Detroit, Michigan.
5. Huang, R., Xi, L., Li, X. *et al.* (2007) Residual life predictions for ball bearings based on self-organizing map and back propagation neural network methods. *Mechanical Systems and Signal Processing*, **21**, 193–207.
6. Teranishi, M., Omatu, S., and Kosaka, T. (2000) Classification of bill fatigue levels by feature-selected acoustic energy pattern using competitive neural network. Proceedings of the International Joint Conference Neural Networks, Como, Italy, pp. 249–252.
7. Castellno, G., Fanelli, A.M., and Roselli, T. (2001) Mining categories of learners by a competitive neural network. Proceedings of the International Joint Conference on Nerual Networks, Washington, DC, pp. 945–950.
8. Yan, J., Guo, C. and Wang, X. (2011) A dynamic multi-scale Markov model based methodology for remaining life prediction. *Mechanical Systems and Signal Processing*, **25** (4), 1364–1376.
9. Das, S., Chattopadhyay, A.B. and Murthy, A.S.R. (1996) Force parameters for on-line tool wear estimation: a neural network approach. *Neural Networks*, **9**, 1639–1645.
10. Li, C., Heinemann, P. and Sherry, R. (2007) Neural network and Bayesian network fusion models to fuse electronic nose and surface acoustic wave sensor data for apple defect detection. *Sensors and Actuators*, **125**, 301–310.
11. Huang, M. and Yang, D. (2001) An efficient fuzzy C-Means clustering algorithm. Proceedings of the First IEEE International Conference on Data Mining, San Jose, CA, pp. 225–232.
12. Pal, N.R., Pal, K., Keller, J.M. *et al.* (2005) A possibilistic fuzzy c-means clustering algorithm. *IEEE Transactions on Fuzzy Systems*, **13**, 517–529.

13. Khanlari, A., Mohammadi, K. and Sohrabi, B. (2008) Prioritizing equipments for preventive maintenance (PM) activities using fuzzy rules. *Computers & Industrial Engineering*, **54** (2), 169–184.
14. Ángel-Bello, F., Álvarez, A., Pacheco, J. *et al.* (2011) A heuristic approach for a scheduling problem with periodic maintenance and sequence-dependent setup times. *Computers & Mathematics with Applications*, **61** (4), 797–808.
15. Park, D.H., Jung, G.M. and Yum, J.K. (2000) Cost minimization for periodic maintenance policy of a system subject to slow degradation. *Reliability Engineering & System Safety*, **68** (2), 105–112.
16. Tian, Z. and Liao, H. (2011) Condition based maintenance optimization for multi-component systems using proportional hazards model. *Reliability Engineering & System Safety*, **96** (5), 581–589.
17. Tian, Z., Jin, T., Wu, B. *et al.* (2011) Condition based maintenance optimization for wind power generation systems under continuous monitoring. *Renewable Energy*, **36** (5), 1502–1509.
18. Radner, R. and Jorgenson, D.W. (1963) Opportunistic replacement of a single part in the presence of several monitored parts. *Management Science*, **10** (1), 70–84.
19. Wang, H. (2002) A survey of maintenance policies of deteriorating systems. *European Journal of Operational Research*, **139** (3), 469–489.
20. Ritchken, P. and Wilson, J.G. (1990) (m, T) group maintenance policies. *Management Science*, **36** (5), 632–639.
21. Sheu, S.H. and Jhang, J.P. (1997) A generalized group maintenance policy. *European Journal of Operational Research*, **96** (2), 232–247.
22. Gertsbakh, I.B. (1984) Optimal group preventive maintenance of a system with observable state parameter. *Advances in Applied Probability*, **16**, 923–925.
23. Abdelhadi, A. (2010) Preventive maintenance grouping using similarity coefficient methodology. PhD in Engineering Dissertation. Industrial and Manufacturing Engineering Department, University of Wisconsin, Milwaukee.
24. Vakharia, A.J. and Wemmerlöv, U. (1995) A comparative investigation of hierarchical clustering techniques and dissimilarity measures applied to the cell formation problem. *Journal of Operations Management*, **13** (2), 117–138.
25. Esbensen, H. and Mazumder, P. (1994) SAGA: a unification of the genetic algorithm with simulated annealing and its application to macro-cell placement. Proceedings of the Seventh International Conference on VLSI Design, 1994, IEEE, January, 1994, pp. 211–214.
26. Yan, J., Hua, D., and Wang, Z. (2011) Reuse oriented group maintenance scheduling based on Hybrid Genetic Algorithm and Tabu Search. 2011 IEEE International Conference on Industrial Engineering and Engineering Management (IEEM), IEEE, December, 2011, pp. 1524–1528.

Index

Machinery Prognostics and Prognosis Oriented Maintenance Management, First Edition. Jihong Yan.